MW00582035

Graphic Reproduction

GRAPHIC MEDICINE

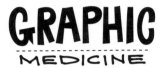

Susan Merrill Squier and Ian Williams, General Editors

Books in the Graphic Medicine series are inspired by a growing awareness of the value of comics as an important resource for communicating about a range of issues broadly termed "medical." For healthcare practitioners, patients, families, and caregivers dealing with illness and disability, graphic narrative enlightens complicated or difficult experience. For scholars in literary, cultural, and comics studies, the genre articulates a complex and powerful analysis of illness, medicine, and disability and a rethinking of the boundaries of "health." The series includes original comics from artists and non-artists alike, such as self-reflective "graphic pathographies" or comics used in medical training and education, as well as monographic studies and edited collections from scholars, practitioners, and medical educators.

OTHER TITLES IN THE SERIES:

MK Czerwiec, Ian Williams, Susan Merrill Squier, Michael J. Green, Kimberly R. Myers, and Scott T. Smith, *Graphic Medicine Manifesto*

Ian Williams, *The Bad Doctor: The Troubled Life and Times of Dr. Iwan James*

Peter Dunlap-Shohl, *My Degeneration: A Journey Through Parkinson's*

Aneurin Wright, *Things to Do in a Retirement Home Trailer Park . . . when You're 29 and Unemployed*

Dana Walrath, *Aliceheimers: Alzheimer's Through the Looking Glass*

Lorenzo Servitje and Sherryl Vint, eds., *The Walking Med: Zombies and the Medical Image*

Henny Beaumont, *Hole in the Heart: Bringing Up Beth*

MK Czerwiec, *Taking Turns: Stories from Unit 371*

Paula Knight, *The Facts of Life*

Gareth Brookes, *A Thousand Coloured Castles*

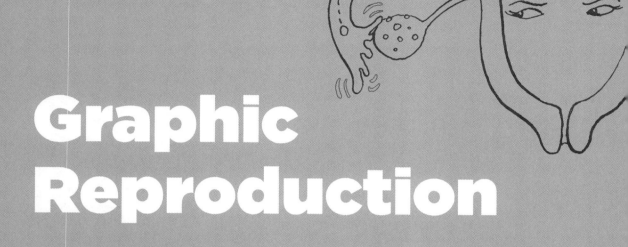

Graphic Reproduction

A Comics Anthology

Edited by Jenell Johnson

Afterword by Susan Merrill Squier

The Pennsylvania State University Press

University Park, Pennsylvania

Spawn of Dykes to Watch Out For © 1993 by Alison Bechdel.

Pushing Back © 2017 by Bethany Doane.

Abortion Eve © 1973 by Joyce Farmer and Lyn Chevli.

Not Funny Ha-Ha © 2015 by Leah Hayes. Published by Fantagraphics Books.

Present / Perfect © 2016 by Jenell Johnson.

Spooky Womb © 2012 by Paula Knight.

X Utero (A Cluster of Comics) © 2013 by Paula Knight.

A Significant Loss © 2014 by Endrené Shepherd.

Pregnant Butch: Nine Long Months Spent in Drag © 2014 by A. K. Summers. Reprinted by permission of Counterpoint.

"Anatomy of a New Mom" © 1988 by Carol Tyler.

"Losing Thomas and Ella: A Father's Story (A Research Comic)" by Marcus B. Weaver-Hightower, *Journal of Medical Humanities*, online first (doi:10.1007/s10912-015-9359-z). With permission of Springer.

Overwhelmed, Anxious, and Angry: Navigating Postpartum Depression, written by Jessica Zucker, illustrated by Ryan Alexander-Tanner.

Library of Congress Cataloging-in-Publication Data

Names: Johnson, Jenell M., 1978- editor.
Title: Graphic reproduction : a comics anthology / edited by Jenell Johnson ; afterword by Susan Merrill Squier.
Other titles: Graphic medicine.
Description: University Park, Pennsylvania : The Pennsylvania State University Press, [2018] | Series: Graphic medicine | Includes bibliographical references.
Summary: "A comics anthology that illustrates the complicated and multiple experiences of human reproduction and explores comics within the growing field of graphic medicine"—Provided by publisher.
Identifiers: LCCN 2017060110 | ISBN 9780271080949 (pbk. : alk. paper)
Subjects: | MESH: Pregnancy | Abortion, Induced | Perinatal Death | Infertility | Maternal Health Services | Parents—psychology | Graphic Novels
Classification: LCC RG525 | NLM WQ 17 | DDC 618.2—dc23
LC record available at https://lccn.loc.gov/2017060110

Title page illustration: Detail from *Spooky Womb* © 2012 by Paula Knight.

For Michael Andrew Xenos

Contents

Acknowledgments

Thanks first and foremost to Sara DiCaglio. Simply put, this book wouldn't exist without Sara, whose inspired vision brought it into being.

I am so grateful to Susan Squier for her pioneering work in graphic medicine, for introducing me to comics scholarship in her grad seminar at Penn State, for writing the wonderful afterword to this book, and, most of all, for her guidance and friendship over the years.

Huge thanks to my editor, Kendra Boileau, who has championed this project for a long time. Kendra encouraged me to include my own comic, and I'm not sure I would have been brave enough to do so without her faith and enthusiasm. Big thanks, too, to Alex Vose for helping with the details and to MK Czerwiec, Erin Heidt-Forsythe, and a third anonymous reviewer, who provided invaluable feedback that helped to tighten the book's focus and organization. Deep thanks to Merryl A. Sloane, my meticulous copyeditor, who softened and sharpened the textual edges of this book in all the right places. And, of course, the biggest thank you of all to the artists and authors (and their publishers) who generously allowed their work to be used in this volume.

I am indebted to the indomitable Lynda Barry and the creative folks in the Applied Comics Kitchen Mellon-Borghesi workshop at the University of Wisconsin–Madison (particularly Ebony Flowers, Katie Zaman, Heather Rosenfeld, Jason Kartez, Liz Anna Kozik, Ife Williams, Kadin Henningsen, KC Councilor, and all of their alter egos). I have learned from Lynda and my ACK! comrades that if you're unsure about what to do next in a comic, an unexpected chicken is usually the answer.

My immeasurable gratitude to KC Councilor. I thought my comics days were far behind me until KC convinced me at exactly the right time to pick up a pen again. He didn't know how much it helped me then, but I hope he knows now.

To my friends, colleagues, and family: your support means everything to me. Thank you.

For Michael Xenos, my beloved partner in this Big Life, "thank you" will not suffice. Mike gave me permission to share our story, even the hard parts, confirmed my memories, and allowed himself to be turned into a cartoon. And yes, he really did give me every one of those injections without flinching.

Introduction

Jenell Johnson

There is a common story about human reproduction that circulates in Western culture. Two (middle- to upper-class, white) people meet, they fall in love, they get married, they have (heterosexual) sex, and then, after a glowing nine months of pregnancy full of ice cream and pickles, a (cisgender) woman has a (healthy, typical-bodied, full-term) baby, maybe two. Maybe two and a half. You know the rest: picket fence, bliss, happy endings, school, college, wedding, grandkids on a porch somewhere, everybody drinking lemonade in glasses tinkling with ice.

To call this narrative a "myth" is an understatement, of course, not only because it's reproduced in nearly every form of media one can imagine, but also because few people have this type of experience with conception, pregnancy, birth, and raising children. A lesbian couple uses donor sperm and conceives via intrauterine insemination. A father spends the first few months of his son's life in the neonatal intensive care unit, anxiously monitoring the vital signs of a tiny human who beeps instead of coos. A single woman gives birth to a baby who dies shortly after birth. A heterosexual couple enters the chutes and ladders of fertility treatment, only to find their way to a dead end. After an uneventful first trimester, a pregnant woman experiences a bad bleed in her second and spends the rest of her pregnancy on bed rest. A gay couple uses in vitro fertilization and a gestational surrogate, who gives birth to twins. A woman spends the first months of her daughter's life in a deep depression. These experiences and many others are not aleatory events that somehow prove the rule of "normal" conception, pregnancy, and birth. Nor do they mark the ways that experiences of conception, pregnancy, and birth are changing in response to social, cultural, medical, and technological changes. They are simply examples of how varied and complex the experience of human reproduction is and has always been. Human reproduction is at once an utterly singular experience and utterly banal: after all, it's happened billions and billions of times.

In humanities books about this subject, this is the point where authors position themselves in the text, drawing on decades of feminist arguments about the role of the personal and private in political and public life and offering a powerful illustration of these arguments. So this is the point where I must note that I do not have any children. And yet while I do not have *children*, I have quite a bit of experience with *reproduction*—or at least the attempt at it. I tried to get pregnant for seven years before finally calling it quits, and I went through just about every possible route to get there.

At some point during this multiyear process, I started keeping an illustrated journal about my experiences, which eventually became the comic *Present / Perfect*. I'm not sure why I started drawing comics about my failed attempts to reproduce, but as I've been working on this book, I discovered why I *kept* drawing them. To put it bluntly: I've never felt more like a body than I did while undergoing fertility treatment. Constantly monitoring and dutifully reporting my bodily processes day after day, month after month, year after year; getting injected, swabbed, poked, prodded, and measured both quantitatively ("this follicle is 3.5") and qualitatively ("your lining is beautiful!"); undergoing invasive procedures and regularly looking at and thinking about my insides (usually with a group of people in the room): when trying to conceive, I was a (female) body first, and, most important, I was a body that didn't work the way I "should." After returning from yet another visit to the gynecologist, reproductive endocrinologist, or obstetrician, there was something thrilling about taking the instruments of representation into my own hands. In the pluripotent space of the comic panel, I had the power to represent not only my body and my experiences, but also my doctors, nurses, friends, and husband. Confronted daily by a pronatalist world that reminded me how abnormal I was, in the constant din of infertility testing and treatment—and then during my pregnancy and the grief that followed its loss—my pencils, pens, paints, and paper offered a quiet place to work out what was happening to me with some measure of critical distance.[1]

French surgeon René Leriche once described health as life lived "in the silence of the organs."[2] Yet as Michel Foucault famously explains in *Birth of the Clinic*, medicine is not just an aural art but a visual one, and the two arts are intimately intertwined. The doctor's silent observation is transubstantiated as speech; clinical observation, Foucault writes, "has the paradoxical ability to *hear a language* as soon as it *perceives a spectacle*." Moreover, the "[precarious] balance between speech and spectacle" underlying medical practice and the scientific impulse to carry this balance forward to create knowledge about the body demand that speech and sight be translated into images.[3]

Medicine makes pictures. Physicians look at and in their patients and craft maps of the body and its processes with X-rays, MRIs, CT scans, ultrasounds, and colonoscopy videos.[4] These pictures, writes Ian Williams, "help construct the illness stereotypes that influence the way in which a condition is viewed by others as well as the patient's experience of the condition."[5] Medical maps of the body, in other words, not only bring the body's territory into being for scientists and doctors; they also represent cultural geographies that shape understanding of our bodies and our very selves.[6] If the twenty-first-century self, as Nikolas Rose has argued, is anchored by a sense of somatic individuality[7]—that is, an understanding of the embodied self filtered through the lens of biomedicine—then this self is given shape through words *and* images. In the intensely visual domain of contemporary medicine, then, to experience health is to enjoy both the privilege of silent organs and the luxury of their invisibility.

The noisy presence of trauma, illness, and pain closely maps onto the experience of even the most typical pregnancy and birth. Many pregnant people (especially pregnant trans people and gender nonconforming folks) feel as though they are on constant display.[8] To be an extraordinary body in the world is to be seen as available for public consumption. As Rosemarie Garland-Thomson writes, "because we come to expect one another to have certain kinds of bodies and behaviors, stares flare up when we glimpse people who look or act in ways that contradict our assumptions by interrupting complacent visual business-as-usual." Staring is "an interrogative gesture that asks what's going on and demands the story," Garland-Thomson explains. "The eyes hang on, working to recognize what seems illegible, order what seems unruly, know what seems strange." This initial interrogatory gesture of staring becomes folded into narrative, which may then be "carried over into engagement," sometimes welcome and sometimes not.[9] As many visibly pregnant people report, the engagement initiated by a look often turns into deeply personal questions and sometimes even direct touch.

As Anne Balsamo writes, "A pregnant woman is divested of ownership of her body, as if to reassert in some primitive way her functional service to the species—she ceases to be an individual, defined through recourse to rights of privacy, *and becomes a biological spectacle*."[10] The pregnant body in the world is first and foremost apprehended as a symbol: a narrative to be deciphered and an image to be seen, consumed, interpreted, and scrutinized.[11] To be visibly pregnant, then, is to lose the privilege of privacy. Even further, visibility, as Peggy Phelan argues, "summons surveillance and the law."[12] A visibly pregnant body not only calls forth stares, advice, and touches, but also judgment, discipline, and control.

Like any other instantiation of power, the regulation of reproduction and the surveillance of pregnant bodies are not distributed equally. The history of reproductive rights in the United States and its territories, for example, is rife with examples in which calls for the individual right to birth control have been transformed into racist practices and eugenic policies of population control. Black, Chicana, Puerto Rican, Indigenous, disabled, and poor women have all been disproportionately subjected to institutionalized fertility control, including involuntary sterilization.[13] As activists and critics have been arguing for generations, human reproduction is a place where the boundaries between biological, social, technological, and political life collapse, even while, as Emily Martin has argued, reproduction is also a site where discourse about the "natural" reigns supreme.[14]

Reproduction is a complicated process of meiosis, if you will—a merging of personal and political, body and ideology, individual and institution, science and technology, joy and pain, nature and culture, sex and gender, humor and horror, seeing and saying.

In this deeply tangled site, *Graphic Reproduction* seeks to intervene. Importantly, we do not aim in this book to unravel the many ways of under-standing reproduction; instead, we investigate their crossings and pull gently on their knots. In other words, this book does *not* seek to resolve the tension that arises among the stories in the following pages. What reproduction means for one artist is not what it means for another. There are (re)productive contradictions and rhetorical contractions throughout the words and images in this volume. The primary function of *Graphic Reproduction* is to provide a discursive and visual forum where the affective, biological, social, and political complexities of repro-duction can exist together in generative uncertainty. The comics in this book offer a rich, multivalent perspective on human reproduction.[15] In the rest of this introduction, I first situate comics about reproduction within the growing field of graphic medicine, with the requisite notes of caution about this positioning. Then, I introduce each comic included here and offer a brief reading of the work to illustrate some of the generative tensions that are revealed.

Graphic Medicine

Defn. of the Field

The field of graphic medicine combines the discourses of medicine with the medium of comics. Scholars and practitioners of graphic medicine explore how comics can effectively represent the many voices and bodies involved in any health-care encounter, and they draw on this multiplicity in productive and unexpected ways. In a landmark essay in the *British Medical Journal*, Michael Green and Kimberly Myers argue that the multiple perspectives of graphic medicine can be used to train more effective and empathetic healthcare providers. "Visual under-standing is intuitive in ways that verbal understanding may not be," they write; comics might assist doctors to communicate effectively with their patients, and graphic pathographies—autobiographical comics about illness—may also help "patients and their families better understand what to expect of a certain disease." Moreover, for medical students and residents, particularly those actively working with patients, these deeply engaging personal accounts of illness and medical care are vivid reminders that "healing a patient involves more than treating a body."[16] In this way, graphic medicine may be viewed as a subset of medical humanities, which is often presented as a method of training more effective doctors and nurses.

While I strongly believe that comics—and the humanities more generally—can and should serve an important function in medical education (and I deeply hope that this book is used that way), there is a risk in viewing comics about

Hidden Knowledge

health and medicine as yet another instrument in a doctor's iconic black case. As Susan Squier argues in *Graphic Medicine Manifesto*, as medical humanities has begun to take a new shape as "health humanities," the field has "expanded from an implicit endorsement of the practitioner's emphasis on medical treatment to a critical incorporation of the caregiver's or patient's experiences, including the social determinants of health and wellbeing."[17] This perspective—the patient's view, the view from below, the view from the table, as it were—is where the *medium* of comics comes to matter a great deal.

As the authors of *Graphic Medicine Manifesto* explain, graphic medicine is "a movement for change that challenges the dominant methods of scholarship in healthcare, offering a more inclusive perspective of medicine, illness, disability, caregiving, and being cared for. . . . [It] arises out of a discomfort with supposed techno-medical progress, working to include those who are not currently represented within its discourse."[18] Comics have long served as a medium to explore taboo subjects. Many of the earliest underground comics, for example, graphically depicted sex and drugs and pushed the legal envelope to the point where several artists, publishers, and comic shops were charged with obscenity. Although the underground comics movement of the 1960s and 1970s was largely dominated by straight white men, there were also many subversive women cartoonists, queer cartoonists, and cartoonists of color whose work was disseminated in political circles.[19] As a medium already on the margins of "proper" literature and culture, then, comics offer an "ideal [forum] for exploring taboo or forbidden areas of illness and healthcare."[20]

And yet, the savvy feminist reader might object, doesn't the very act of categorizing comics about conception, pregnancy, and childbirth as graphic "medicine" reinforce the medicalization of reproduction, an issue that has become its own cottage industry within feminist scholarship?[21] This is a point well taken. However, there is no question that most pregnancies and births in the West have a medical component, even if only a resistance to the medicalization of reproduction. Notably, many comics in this book directly challenge medicine's authority over pregnancy and childbirth, and it is their critique of medicalization that makes them ideal exemplars of the genre of graphic medicine. Many works of graphic medicine, such as David Small's award-winning *Stitches* and John Porcellino's *The Hospital Suite*, object to the common assumption that medical treatment is always the answer to our health troubles and explore how medical treatment may also create issues of its own. In the seemingly simple act of privileging the patient's experience, graphic medicine offers a direct challenge to the authorship of the narrative that characterizes the medical encounter and shakes the subject-object relationship in which "agent" is applied only to the healthcare provider and "patient" is applied to, well, the patient.

The visual presentation of the embodied self by "autographic" artists offers many other critical affordances.[22] Although all forms of autobiography require a presentation of self, that presentation in graphic form requires an attention to temporal embodiment utterly unique to the genre. According to Elisabeth El Refaie, the "requirement to produce multiple drawn versions of one's self necessarily involves an intense engagement with embodied aspects of identity."[23] The "multiple" aspects of what El Refaie calls "pictorial embodiment" also reflect a feature of comics that has long captivated scholars of the medium: the relationship that comics present between time and space.[24]

As the sighted reader's eye moves across the page, narrative emerges from one panel to the next, but also in the spaces between them, or what is known as the "gutter." To appreciate the power of comics is to understand the hermeneutic interplay between time, space, and the reader, who fills in the semantic and temporal gaps in a process Scott McCloud describes as "closure," which "allows us to connect these moments and mentally construct a unified reality."[25] All arts rely on closure in some way—the reader of a novel supplies information between chapters, the viewer of a painting relies on context and clues from visual culture—but comics use closure "like no other" art form does, McCloud argues emphatically. The audience of a comic is not just a passive recipient of the narrative but its active co-creator: "in the limbo of the gutter, human imagination takes two separate images and transforms them into a single idea."[26] This relationship between time and space, McCloud argues, is the very "essence" of comics: in comics, time *equals* space.[27]

In this way, a gutter functions as what scholars of rhetoric would call an enthymeme, a form of reasoning in which the audience supplies an unstated premise.[28] For example, if I explain that people enjoy comics because they are drawn in and moved by them, I assume that my reader believes that *people enjoy things they are drawn in and moved by.* As Cara Finnegan explains, "The power of the enthymeme lies in the fiction that its unstated premise, at once invisible and transparent, is 'natural' rather than context-bound; it is simply something that 'everybody knows.' In addition, enthymemes are powerful because they grant audiences agency. The audience is not merely a witness to the argument, but a participant in its creation."[29] Yet while the enthymematic process of co-creating meaning makes comics a rhetorically powerful art form, it also makes the medium highly unstable. Two people might read a comic in two radically different ways, depending on how they have filled in the space/time between the panels. The power of the enthymeme is in what it assumes of its audience, yet it is the radical contingency of closure, not its universality, that makes the medium of comics so generative. You can test this: find two sequential panels in the comics that follow and ask a group of people to describe—or, better yet, draw—the action that takes place off the page. I suspect you will get a host of different answers, each of which pulls the reader's experience into the artwork. Despite the fact that the hermeneutic flexibility of comics might be risky in some respects (in that a comic does not communicate its meaning without remainder and is subject to

enthymeme

misreading), the plasticity and polysemy they allow is one of the most engaging aspects of the medium since readers are required to become directly involved in the story that unfolds over the panels.[30]

While most of the comics in this collection can be understood as graphic medicine, even in their challenges to the medicalization of reproduction, I want to make clear that most of the comics included here do not fall into the category of graphic pathography, a genre that explores the pictorial embodiment of illness.[31] While there is quite a bit of medicine in the pages that follow, and quite a bit of physical and emotional pain, there is very little illness. I make this distinction not to distinguish pregnancy from illness or disability in a way that devalues people with an illness or disability,[32] but to uphold the critical voice at the core of these narratives. As Marika Seigel argues, "How we define the work of pregnancy has material consequences on women's bodies and ways of living."[33] While pregnancy may sometimes involve negative health effects, and childbirth involves pain, pregnancy is not de facto an illness, and childbirth is not de facto a medical emergency.

Exploring This Book

The comics in this anthology offer a multitude of perspectives on the experience of getting pregnant and being pregnant and on the ending of pregnancy, and they all represent the experiences of everyday people. There are no superheroes here (although superheroes, too, can get pregnant).[34] This variety includes the artists themselves. Some (Farmer and Chevli, Summers, Knight, Tyler, Bechdel) are well-established, award-winning cartoonists. Some, like me, have little artistic training. Some (Summers, Shepherd, Doane) write about their own experiences, while others seek to represent the experiences of others, both real (Alexander-Tanner, Hayes, Weaver-Hightower, and Zucker) and fictional (Farmer and Chevli, Bechdel). What all of these comics share, however, are narratives about reproduction that preserve and highlight its messiness, complexity, and ambiguity.

The collection begins with *Abortion Eve*, drawn by legendary feminist cartoonists Joyce Farmer and Lyn Chevli. In 1972 Farmer and Chevli published *Tits and Clits Comix*, one of the first comics written, drawn, and published by women. In 1973, writing under pseudonyms, they collaborated on the comic *Abortion Eve*, which chronicles five fictional women (whose names are all variants on "Eve") and their experiences obtaining legal abortions shortly after *Roe v. Wade*. The comic was inspired in part by Farmer's decision to get an abortion in 1970. After consulting with a psychiatrist (a requirement for the procedure under California law pre-*Roe*), Farmer was initially denied because the psychiatrist found her "mentally fit" to bear children. After she stated that she would then do the procedure herself, the psychiatrist declared Farmer to be "suicidal" and therefore unfit to be a mother. "Thus began my radicalization," Farmer explains. "I was astounded that I had to prove to the state that I was suicidal, when all I wanted was an abortion, clean and safe."[35]

Produced at a time when the very idea of abortion without apology was a radical perspective, *Abortion Eve* pushes boundaries in both form and content—to the point where Planned Parenthood resisted distributing it because of the graphic artwork it contained.[36] The comic doesn't shy away from the complex questions and emotions that sometimes accompany abortion, although it does work to contain them in service to its narrative. Presenting a diverse cast of characters with multiple reasons for seeking abortion (and employing some racial stereotypes, it must be noted, to differentiate those characters) and peppered with the language ("Far out!") and fashions of the moment and expressions of sisterhood, *Abortion Eve* offers a compelling snapshot of the personal dimension of reproductive rights during the radical U.S. women's health movement of the 1970s.

Leah Hayes provides a more contemporary look at abortion in *Not Funny Ha-Ha*, which, like *Abortion Eve*, is designed as a handbook. In this illustrated guide, Hayes uses second-person pronouns, colloquial language, and simple illustrations to walk women through the different types of abortion and what they can expect afterward, both physically and emotionally, and it is here that her comic departs a bit from Farmer and Chevli's. Hayes centers emotions in these excerpts from the longer book, but departing from the narrative form of *Abortion Eve*, *Not Funny* allows complex, contradictory emotions to remain without forcing resolution. "Remember," Hayes explains, "this is not an easy thing to go through. Don't be afraid to talk to someone (or someones!) about what you're feeling." Although the text is vague regarding the specific feelings one might expect after the procedure, the illustrations provide some examples: the woman in the full-page illustration on the penultimate page cries, and the women on the final page wear a collection of different expressions—some seem to express sadness, some a sort of blankness, some relief and happiness, and, most interestingly, some display a combination of all of these. Produced more than forty years apart—in 1973, just a few months after abortion was first made legal and widely available, and in 2015, when numerous state laws have sought to curtail its legality and availability—these two handbooks offer views of the procedure from the perspective of the women who are seeking it.

The next three comics make visible two common experiences with reproduction that, like abortion, are rarely represented in visual culture: infertility and miscarriage.[37] Although 10–15 percent of people seeking to reproduce struggle with infertility, and although 10–20 percent of pregnancies end in miscarriage,[38] these experiences are rarely discussed with others, even family and friends. The strong cultural mandate to reproduce and the thick ideological bands that tie reproductive capacity to the proper performance of gender roles often result in stigma and shame, particularly for women.[39] The invisibility of miscarriage specifically is mirrored (if not produced) by medical and popular advice to keep a pregnancy secret until it becomes visible on the body, lest one go through the uncomfortable social work of retracting a pregnancy announcement. Because of this secrecy and shame, these common experiences have been rendered almost entirely invisible. They are rarely depicted in popular culture, and in the few cases that either infertility or miscarriage do make an appearance, it is almost always to support a narrative that ends with a baby. The comics in this collection by Knight, Johnson, and Shepherd not only make infertility and miscarriage visible, but they also challenge the typical move to contain those experiences as merely a more dramatic version of that familiar cultural narrative: a rockier road that always ends with successful reproduction.

Paula Knight's *Spooky Womb* personifies Knight's relationship with her reproductive body, which takes form as a separate entity that follows her around. Beginning the narrative with an hourglass and her thirtieth birthday, Knight shows her womb as a symbol of a biological clock; it pops in and out of her awareness to gently pester her with a demand to get pregnant. After a few years, the womb's requests are answered ("I'll see what I can do," Knight tells it) by a pregnancy, which is lost. After the miscarriage, the dynamic of the comic changes, as Knight blames the spooky womb, shaking her finger in anger until it disappears with a puff. In the next panels, however, the womb returns to her consciousness, the two reconcile, and they walk hand-in-fallopian-tube toward an uncertain future: "What now?" Knight wonders. In *X Utero*, "a cluster of comics" from Knight, she confronts the issues of infertility and miscarriage but without the frame of an overarching narrative. The images, some of which draw on mixed-media collages of her medical documents, family pictures, and representations of DNA and genetics, illustrate some of the existential questions of genetic kinship that infertility and pregnancy loss often provoke: Who am I? What or who have I lost? Where have I been? Where am I going? In one series of images, Knight documents the unique traits of her family members in a collaged photo album and then affixes this diachronic embodied kinship to her singular body in the present moment. "These things will be forever mine," she writes, "because I'll never pass them on. I'm the end of the line. So this album is redundant; a finite book—unless you'd care to take a look?"

The emphasis on temporality in Knight's work is also seen in my comic *Present / Perfect*, which depicts the many years I spent dealing with unexplained infertility. Like Knight, I grapple with the complex emotions that accompany difficulties with reproduction, with a focus on the processes of infertility treatment and the queer temporality that accompanies infertility and miscarriage. Like many pieces in this collection, my comic does not end on a note of triumph, but with uncertainty. It leaves the reader to ponder what it means to accept a non-normative life in the present and to consider the possibilities of a future untethered to a cultural script.

This section of the volume ends with Endrené Shepherd's *A Significant Loss*, which details her story of becoming pregnant and having a "missed" miscarriage at nine weeks. Shepherd's comic illustrates a common medical quandary rarely discussed regarding miscarriage: the decision about whether to have a surgical abortion or a "natural" miscarriage at home. "Natural is better, right?" Shepherd thinks, and then endures what she calls a "real horror-show, painful, bloody & terrifying." Shepherd's nuanced portrayal of her physical pain is matched by her description of the psychological pain of miscarriage, as different everyday events—from hearing a baby cry to "too much sympathy"—triggered waves of grief. Like the comics by Knight and Johnson, this one also ends with the acceptance of an uncertain future. "I'd still like to have kids," Shepherd explains, "but it's OK if it's not in the cards. Who knows, right? I'll be OK."

These three comics each illustrate a slightly different approach to representing the artist's connection to the embryo and/or fetus. "It was only a cluster of cells," says Knight about an early pregnancy loss, "but it was MY cluster of cells!" My comic explains that although my husband and I did not imbue our frozen embryos with personhood, we nonetheless gave each a fictional name to keep track of them. Shepherd uses the word "baby" to describe her lost fetus and uses masculine pronouns to mark the singularity of the pregnancy: "I'll always be sad to have lost that baby. That specific baby. I'm not in a hurry to replace him." These differences in fetal representation illustrate a common tension regarding how to characterize the strange grief of miscarriage. What, exactly, is one grieving? Are we mourning what has been lost or what will never be?

Grief also comes to the fore in Marcus Weaver-Hightower's narrative "Losing Thomas and Ella," which presents a situation even more rare than infertility and miscarriage: perinatal loss. Weaver-Hightower's project initially began as a qualitative study of the experiences that a man named Paul and his wife, Jenna, had during and after the loss of premature twins. However, after combing through his interview notes, Weaver-Hightower found that traditional academic discourse did not sufficiently capture the richness of Paul's narrative, so he turned to a visual medium. Incorporating techniques from qualitative research methods (member checking, for example, which required that he share the comic with Paul as it developed in order to solicit feedback), Weaver-Hightower's comic presents scholarly research in a new mode and also uses that mode to reimagine the processes and boundaries of qualitative research itself. As Weaver-Hightower puts it, "Comics afford their creators sights, motion, sound effects, the elapsing of time, and even glimpses into places where normal, unaided vision cannot go, like inside the body."[40] The result is a multitextured window onto perinatal loss that brings to our attention some elements of the experience that might have fallen into the background of a traditional study: the everyday (such as the pulled pork sandwiches eaten in grief, the forbidden bologna and soft cheese of pregnancy), the endless, boring days in the hospital, the collision of past trauma and present anxiety (vividly pictured in a panel by positioning one of the lost babies next to Jenna's current pregnancy), and, perhaps most striking, the deep-seated feelings of unease that follow pregnancy loss and infant death. Much like the question marks that conclude the previous comics about infertility and miscarriage, even though Paul and Jenna become pregnant again, the comic ends with uncertainty. "You like to think that there's some guarantees that are going to come out of it or some sort of lesson," Paul explains. "Well, you can't do anything really. You can just kind of hope that you're not going to get the bad call next time." In the pen-ultimate panel, Paul looks silently toward the last panel: a black box, an unknown future.

If one of the unique affordances of comics is the capacity to depict embodiment over time, closely related is the power of comics to depict the complexity of emotions at a single moment. Comics draw on established cultural iconography to make emotions visible on the body (facial expressions, posture) and on iconographies specific to the medium (such as emanata, the swirls and lines that convey anxiety, anger, and sadness; or using light and shadow to set a mood), as well as more idiosyncratic representations of emotion that help to communicate "the raw veracity of lived experience."[41] Particularly powerful in this regard is the capacity of comics to depict multiple emotions at once. Emotions are usually discussed in isolation from one another, but many comics in this collection illustrate their characters experiencing simultaneous, and sometimes contradictory, emotions: the joy/pain of hearing about others' pregnancies during infertility or after miscarriage, the excitement/anxiety of a new pregnancy after infant loss, the exhilaration/exhaustion of being a new parent.

The next two comics in this volume address the diverse experiences of pregnancy care and the relationship between institutional medicine and midwifery, and they both illustrate the power of graphic medicine to challenge the medical status quo. In A. K. Summers's *Pregnant Butch*, based on her experience reconciling pregnancy with her gender identity, we see her character, Teek, confront the insistently heterosexual, gender-dimorphic discourses of obstetrics, midwifery, and childbirth education. This tension builds to a fantasy resolution, as Teek imagines a "dream [childbirth] class" filled with a "hot single," a "bearded lady," pregnant butches, "birth givers," "birth partners," "some highly idiosyncratic classifications," and "at least one threesome." This section of the comic ends in a marvelously queer pyramid, a fantasy of community and support.

In Bethany Doane's *Pushing Back*, we see another challenge to institutionalized medicine and to the state interests with which it is entangled. Doane and her husband, Jeff, choose to have a home birth assisted by a midwife. The birth is free from complications, save a tear that Doane's midwife recommends she have stitched at a local hospital. After Doane is admitted, she is treated by "intrusive," "judgmental" hospital staff, who wonder where her baby is and demand that she provide information about her "care provider." To calm them, Doane tells

"the about to die moment"

the experience of reading the comic is different than reading text the nurses that her home birth was an accident, but the staff do not believe her; as she is receiving treatment, the police and fire department both appear at her house, frightening her husband. The next day, she and her husband are visited by Child Protective Services.

The next two comics focus on the difficult and sometimes overwhelming months immediately following childbirth. The first, *Overwhelmed, Anxious, and Angry*, written by Jessica Zucker, a clinical psychologist, and illustrated by Ryan Alexander-Tanner, chronicles women's experiences with postpartum depression. Though fictionalized, the narratives are based on the stories of real women, and the resulting comic not only sheds light on a difficult topic, but also—like the comics about abortion and perinatal loss—uses the comic form for a pedagogical purpose, to educate readers about the "most common complication associated with childbirth." The featured women confess to ambivalence, resentment, anger, trauma, failure, and guilt about feeling anything other than joy and excitement about motherhood. The comic builds toward a medicalized understanding of postpartum depression that seeks to show how common the condition is and, most important, emphasizes that it is often treatable. This is the only comic in the collection that privileges the voice of a medical provider—a therapist. This comic is paired with Carol Tyler's single-panel "Anatomy of a New Mom," which provides a tongue-in-cheek guide to a mother's mind and body in the first few months after giving birth.

Graphic Reproduction concludes with a selection from Alison Bechdel's celebrated comic *Dykes to Watch Out For*, in which the fictional Toni and Clarice experience a midwife-assisted homebirth attended by their friends. The excerpt begins with the characters musing on the changing norms of parenthood in queer communities. "Used to be," remarks Ginger, "being a dyke got you off the hook. No one expected you to make babies." Acerbic Mo agrees: "What I want to know is, how much is this lesbian baby boom just a ticket to being socially acceptable—a way for dykes to prove they're 'real women' in a culture that equates womanhood with motherhood?" Even as the characters argue about what motherhood means to their community, they have showed up en masse to support Toni and Clarice, and the final birth scene is a joyous celebration of the community that sustains the new parents. Bechdel's comic offers a very different picture of reproduction than the typical cultural narrative that circulates in the Western world. With an emphasis on community and an extended meaning of kinship that draws the line of family beyond blood and genetics; a celebration of pregnant embodiment that does not portray birth as an agonizing, thoroughly medicalized, and technologized process; and a carefully considered perspective on the personal and political meaning of parenthood (and, if one continues reading this particular story line through the series, a full exploration of the impact of children on a relationship), Bechdel's comic summarizes the many tensions that characterize the comics in this volume. "What a wonderful atmosphere to be born into!" the romantic Sparrow exclaims toward the end of Bechdel's comic. "He might not even need therapy when he grows up!"

As Ian Williams argues, "Images do not just 'mirror' the world; they help to build it."[42] Comics do not just portray different perspectives on the world we live in; they also have the potential to imagine new worlds. In the case of reproduction, comics offer a window onto a future world that grapples seriously with the personal and political meanings of conception, pregnancy, and childbirth, as well as their contradictions; a world that faces honestly the many struggles that people have with conception, pregnancy, and birth with the hope of ameliorating stigma, shame, grief, and loneliness; a world that looks candidly at the complex emotions that accompany any act of reproduction; and even a world that considers a life without children to be as rich and meaningful as a life with them. By presenting this multiplicity without yielding to the demand for a neat narrative, a perfect resolution, or a singular meaning, the comics of *Graphic Reproduction* demonstrate that these potential worlds might be found in the cracks of the world we already live in. That is, as Paula Knight puts it, if "you'd care to take a look."

NOTES

1. For an exploration of how making comics may serve a therapeutic function (and the limits of this association), see Ian Williams, "Autography as Auto-Therapy: Psychic Pain and the Graphic Memoir," *Journal of Medical Humanities* 32, no. 4 (2011): 353–66.

2. Quoted in Georges Canguilhem, *The Normal and the Pathological* (New York: Zone, 1989).

3. Michel Foucault, *The Birth of the Clinic*, trans. A. M. Sheridan Smith (New York: Vintage, 1973), 108 (emphases in original), 115.

4. See, for example, Kelly Ann Joyce, *Magnetic Appeal: MRI and the Myth of Transparency* (Ithaca: Cornell University Press, 2008).

5. Ian Williams, "Comics and the Iconography of Illness," in MK Czerwiec, Ian Williams, Susan Merrill Squier, Michael J. Green, Kimberly R. Myers, and Scott T. Smith, *Graphic Medicine Manifesto* (University Park: Penn State University Press, 2015), 118.

6. See Elizabeth Wilson's work on this metaphor of mapping in her *Neural Geographies: Feminism and the Microstructure of Cognition* (New York: Routledge, 1998).

7. Nikolas Rose, *The Politics of Life Itself* (Princeton: Princeton University Press, 2009).

8. I am thinking here about the huge rush of publicity and interest in Thomas Beatie's pregnancies. For more on the circulating meaning around Beatie's pregnancies, see J. Halberstam, "The Pregnant Man," *Velvet Light Trap* 65, no. 1 (2010): 77–78.

9. Rosemarie Garland-Thomson, *Staring: How We Look* (Oxford: Oxford University Press, 2009), 3–4.

10. Anne Balsamo, "Public Pregnancies and Cultural Narratives of Surveillance," in *Revisioning Women, Health, and Healing: Feminist, Cultural, and Technoscience Perspectives*, ed. Adele E. Clarke and Virginia Olesen (New York: Routledge, 1999), 231–53, 231, my emphasis.

11. Many feminist scholars have written about how the collision of pregnant embodiment and visual culture impacts the construction of maternal and fetal subjectivity, and it would take an encyclopedia to list them all. For foundational studies on the subject, see Rosalind Pollack Petchesky, "Foetal Images: The Power of Visual Culture in the Politics of Reproduction," in *Reproductive*

Technologies: Gender, Motherhood, and Medicine, ed. Michelle Stanworth (Minneapolis: University of Minnesota Press, 1987); Carol A. Stabile, "Shooting the Mother: Fetal Photography and the Politics of Disappearance," *Camera Obscura* 10, no. 128 (1992): 178–205; Susan Merrill Squier, *Babies in Bottles: Twentieth-Century Visions of Reproductive Technologies* (New Brunswick: Rutgers University Press, 1994); and especially Barbara Duden's classic *Disembodying Women: Perspectives on Pregnancy and the Unborn* (Cambridge: Harvard University Press, 1993).

12. Peggy Phelan, *Unmarked: The Politics of Performance* (London: Routledge, 2003), 6–7. For a detailed discussion of visibility and pregnancy, see 130–45.

13. See, for example, Angela Y. Davis, *Women, Race, and Class* (1981; repr., New York: Vintage, 2011), esp. 202–21; Inés Hernández-Avila, "In Praise of Insubordination; or, What Makes a Good Woman Go Bad?" in *Transforming a Rape Culture*, ed. Emilie Buchwald, Pamela R. Fletcher, and Martha Roth (Minneapolis: Milkweed, 1993), 323–42; Virginia Espino, "Women Sterilized as They Give Birth: Forced Sterilization and the Chicana Resistance in the 1970s," in *Las Obreras: Chicana Politics of Work and Family*, ed. Vicki Ruiz (Los Angeles: UCLA Chicano Studies Research Center Publications, 2000), 65–82; Jessica Enoch, "Survival Stories: Feminist Historiographic Approaches to Chicana Rhetorics of Sterilization Abuse," *Rhetoric Society Quarterly* 35, no. 3 (2005): 5–30; Dorothy Roberts, *Killing the Black Body: Race, Reproduction, and the Meaning of Liberty* (New York: Vintage, 2014); and Loretta Ross, Elena Gutiérrez, Marlene Gerber, and Jael Silliman, eds., *Undivided Rights: Women of Color Organizing for Reproductive Justice* (New York: Haymarket, 2016).

14. Emily Martin, *The Woman in the Body: A Cultural Analysis of Reproduction* (New York: Beacon, 2001).

15. There are significant limits to the volume's scope and any claims to representation, particularly since it does not include comics by artists of color. The collection unfortunately had to be limited to extant comics—none could be commissioned— and only includes comics for which I was able to secure the rights to reprint. I hope that as the field of comics keeps growing, this volume is not the only one dedicated to graphic approaches to reproduction, merely the first. For scholarship on the intersection of race and comics, see Jeffrey A. Brown, *Black Superheroes, Milestone Comics, and Their Fans* (Oxford: University of Mississippi Press, 2001); Héctor Fernández L'Hoeste and Juan Poblete, eds., *Redrawing the Nation: National Identity in Latin/o American Comics* (London: Springer, 2009); and Deborah Elizabeth Whaley, *Black Women in Sequence: Re-Inking Comics, Graphic Novels, and Anime* (Seattle: University of Washington Press, 2015).

16. Michael J. Green and Kimberly Myers, "Graphic Medicine: Use of Comics in Medical Education and Patient Care," *British Medical Journal* 340 (2010): 574–77, 576.

17. Susan Merrill Squier, "The Uses of Graphic Medicine for Engaged Scholarship," in Czerwiec et al., *Graphic Medicine Manifesto*, 41–66, 48. See also Catherine Belling, "Toward a Harder Humanities in Medicine," *Atrium* 3 (2006): 1–5.

18. Czerwiec et al., *Graphic Medicine Manifesto*, 2–3.

19. For more on the politics of difference in mainstream comics, see Ramzi Fawaz, *The New Mutants: Superheroes and the Radical Imagination of American Comics* (New York: New York University Press, 2016).

20. Czerwiec et al., *Graphic Medicine Manifesto*, 3.

21. For a sample of the many feminist challenges to the medicalization of pregnancy, see Judith Walzer Leavitt, *Brought to Bed: Childbearing in America, 1750 to 1950* (New York: Oxford University Press, 1986); Kristin K. Barker, "A Ship upon a Stormy Sea: The Medicalization of Pregnancy," *Social Science and Medicine* 47, no. 8 (1998): 1067–76; Robbie E. Davis-Floyd, *Birth as an American*

Rite of Passage (Berkeley: University of California Press, 2004); Sheila Kitzniger, *Birth Crisis* (New York: Routledge, 2006); and Marika Seigel, *The Rhetoric of Pregnancy* (Chicago: University of Chicago Press, 2013).

22. Gilliam Whitlock, "Autographics: The Seeing 'I' of Comics," *MFS: Modern Fiction Studies* 52, no. 4 (2006): 965–79, 966.

23. Elisabeth El Refaie, *Autobiographical Comics: Life-Writing in Pictures* (Oxford: University of Mississippi Press, 2012), 4.

24. El Refaie, *Autobiographical Comics*, 51.

25. Scott McCloud, *Understanding Comics: The Invisible Art* (New York: HarperCollins, 1993), 67.

26. McCloud, *Understanding Comics*, 66.

27. "Round and Round with Scott McCloud: Interview by R. C. Harvey," *Comics Journal* 179 (1995): 52–81. See also Scott McCloud, *Reinventing Comics* (New York: Paradox, 2000). For a complication of the cognitive elements at play in McCloud's argument, see Neil Cohn, "The Limits of Time and Transitions: Challenges to Theories of Sequential Image Comprehension," *Studies in Comics* 1, no. 1 (2010): 127–47.

28. Robert Dennis Watkins, "Sequential Rhetoric: Teaching Comics as Visual Rhetoric" (Ph.D. diss., University of Iowa, 2014), 57. For more on the rhetorical function of gutters, see Joshua C. Hilst, "Gutter Talk: (An)Other Idiom," *JAC: A Journal of Rhetoric, Culture, and Politics* 31, nos. 1–2 (2011): 153–76, and the subsequent response from Jeff Rice, "Guttered Anecdotes," *JAC* 32, nos. 1–2 (2012): 362–72.

29. Cara A. Finnegan, "Recognizing Lincoln: Image Vernaculars in Nineteenth-Century Visual Culture," *Rhetoric and Public Affairs* 8, no. 1 (2005): 31–57, 34.

30. For more on polysemy, see Leah Ceccarelli, "Polysemy: Multiple Meanings in Rhetorical Criticism," *Quarterly Journal of Speech* 84, no. 4 (1998): 395–415.

31. Green and Myers, "Graphic Medicine." There is a great deal of semantic wrangling over what to call the emerging genre of autobiographical comics that don't fit comfortably into the dominant category of graphic novels. Some scholars prefer the terms "autobiographical comics," "graphic memoirs," and "graphic life writing." See, for example, David Herman, "Multimodal Storytelling and Identity Construction in Graphic Narratives," in *Telling Stories: Language, Narrative, and Social Life*, ed. Deborah Schiffrin, Anna De Fina, and Anastasia Nylund (Washington, D.C.: Georgetown University Press, 2010), 195–208. Others prefer the term "autography," such as Whitlock, "Autographics"; Gilliam Whitlock and Anna Poletti, "Self-Regarding Art," *Biography* 31, no. 1 (2008): v–xxiii; and Williams, "Autography as Auto-Therapy."

32. See Douglas C. Baynton, "Disability and the Justification of Inequality in American History," in *The New Disability History: American Perspectives*, ed. Paul K. Longmore and Lauri Umansky (New York: New York University Press, 2001), 33–57.

33. Seigel, *Rhetoric of Pregnancy*, 6.

34. Jeffrey A. Brown, "Supermoms? Maternity and the Monstrous-Feminine in Superhero Comics," *Journal of Graphic Novels and Comics* 2, no. 1 (2011): 77–87.

35. Sam Meier, "The Comic Book That Guided Women Through Abortion Months After 'Roe.'" *Rewire*, June 8, 2016, https://rewire.news/article/2016/06/08/comic-book-abortion-after-roe.

36. Desmond Cole, "Comic Relief," *Canadian Medical Journal* 184, no. 16 (2012): E879–80, E880.

37. For perspectives on art related to infertility and miscarriage, see Maria Novotny, "Craft as a Memorializing Rhetoric," *Harlot* 14 (2015), http://harlotofthehearts.org/index.php/harlot/article/view/247/172.

38. "Infertility," Mayo Clinic, http://www.mayoclinic.org/diseases-conditions/infertility/home/ovc-20228734; and "Miscarriage," Mayo Clinic, http://www.mayoclinic.org/diseases-conditions/pregnancy-loss-miscarriage/home/ovc-20213664 (both accessed June 6, 2017).

39. For an excellent history of the shifting meanings of infertility in the scientific

and popular imaginations, see Robin E. Jensen, *Infertility: Tracing the History of a Transformative Term* (University Park: Penn State University Press, 2016).

40. Marcus B. Weaver-Hightower, "Losing Thomas and Ella: A Father's Story (A Research Comic)," *Journal of Medical Humanities* 38, no. 3 (2015): 1–16, 14.

41. Williams, "Comics and the Iconography of Illness," 119.

42. Williams, "Comics and the Iconography of Illness," 119.

Abortion Eve

(1973)

Joyce Farmer and Lyn Chevli

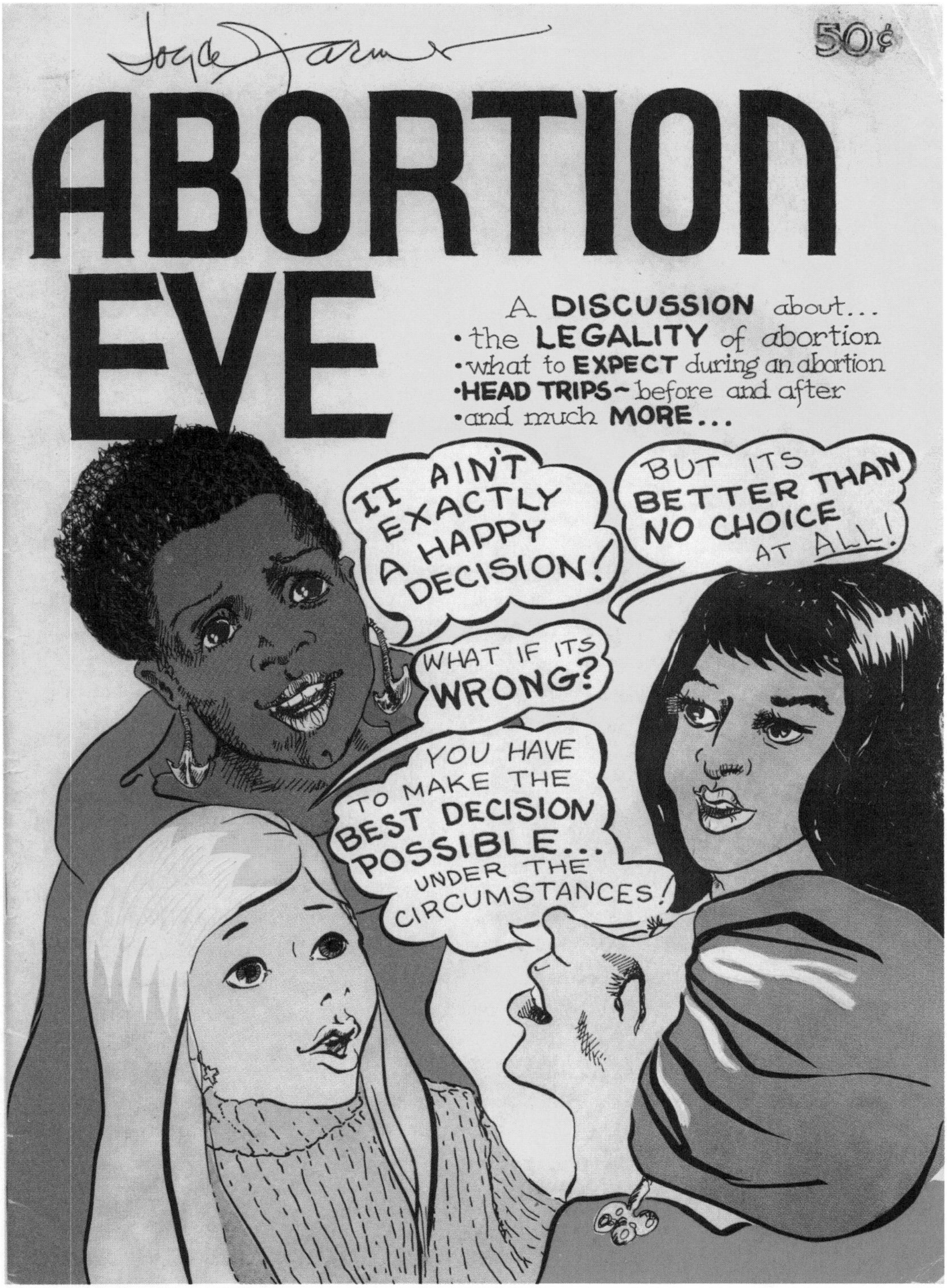
50¢
ABORTION EVE
A DISCUSSION about...
• the LEGALITY of abortion
• what to EXPECT during an abortion
• HEAD TRIPS ~ before and after
• and much MORE...
IT AIN'T EXACTLY A HAPPY DECISION!
BUT ITS BETTER THAN NO CHOICE AT ALL!
WHAT IF ITS WRONG?
YOU HAVE TO MAKE THE BEST DECISION POSSIBLE... UNDER THE CIRCUMSTANCES!

Are some people more likely to suffer from "UNWANTED PREGNANCY" than others?

Yes!

Scientific research shows that certain groups of people are immune to this dread affliction. For example: not one President of the United States has ever been known to suffer from it. In all the wars which our proud country has known, not one General of the Army, Admiral of the Navy or even a lowly helicopter pilot has ever contracted this malignant plague. Bank presidents, nuclear physicists, pipe fitters and sanitary engineers are also statistically "clean".

sexism

You may well ask who, then, is it that suffers the most? For some strange reason typists do, as well as nurses, secretaries welfare mothers and sopranos. Even some well-known actresses and athletes have fallen victim to it. Extensive analysis shows the one common denominator in people who have an unwanted pregnancy is:

THEY ARE ALL FEMALE!

The effective way for women to avoid this cursed plague is to practise Birth Control every day - like good diet or exercise. You will be delighted how rewarding it is!

THIS BOOK COULD NOT HAVE BEEN WRITTEN WITHOUT CREATIVE CONTACT WITH WOMENS GROUPS, FREE CLINICS, SCHOOLS, YOUNG-PEOPLE, REFERRAL AGENCIES, HOSPITALS AND DOCTORS. WE WELCOME MORE EXCHANGE WITH ALL THESE GROUPS. WE WOULD BE HAPPY TO DISCUSS SPECIAL RATES FOR ORDERS OVER 25 COPIES, AND THE POSSIBILITY OF INCLUDING YOUR AD.

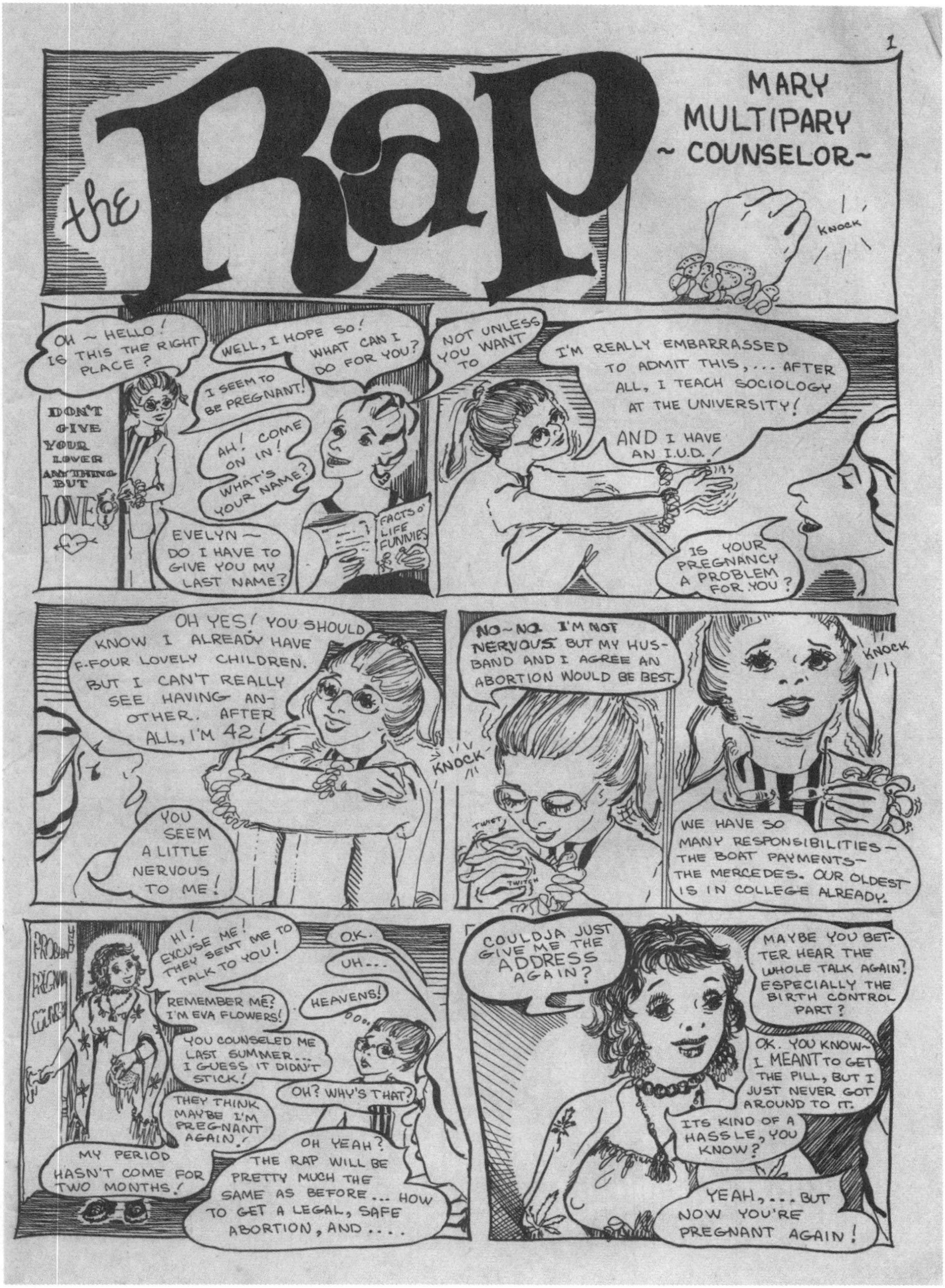
1
the Rap
MARY MULTIPARY ~COUNSELOR~
KNOCK
OH ~ HELLO! IS THIS THE RIGHT PLACE?
WELL, I HOPE SO! WHAT CAN I DO FOR YOU?
I SEEM TO BE PREGNANT!
AH! COME ON IN! WHAT'S YOUR NAME?
EVELYN — DO I HAVE TO GIVE YOU MY LAST NAME?
DON'T GIVE YOUR LOVER ANYTHING BUT LOVE
FACTS O' LIFE FUNNIES
NOT UNLESS YOU WANT TO
I'M REALLY EMBARRASSED TO ADMIT THIS, ... AFTER ALL, I TEACH SOCIOLOGY AT THE UNIVERSITY!
AND I HAVE AN I.U.D.!
IS YOUR PREGNANCY A PROBLEM FOR YOU?
OH YES! YOU SHOULD KNOW I ALREADY HAVE F-FOUR LOVELY CHILDREN. BUT I CAN'T REALLY SEE HAVING AN-OTHER. AFTER ALL, I'M 42!
YOU SEEM A LITTLE NERVOUS TO ME!
KNOCK
NO~NO. I'M NOT NERVOUS. BUT MY HUS-BAND AND I AGREE AN ABORTION WOULD BE BEST.
TWIST
TWITCH
KNOCK
WE HAVE SO MANY RESPONSIBILITIES— THE BOAT PAYMENTS— THE MERCEDES. OUR OLDEST IS IN COLLEGE ALREADY.
HI! EXCUSE ME! THEY SENT ME TO TALK TO YOU!
O.K.
UH...
REMEMBER ME? I'M EVA FLOWERS!
HEAVENS!
YOU COUNSELED ME LAST SUMMER... I GUESS IT DIDN'T STICK!
OH? WHY'S THAT?
THEY THINK MAYBE I'M PREGNANT AGAIN!
MY PERIOD HASN'T COME FOR TWO MONTHS!
OH YEAH? THE RAP WILL BE PRETTY MUCH THE SAME AS BEFORE... HOW TO GET A LEGAL, SAFE ABORTION, AND....
COULDJA JUST GIVE ME THE ADDRESS AGAIN?
MAYBE YOU BET-TER HEAR THE WHOLE TALK AGAIN? ESPECIALLY THE BIRTH CONTROL PART?
OK. YOU KNOW— I MEANT TO GET THE PILL, BUT I JUST NEVER GOT AROUND TO IT.
ITS KIND OF A HASSLE, YOU KNOW?
YEAH, ... BUT NOW YOU'RE PREGNANT AGAIN!

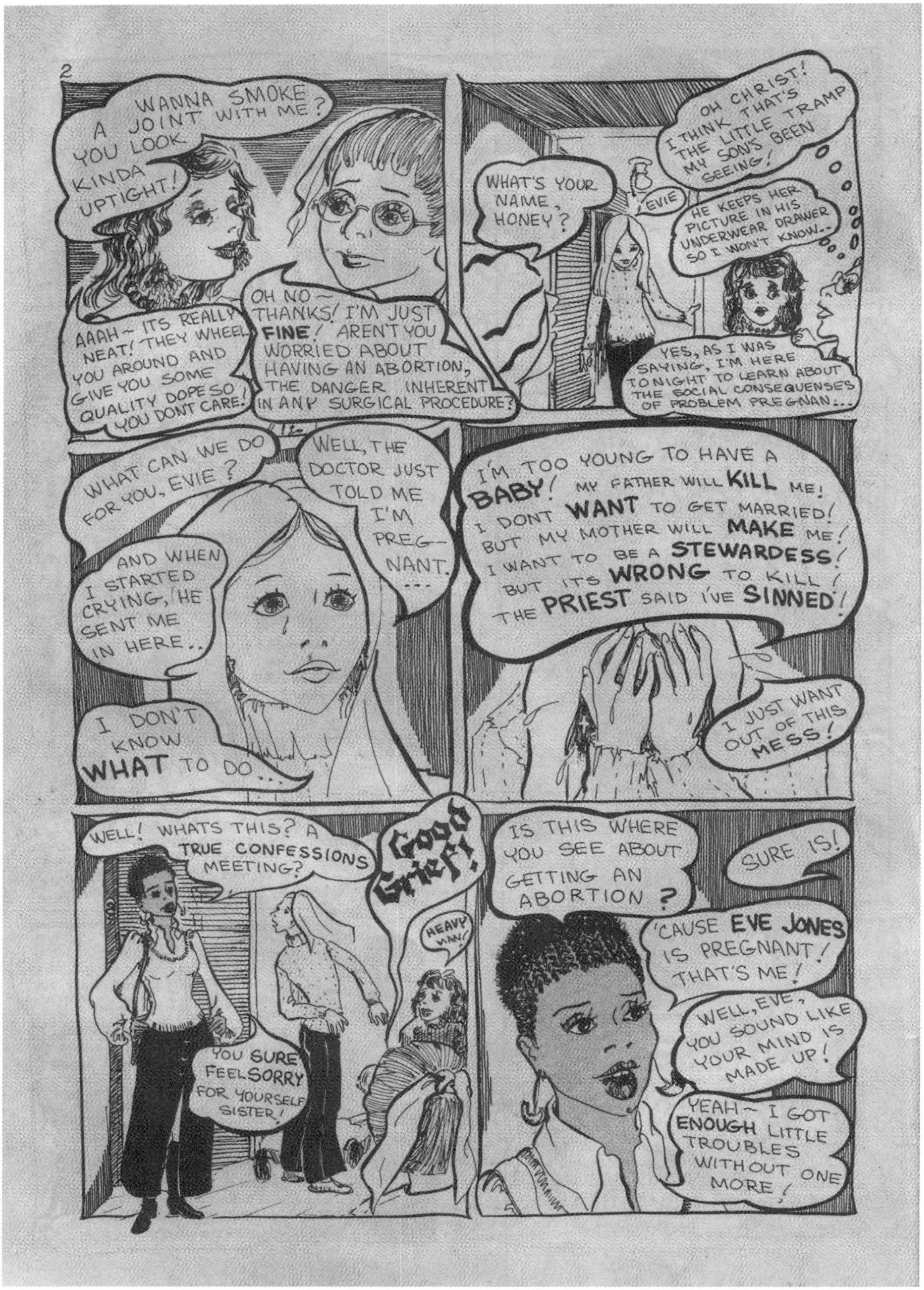
2
A WANNA SMOKE JOINT WITH ME? YOU LOOK KINDA UPTIGHT!
AAAH~ ITS REALLY NEAT! THEY WHEEL YOU AROUND AND GIVE YOU SOME QUALITY DOPE SO YOU DONT CARE!
OH NO~ THANKS! I'M JUST FINE! AREN'T YOU WORRIED ABOUT HAVING AN ABORTION, THE DANGER INHERENT IN ANY SURGICAL PROCEDURE?
OH CHRIST! I THINK THAT'S THE LITTLE TRAMP MY SON'S BEEN SEEING!
HE KEEPS HER PICTURE IN HIS UNDERWEAR DRAWER SO I WON'T KNOW..
WHAT'S YOUR NAME, HONEY?
EVIE
YES, AS I WAS SAYING, I'M HERE TONIGHT TO LEARN ABOUT THE SOCIAL CONSEQUENSES OF PROBLEM PREGNAN...
WHAT CAN WE DO FOR YOU, EVIE?
WELL, THE DOCTOR JUST TOLD ME I'M PREG-NANT...
AND WHEN I STARTED CRYING, HE SENT ME IN HERE..
I DON'T KNOW WHAT TO DO...
I'M TOO YOUNG TO HAVE A BABY! MY FATHER WILL KILL ME! I DONT WANT TO GET MARRIED! BUT MY MOTHER WILL MAKE ME! I WANT TO BE A STEWARDESS! BUT ITS WRONG TO KILL! THE PRIEST SAID I'VE SINNED!
I JUST WANT OUT OF THIS MESS!
WELL! WHATS THIS? A TRUE CONFESSIONS MEETING?
Good Grief!
HEAVY MAN!
YOU SURE FEEL SORRY FOR YOURSELF SISTER!
IS THIS WHERE YOU SEE ABOUT GETTING AN ABORTION?
SURE IS!
'CAUSE EVE JONES IS PREGNANT! THAT'S ME!
WELL, EVE, YOU SOUND LIKE YOUR MIND IS MADE UP!
YEAH~ I GOT ENOUGH LITTLE TROUBLES WITHOUT ONE MORE!

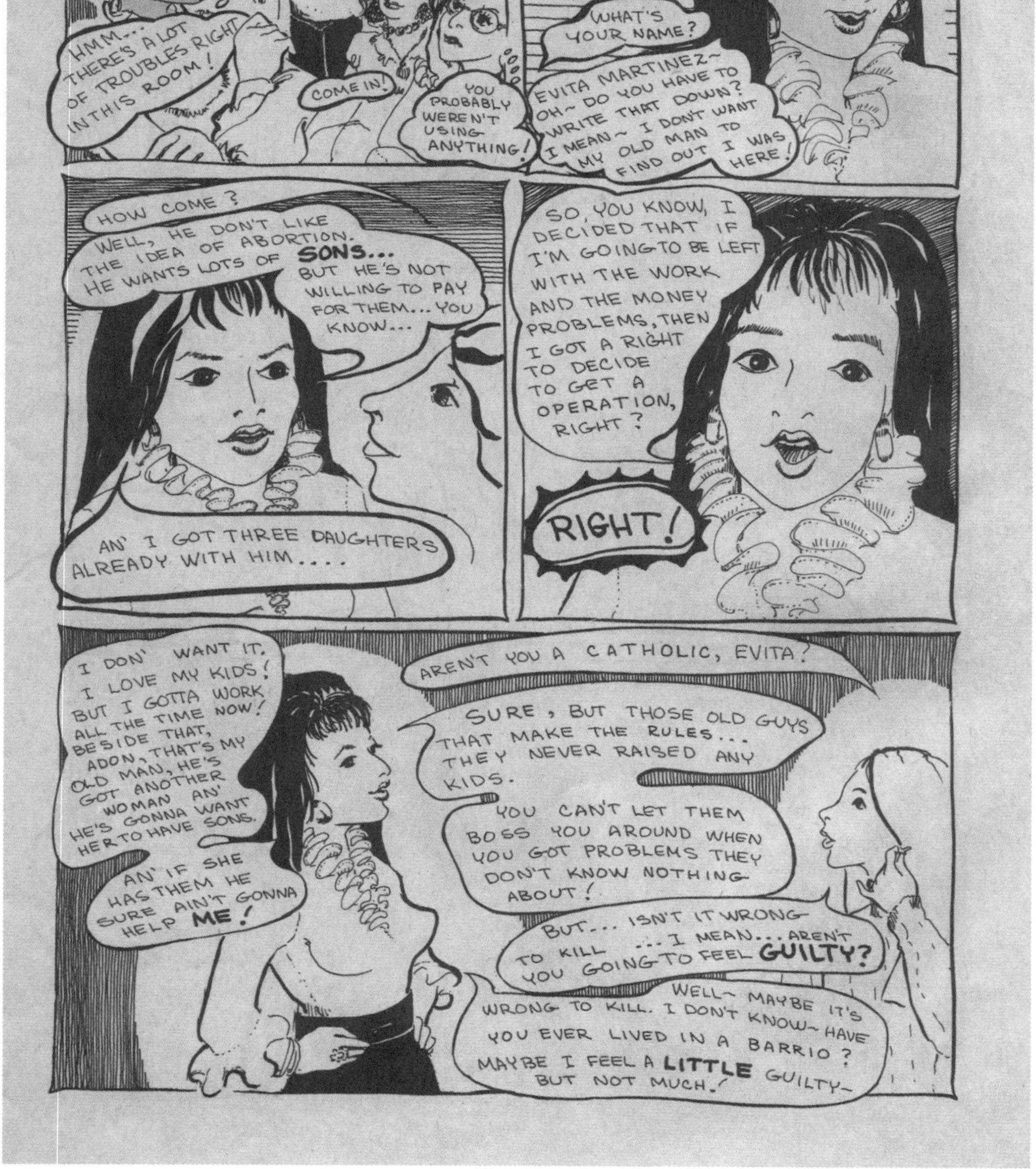
3
KNOCK KNOCK
HMM... THERE'S A LOT OF TROUBLES RIGHT IN THIS ROOM!
GOSH, EVERYBODY HERE HAS THE SAME PROBLEM!
OH EVIE! YOU DUMB KID!
COME IN!
YOU PROBABLY WEREN'T USING ANYTHING!
HELLO! IS THIS THE RIGHT PLACE TO TALK ABOUT A "PROBLEM PREGNANCY"?
SURE! COME ON IN!
WHAT'S YOUR NAME?
EVITA MARTINEZ~ OH~ DO YOU HAVE TO WRITE THAT DOWN? I MEAN~ I DON'T WANT MY OLD MAN TO FIND OUT I WAS HERE!
HOW COME?
WELL, HE DON'T LIKE THE IDEA OF ABORTION. HE WANTS LOTS OF SONS... BUT HE'S NOT WILLING TO PAY FOR THEM... YOU KNOW...
AN' I GOT THREE DAUGHTERS ALREADY WITH HIM....
SO, YOU KNOW, I DECIDED THAT IF I'M GOING TO BE LEFT WITH THE WORK AND THE MONEY PROBLEMS, THEN I GOT A RIGHT TO DECIDE TO GET A OPERATION, RIGHT?
RIGHT!
I DON' WANT IT. I LOVE MY KIDS! BUT I GOTTA WORK ALL THE TIME NOW! BESIDE THAT, ADON, THAT'S MY OLD MAN, HE'S GOT ANOTHER WOMAN AN' HE'S GONNA WANT HER TO HAVE SONS.
AN' IF SHE HAS THEM HE SURE AIN'T GONNA HELP ME!
AREN'T YOU A CATHOLIC, EVITA?
SURE, BUT THOSE OLD GUYS THAT MAKE THE RULES... THEY NEVER RAISED ANY KIDS.
YOU CAN'T LET THEM BOSS YOU AROUND WHEN YOU GOT PROBLEMS THEY DON'T KNOW NOTHING ABOUT!
BUT... ISN'T IT WRONG TO KILL ... I MEAN... AREN'T YOU GOING TO FEEL GUILTY?
WELL~ MAYBE IT'S WRONG TO KILL. I DON'T KNOW~ HAVE YOU EVER LIVED IN A BARRIO? MAYBE I FEEL A LITTLE GUILTY~ BUT NOT MUCH!

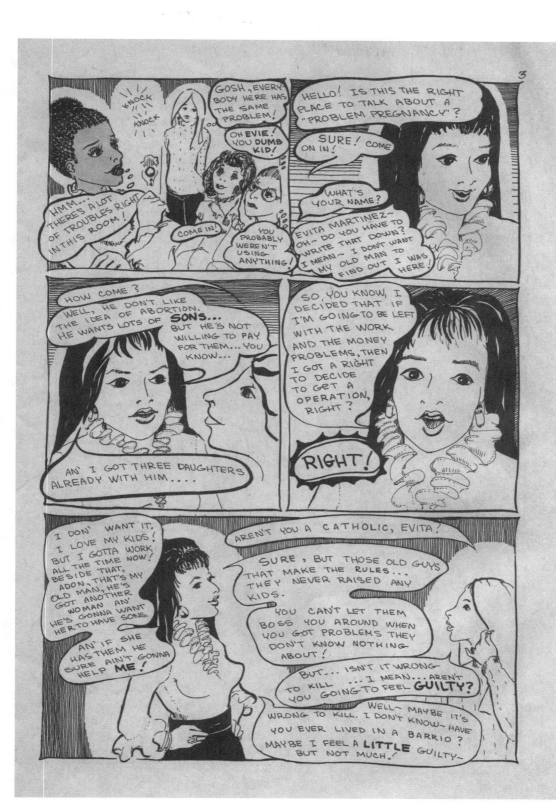

So much is happening - mirroring confusion?

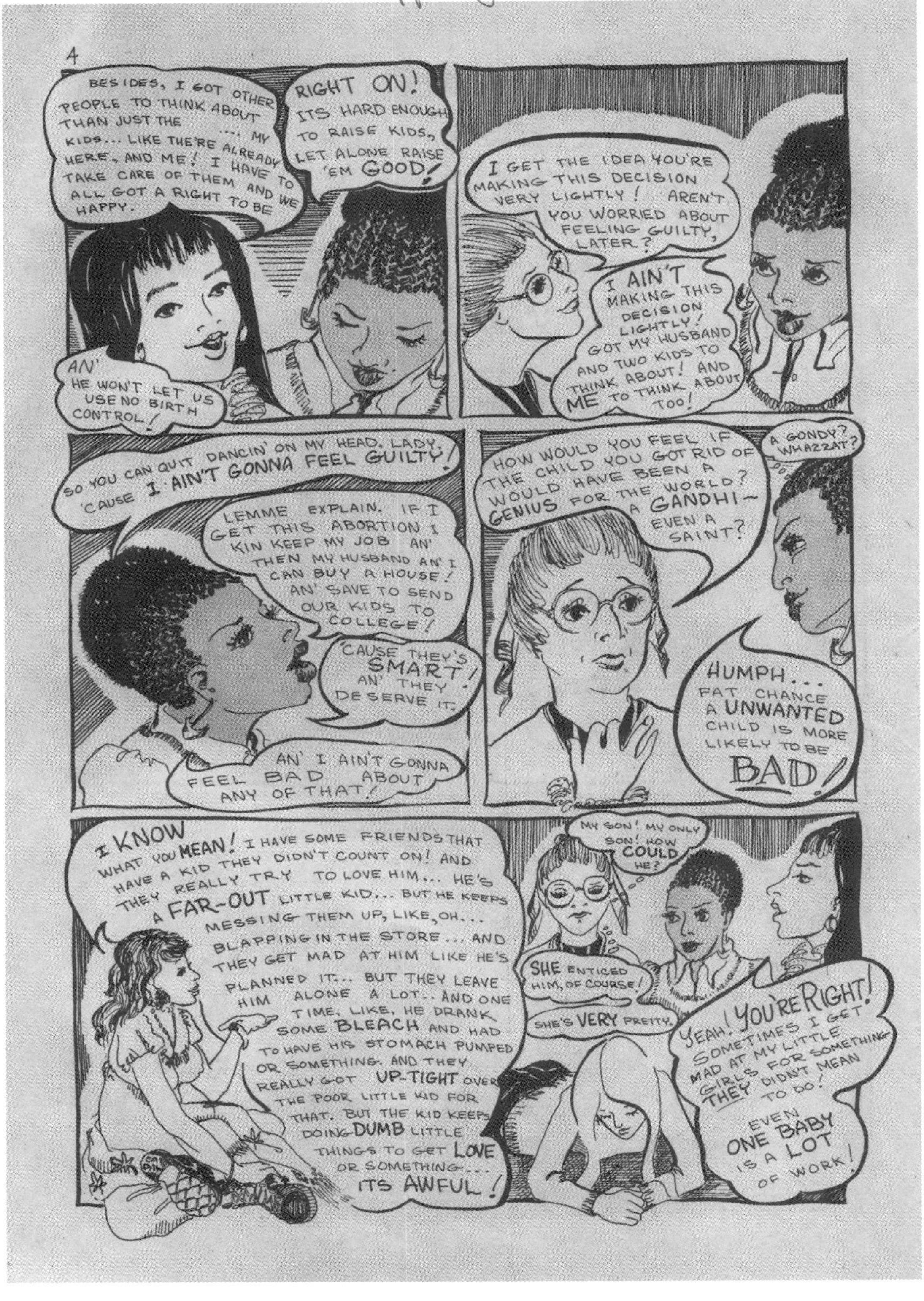
4
BESIDES, I GOT OTHER PEOPLE TO THINK ABOUT THAN JUST THE .... MY KIDS... LIKE THE'RE ALREADY HERE, AND ME! I HAVE TO TAKE CARE OF THEM AND WE ALL GOT A RIGHT TO BE HAPPY.
RIGHT ON! ITS HARD ENOUGH TO RAISE KIDS, LET ALONE RAISE 'EM GOOD!
AN' HE WON'T LET US USE NO BIRTH CONTROL!
I GET THE IDEA YOU'RE MAKING THIS DECISION VERY LIGHTLY! AREN'T YOU WORRIED ABOUT FEELING GUILTY, LATER?
I AIN'T MAKING THIS DECISION LIGHTLY! GOT MY HUSBAND AND TWO KIDS TO THINK ABOUT! AND ME TO THINK ABOUT TOO!
SO YOU CAN QUIT DANCIN' ON MY HEAD, LADY, 'CAUSE I AIN'T GONNA FEEL GUILTY!
LEMME EXPLAIN. IF I GET THIS ABORTION I KIN KEEP MY JOB AN' THEN MY HUSBAND AN' I CAN BUY A HOUSE! AN' SAVE TO SEND OUR KIDS TO COLLEGE!
'CAUSE THEY'S SMART! AN' THEY DESERVE IT.
AN' I AIN'T GONNA FEEL BAD ABOUT ANY OF THAT!
HOW WOULD YOU FEEL IF THE CHILD YOU GOT RID OF WOULD HAVE BEEN A GENIUS FOR THE WORLD? A GANDHI~ EVEN A SAINT?
A GONDY? WHAZZAT?
HUMPH... FAT CHANCE A UNWANTED CHILD IS MORE LIKELY TO BE BAD!
I KNOW WHAT YOU MEAN! I HAVE SOME FRIENDS THAT HAVE A KID THEY DIDN'T COUNT ON! AND THEY REALLY TRY TO LOVE HIM... HE'S A FAR-OUT LITTLE KID... BUT HE KEEPS MESSING THEM UP, LIKE, OH... BLAPPING IN THE STORE... AND THEY GET MAD AT HIM LIKE HE'S PLANNED IT... BUT THEY LEAVE HIM ALONE A LOT.. AND ONE TIME, LIKE, HE DRANK SOME BLEACH AND HAD TO HAVE HIS STOMACH PUMPED OR SOMETHING. AND THEY REALLY GOT UP-TIGHT OVER THE POOR LITTLE KID FOR THAT. BUT THE KID KEEPS DOING DUMB LITTLE THINGS TO GET LOVE OR SOMETHING... ITS AWFUL!
MY SON! MY ONLY SON! HOW COULD HE?
SHE ENTICED HIM, OF COURSE!
SHE'S VERY PRETTY.
YEAH! YOU'RE RIGHT! SOMETIMES I GET MAD AT MY LITTLE GIRLS FOR SOMETHING THEY DIDN'T MEAN TO DO!
EVEN ONE BABY IS A LOT OF WORK!

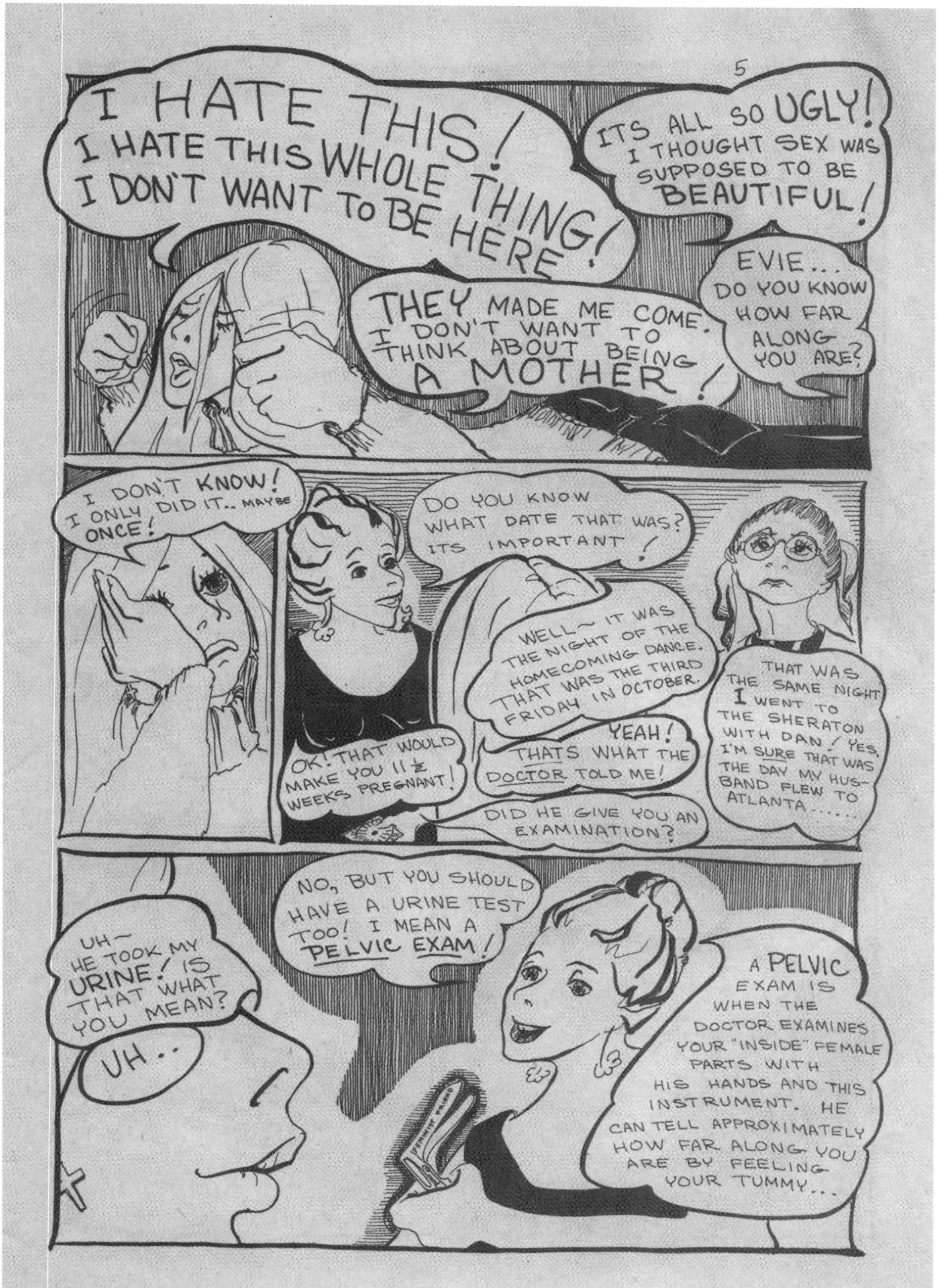
5
I HATE THIS! I HATE THIS WHOLE THING! I DON'T WANT TO BE HERE
ITS ALL SO UGLY! I THOUGHT SEX WAS SUPPOSED TO BE BEAUTIFUL!
THEY MADE ME COME. I DON'T WANT TO THINK ABOUT BEING A MOTHER!
EVIE... DO YOU KNOW HOW FAR ALONG YOU ARE?
I DON'T KNOW! I ONLY DID IT.. MAYBE ONCE!
DO YOU KNOW WHAT DATE THAT WAS? ITS IMPORTANT!
WELL~ IT WAS THE NIGHT OF THE HOMECOMING DANCE. THAT WAS THE THIRD FRIDAY IN OCTOBER.
THAT WAS THE SAME NIGHT I WENT TO THE SHERATON WITH DAN! YES, I'M SURE THAT WAS THE DAY MY HUSBAND FLEW TO ATLANTA......
OK! THAT WOULD MAKE YOU 11½ WEEKS PREGNANT!
YEAH! THATS WHAT THE DOCTOR TOLD ME!
DID HE GIVE YOU AN EXAMINATION?
UH~ HE TOOK MY URINE! IS THAT WHAT YOU MEAN?
NO, BUT YOU SHOULD HAVE A URINE TEST TOO! I MEAN A PELVIC EXAM!
UH..
A PELVIC EXAM IS WHEN THE DOCTOR EXAMINES YOUR "INSIDE" FEMALE PARTS WITH HIS HANDS AND THIS INSTRUMENT. HE CAN TELL APPROXIMATELY HOW FAR ALONG YOU ARE BY FEELING YOUR TUMMY...
FEMINIST FRIEND

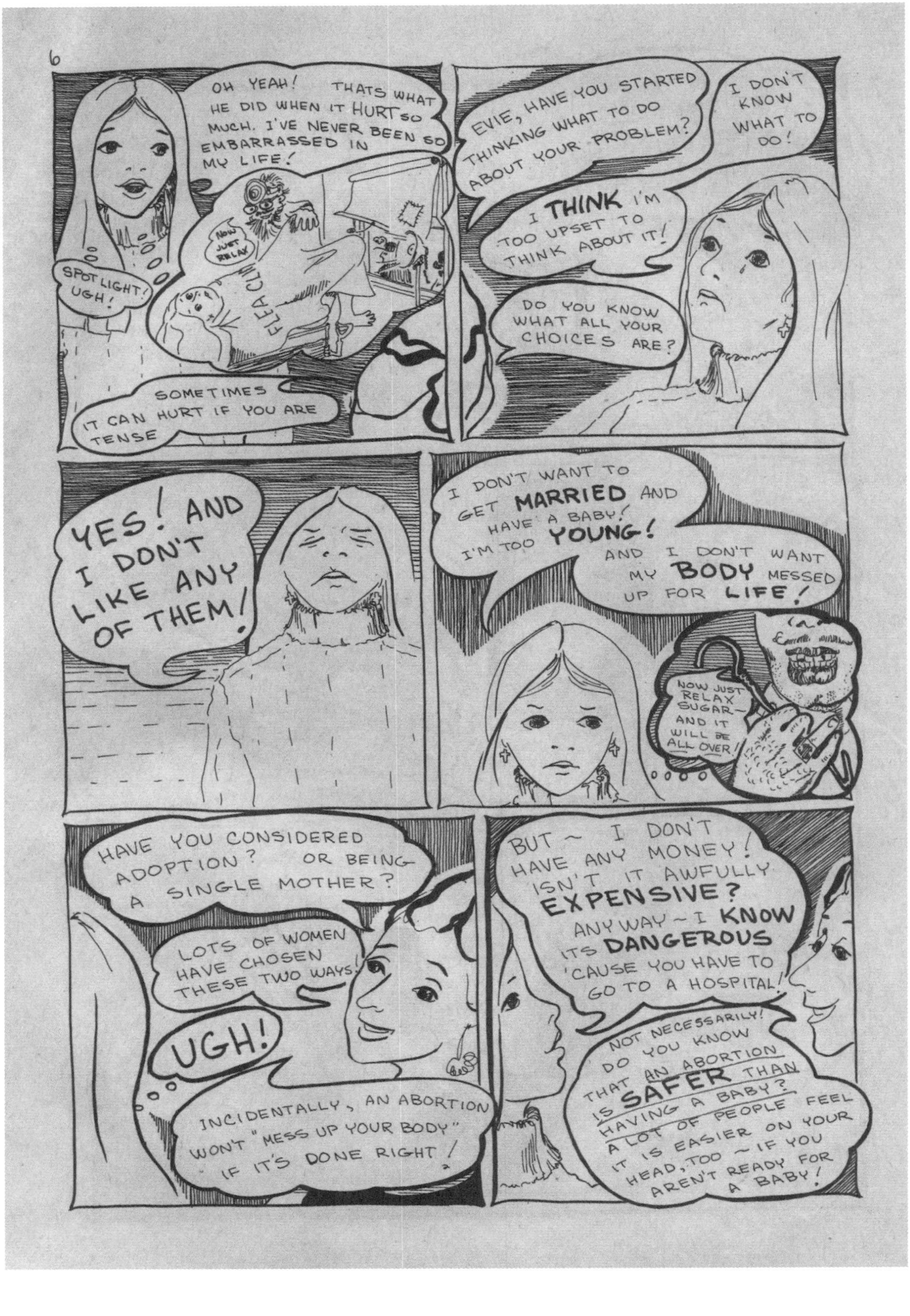
6
OH YEAH! THATS WHAT HE DID WHEN IT HURT SO MUCH. I'VE NEVER BEEN SO EMBARRASSED IN MY LIFE!
NOW JUST RELAX
FLEA CLI
SPOT LIGHT! UGH!
SOMETIMES IT CAN HURT IF YOU ARE TENSE
EVIE, HAVE YOU STARTED THINKING WHAT TO DO ABOUT YOUR PROBLEM?
I DON'T KNOW WHAT TO DO!
I THINK I'M TOO UPSET TO THINK ABOUT IT!
DO YOU KNOW WHAT ALL YOUR CHOICES ARE?
YES! AND I DON'T LIKE ANY OF THEM!
I DON'T WANT TO GET MARRIED AND HAVE A BABY! I'M TOO YOUNG!
AND I DON'T WANT MY BODY MESSED UP FOR LIFE!
NOW JUST RELAX SUGAR AND IT WILL BE ALL OVER!
HAVE YOU CONSIDERED ADOPTION? OR BEING A SINGLE MOTHER?
LOTS OF WOMEN HAVE CHOSEN THESE TWO WAYS.
UGH!
INCIDENTALLY, AN ABORTION WON'T "MESS UP YOUR BODY" IF IT'S DONE RIGHT!
BUT ~ I DON'T HAVE ANY MONEY! ISN'T IT AWFULLY EXPENSIVE?
ANY WAY ~ I KNOW ITS DANGEROUS 'CAUSE YOU HAVE TO GO TO A HOSPITAL!
NOT NECESSARILY! DO YOU KNOW THAT AN ABORTION IS SAFER THAN HAVING A BABY?
A LOT OF PEOPLE FEEL IT IS EASIER ON YOUR HEAD, TOO ~ IF YOU AREN'T READY FOR A BABY!

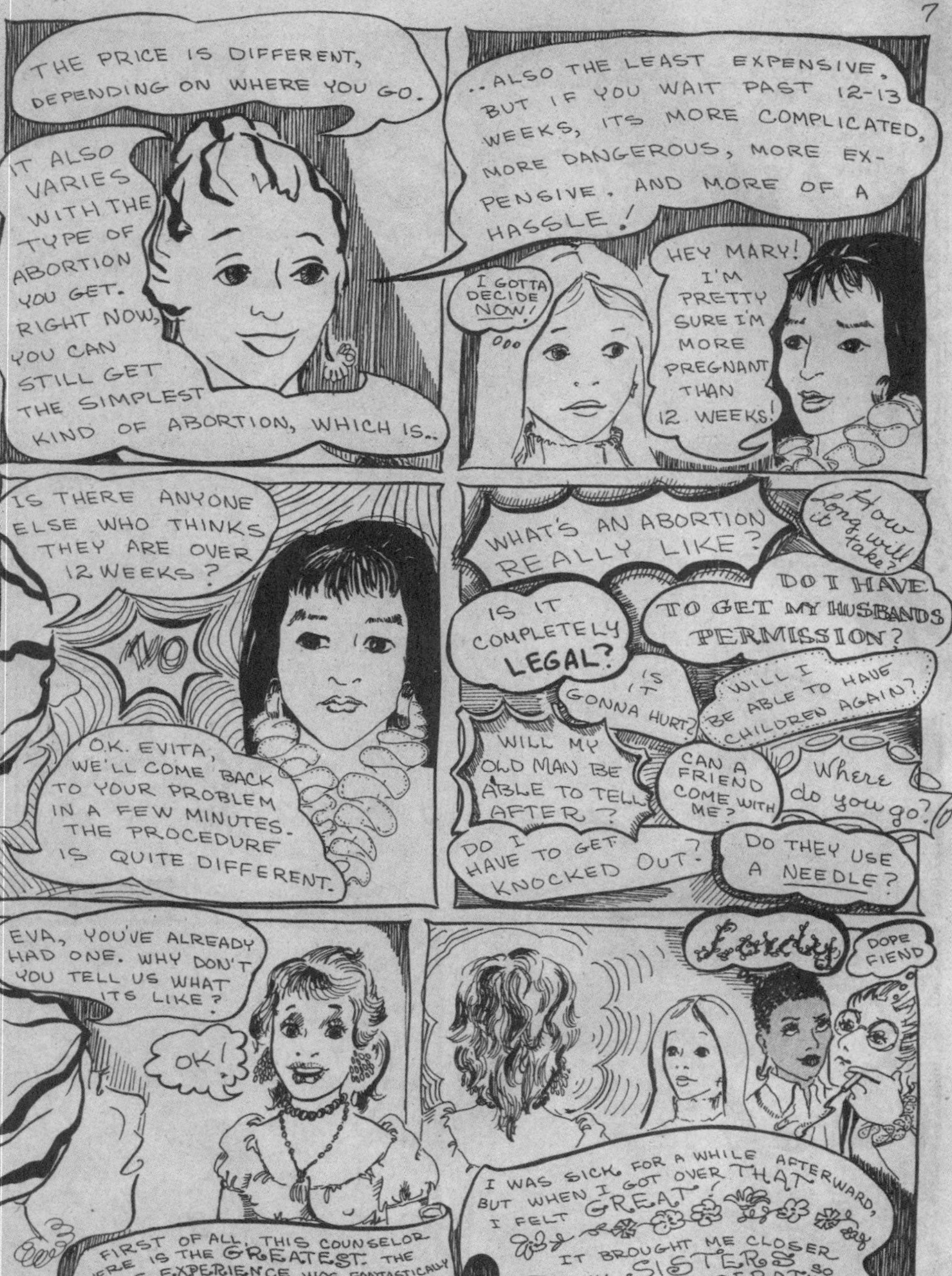
7
THE PRICE IS DIFFERENT, DEPENDING ON WHERE YOU GO.
IT ALSO VARIES WITH THE TYPE OF ABORTION YOU GET. RIGHT NOW, YOU CAN STILL GET THE SIMPLEST KIND OF ABORTION, WHICH IS..
..ALSO THE LEAST EXPENSIVE, BUT IF YOU WAIT PAST 12-13 WEEKS, ITS MORE COMPLICATED, MORE DANGEROUS, MORE EX-PENSIVE. AND MORE OF A HASSLE!
I GOTTA DECIDE NOW!
HEY MARY! I'M PRETTY SURE I'M MORE PREGNANT THAN 12 WEEKS!
IS THERE ANYONE ELSE WHO THINKS THEY ARE OVER 12 WEEKS?
NO
O.K. EVITA, WE'LL COME BACK TO YOUR PROBLEM IN A FEW MINUTES. THE PROCEDURE IS QUITE DIFFERENT.
WHAT'S AN ABORTION REALLY LIKE?
How long will it take?
DO I HAVE TO GET MY HUSBANDS PERMISSION?
IS IT COMPLETELY LEGAL?
IS IT GONNA HURT?
WILL I BE ABLE TO HAVE CHILDREN AGAIN?
WILL MY OLD MAN BE ABLE TO TELL AFTER?
CAN A FRIEND COME WITH ME?
Where do you go?
DO I HAVE TO GET KNOCKED OUT?
DO THEY USE A NEEDLE?
EVA, YOU'VE ALREADY HAD ONE. WHY DON'T YOU TELL US WHAT ITS LIKE?
OK!
FIRST OF ALL, THIS COUNSELOR HERE IS THE GREATEST. THE WHOLE EXPERIENCE WAS FANTASTICALLY DREAMY.... THEY GAVE ME A BUNCH OF TESTS...EVERY-BODY WAS LOVING AND KIND... AND I REALLY DUG THE DRUG TRIP...
Lordy
DOPE FIEND
I WAS SICK FOR A WHILE AFTERWARD, BUT WHEN I GOT OVER THAT I FELT GREAT! IT BROUGHT ME CLOSER TO MY SISTERS SO IT REALLY WAS LIBERATING IN THAT WAY... KIND OF COSMICALLY LIBERATED, YOU KNOW?

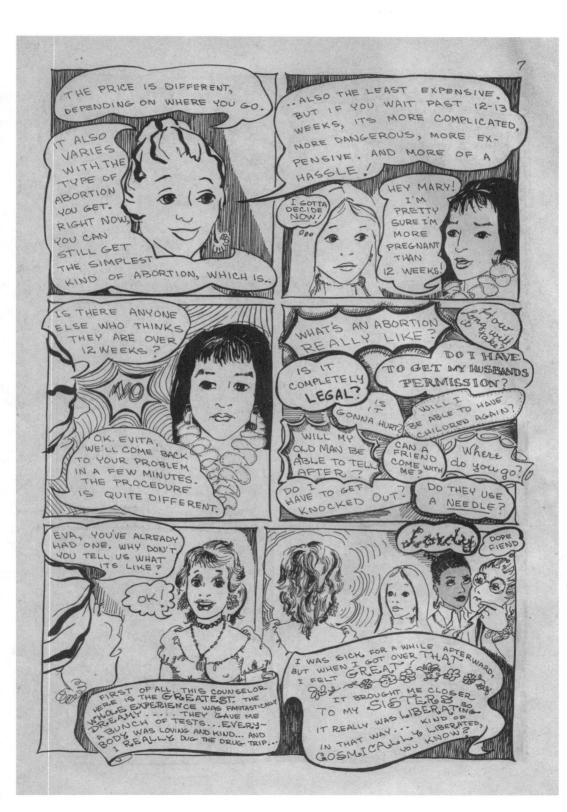

Doctor is a "he"

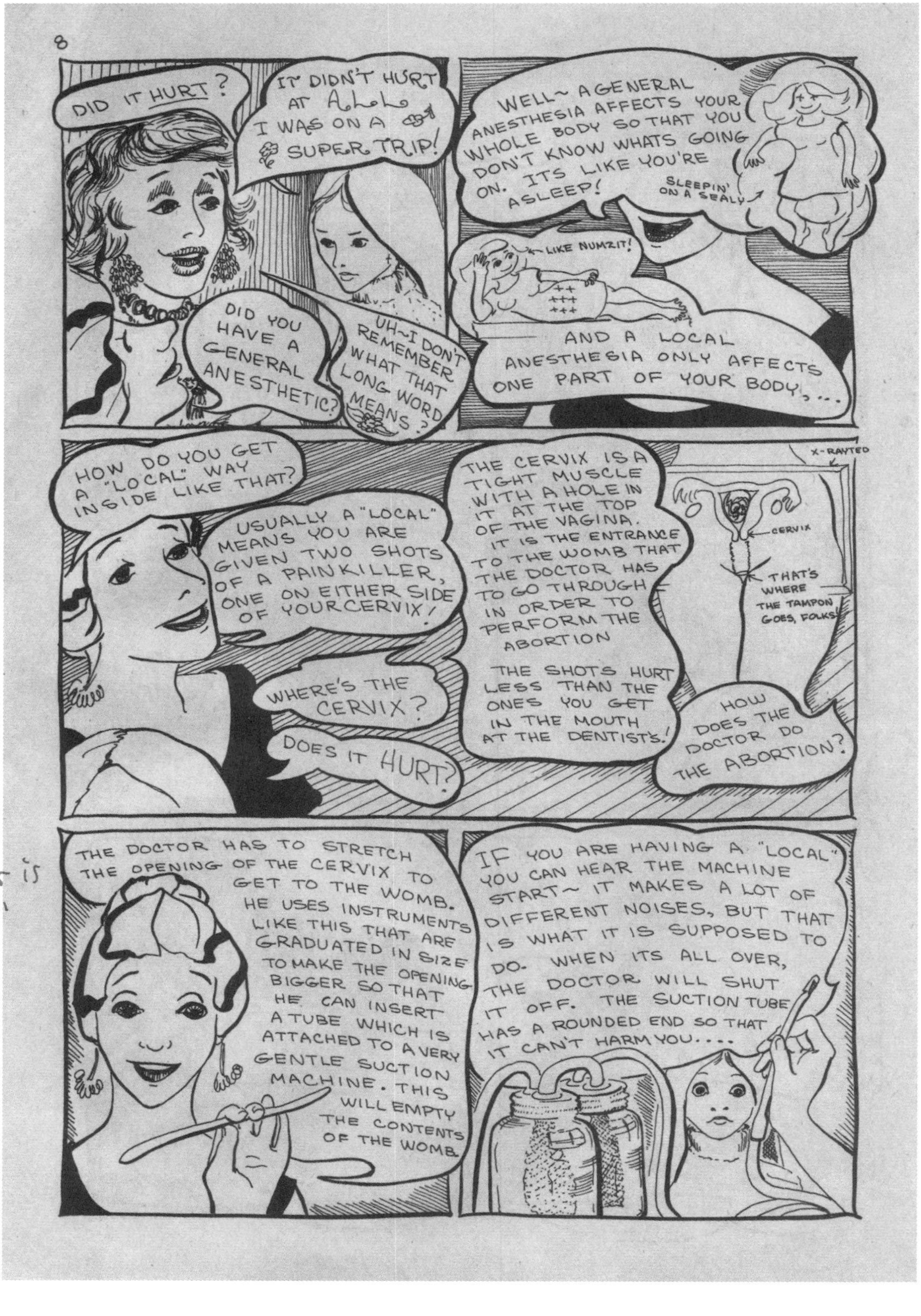
8
DID IT HURT?
IT DIDN'T HURT AT ALL I WAS ON A SUPER TRIP!
WELL~ A GENERAL ANESTHESIA AFFECTS YOUR WHOLE BODY SO THAT YOU DON'T KNOW WHATS GOING ON. ITS LIKE YOU'RE ASLEEP!
SLEEPIN' ON A SEALY
LIKE NUMZIT!
DID YOU HAVE A GENERAL ANESTHETIC?
UH~I DON'T REMEMBER WHAT THAT LONG WORD MEANS?
AND A LOCAL ANESTHESIA ONLY AFFECTS ONE PART OF YOUR BODY, . . .
HOW DO YOU GET A "LOCAL" WAY INSIDE LIKE THAT?
USUALLY A "LOCAL" MEANS YOU ARE GIVEN TWO SHOTS OF A PAINKILLER, ONE ON EITHER SIDE OF YOUR CERVIX!
WHERE'S THE CERVIX?
DOES IT HURT?
THE CERVIX IS A TIGHT MUSCLE WITH A HOLE IN IT AT THE TOP OF THE VAGINA. IT IS THE ENTRANCE TO THE WOMB THAT THE DOCTOR HAS TO GO THROUGH IN ORDER TO PERFORM THE ABORTION
THE SHOTS HURT LESS THAN THE ONES YOU GET IN THE MOUTH AT THE DENTIST'S!
X-RAYTED
CERVIX
THAT'S WHERE THE TAMPON GOES, FOLKS!
HOW DOES THE DOCTOR DO THE ABORTION?
THE DOCTOR HAS TO STRETCH THE OPENING OF THE CERVIX TO GET TO THE WOMB. HE USES INSTRUMENTS LIKE THIS THAT ARE GRADUATED IN SIZE TO MAKE THE OPENING BIGGER SO THAT HE CAN INSERT A TUBE WHICH IS ATTACHED TO A VERY GENTLE SUCTION MACHINE. THIS WILL EMPTY THE CONTENTS OF THE WOMB.
IF YOU ARE HAVING A "LOCAL" YOU CAN HEAR THE MACHINE START~ IT MAKES A LOT OF DIFFERENT NOISES, BUT THAT IS WHAT IT IS SUPPOSED TO DO. WHEN ITS ALL OVER, THE DOCTOR WILL SHUT IT OFF. THE SUCTION TUBE HAS A ROUNDED END SO THAT IT CAN'T HARM YOU. . . .

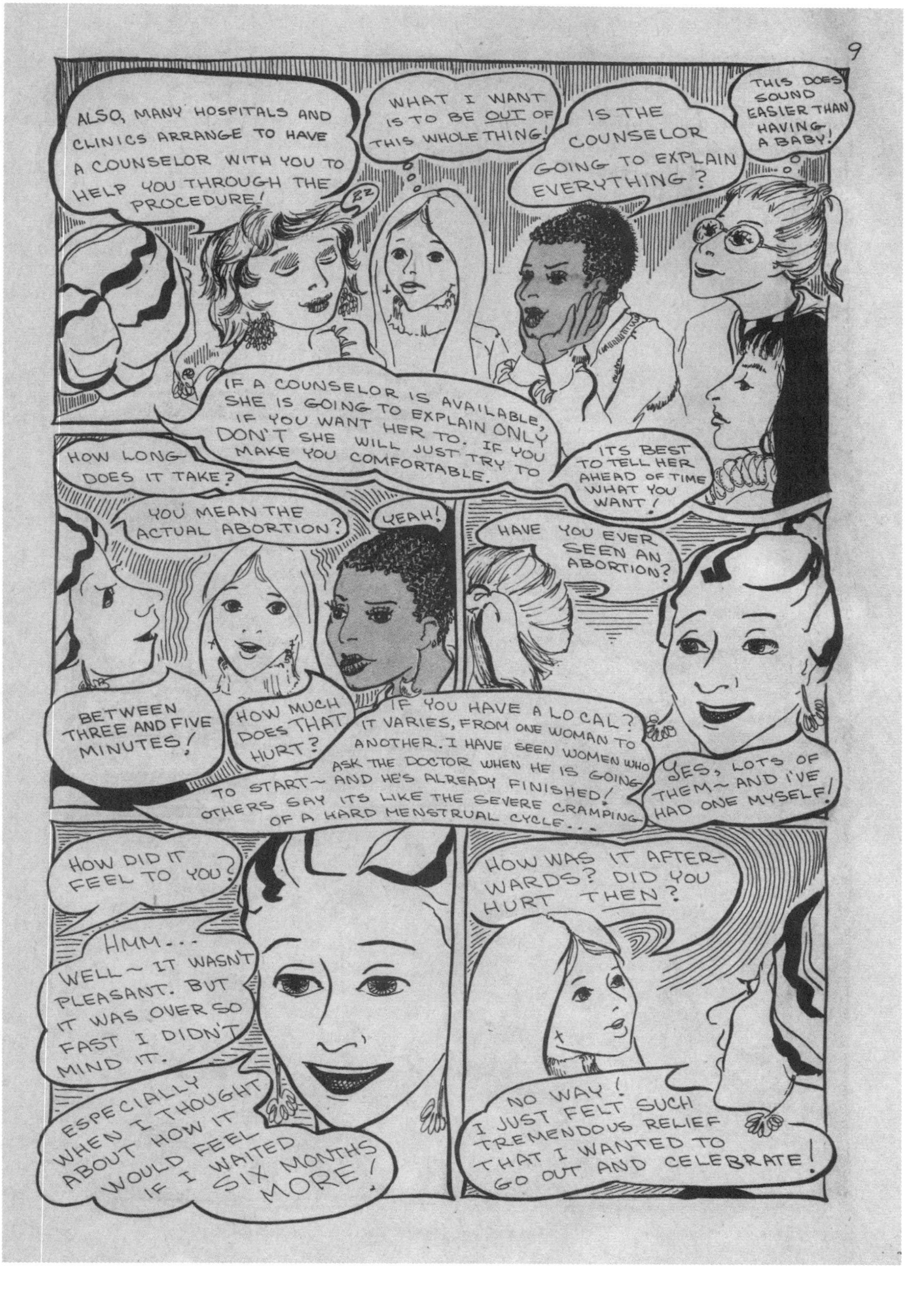
9
ALSO, MANY HOSPITALS AND CLINICS ARRANGE TO HAVE A COUNSELOR WITH YOU TO HELP YOU THROUGH THE PROCEDURE!
ZZ
WHAT I WANT IS TO BE OUT OF THIS WHOLE THING!
IS THE COUNSELOR GOING TO EXPLAIN EVERYTHING?
THIS DOES SOUND EASIER THAN HAVING A BABY!
IF A COUNSELOR IS AVAILABLE, SHE IS GOING TO EXPLAIN ONLY IF YOU WANT HER TO. IF YOU DON'T SHE WILL JUST TRY TO MAKE YOU COMFORTABLE.
ITS BEST TO TELL HER AHEAD OF TIME WHAT YOU WANT!
HOW LONG DOES IT TAKE?
YOU MEAN THE ACTUAL ABORTION?
YEAH!
BETWEEN THREE AND FIVE MINUTES!
HAVE YOU EVER SEEN AN ABORTION?
YES, LOTS OF THEM~ AND I'VE HAD ONE MYSELF!
HOW MUCH DOES THAT HURT?
IF YOU HAVE A LOCAL? IT VARIES, FROM ONE WOMAN TO ANOTHER. I HAVE SEEN WOMEN WHO ASK THE DOCTOR WHEN HE IS GOING TO START~ AND HE'S ALREADY FINISHED! OTHERS SAY ITS LIKE THE SEVERE CRAMPING OF A HARD MENSTRUAL CYCLE...
HOW DID IT FEEL TO YOU?
HMM... WELL~ IT WASN'T PLEASANT. BUT IT WAS OVER SO FAST I DIDN'T MIND IT.
ESPECIALLY WHEN I THOUGHT ABOUT HOW IT WOULD FEEL IF I WAITED SIX MONTHS MORE!
HOW WAS IT AFTERWARDS? DID YOU HURT THEN?
NO WAY! I JUST FELT SUCH TREMENDOUS RELIEF THAT I WANTED TO GO OUT AND CELEBRATE!

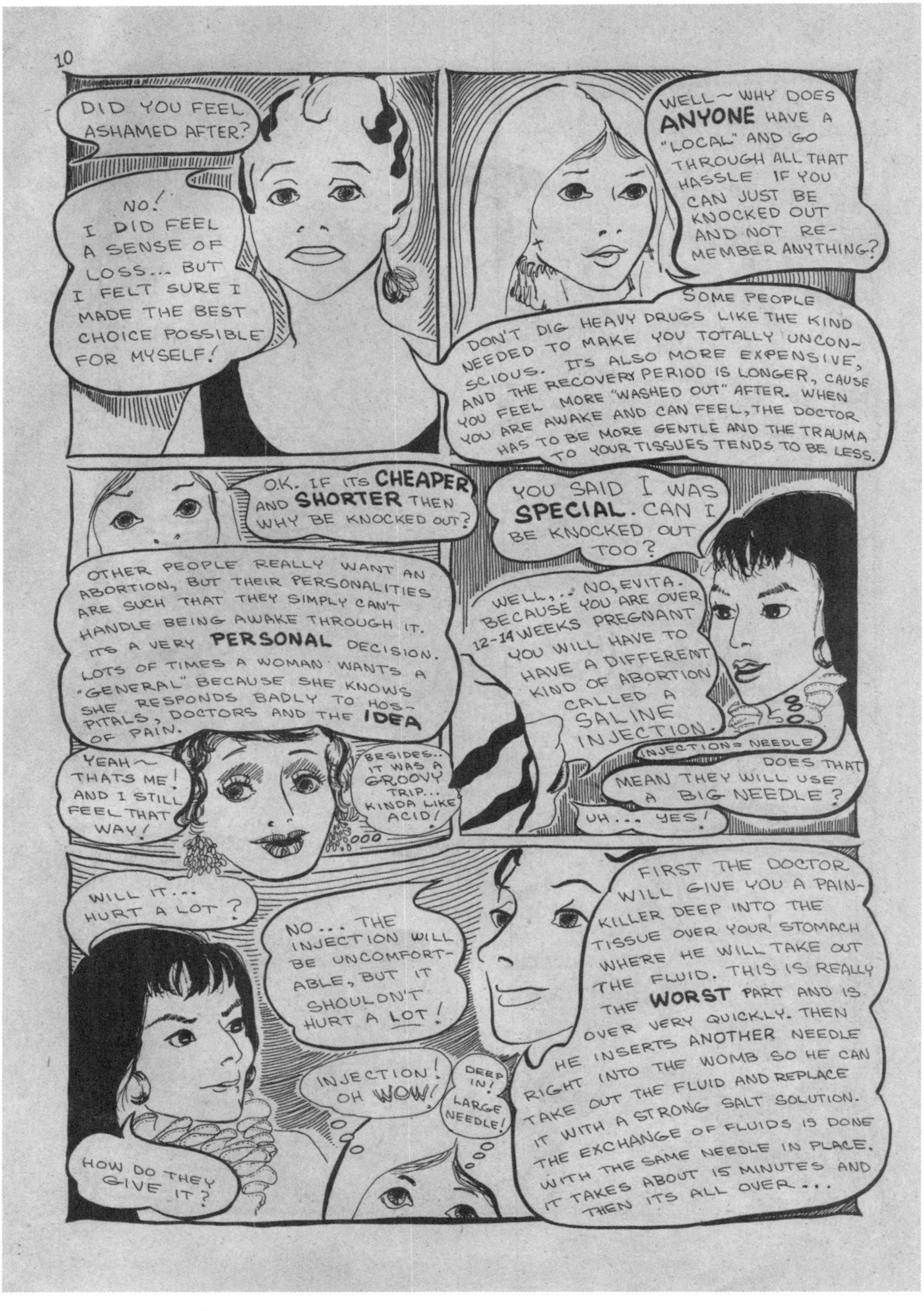
10
DID YOU FEEL ASHAMED AFTER?
NO! I DID FEEL A SENSE OF LOSS... BUT I FELT SURE I MADE THE BEST CHOICE POSSIBLE FOR MYSELF!
WELL ~ WHY DOES ANYONE HAVE A "LOCAL" AND GO THROUGH ALL THAT HASSLE IF YOU CAN JUST BE KNOCKED OUT AND NOT REMEMBER ANYTHING?
SOME PEOPLE DON'T DIG HEAVY DRUGS LIKE THE KIND NEEDED TO MAKE YOU TOTALLY UNCONSCIOUS. ITS ALSO MORE EXPENSIVE, AND THE RECOVERY PERIOD IS LONGER, CAUSE YOU FEEL MORE "WASHED OUT" AFTER. WHEN YOU ARE AWAKE AND CAN FEEL, THE DOCTOR HAS TO BE MORE GENTLE AND THE TRAUMA TO YOUR TISSUES TENDS TO BE LESS.
O.K. IF ITS CHEAPER AND SHORTER THEN WHY BE KNOCKED OUT?
OTHER PEOPLE REALLY WANT AN ABORTION, BUT THEIR PERSONALITIES ARE SUCH THAT THEY SIMPLY CAN'T HANDLE BEING AWAKE THROUGH IT. ITS A VERY PERSONAL DECISION. LOTS OF TIMES A WOMAN WANTS A "GENERAL" BECAUSE SHE KNOWS SHE RESPONDS BADLY TO HOSPITALS, DOCTORS AND THE IDEA OF PAIN.
YEAH ~ THATS ME! AND I STILL FEEL THAT WAY!
BESIDES.. IT WAS A GROOVY TRIP... KINDA LIKE ACID!
YOU SAID I WAS SPECIAL. CAN I BE KNOCKED OUT TOO?
WELL,.. NO, EVITA. BECAUSE YOU ARE OVER 12-14 WEEKS PREGNANT YOU WILL HAVE TO HAVE A DIFFERENT KIND OF ABORTION CALLED A SALINE INJECTION.
INJECTION = NEEDLE
DOES THAT MEAN THEY WILL USE A BIG NEEDLE?
UH... YES!
WILL IT... HURT A LOT?
NO... THE INJECTION WILL BE UNCOMFORTABLE, BUT IT SHOULDN'T HURT A LOT!
INJECTION! OH WOW!
DEEP IN! LARGE NEEDLE!
HOW DO THEY GIVE IT?
FIRST THE DOCTOR WILL GIVE YOU A PAIN-KILLER DEEP INTO THE TISSUE OVER YOUR STOMACH WHERE HE WILL TAKE OUT THE FLUID. THIS IS REALLY THE WORST PART AND IS OVER VERY QUICKLY. THEN HE INSERTS ANOTHER NEEDLE RIGHT INTO THE WOMB SO HE CAN TAKE OUT THE FLUID AND REPLACE IT WITH A STRONG SALT SOLUTION. THE EXCHANGE OF FLUIDS IS DONE WITH THE SAME NEEDLE IN PLACE. IT TAKES ABOUT 15 MINUTES AND THEN ITS ALL OVER...

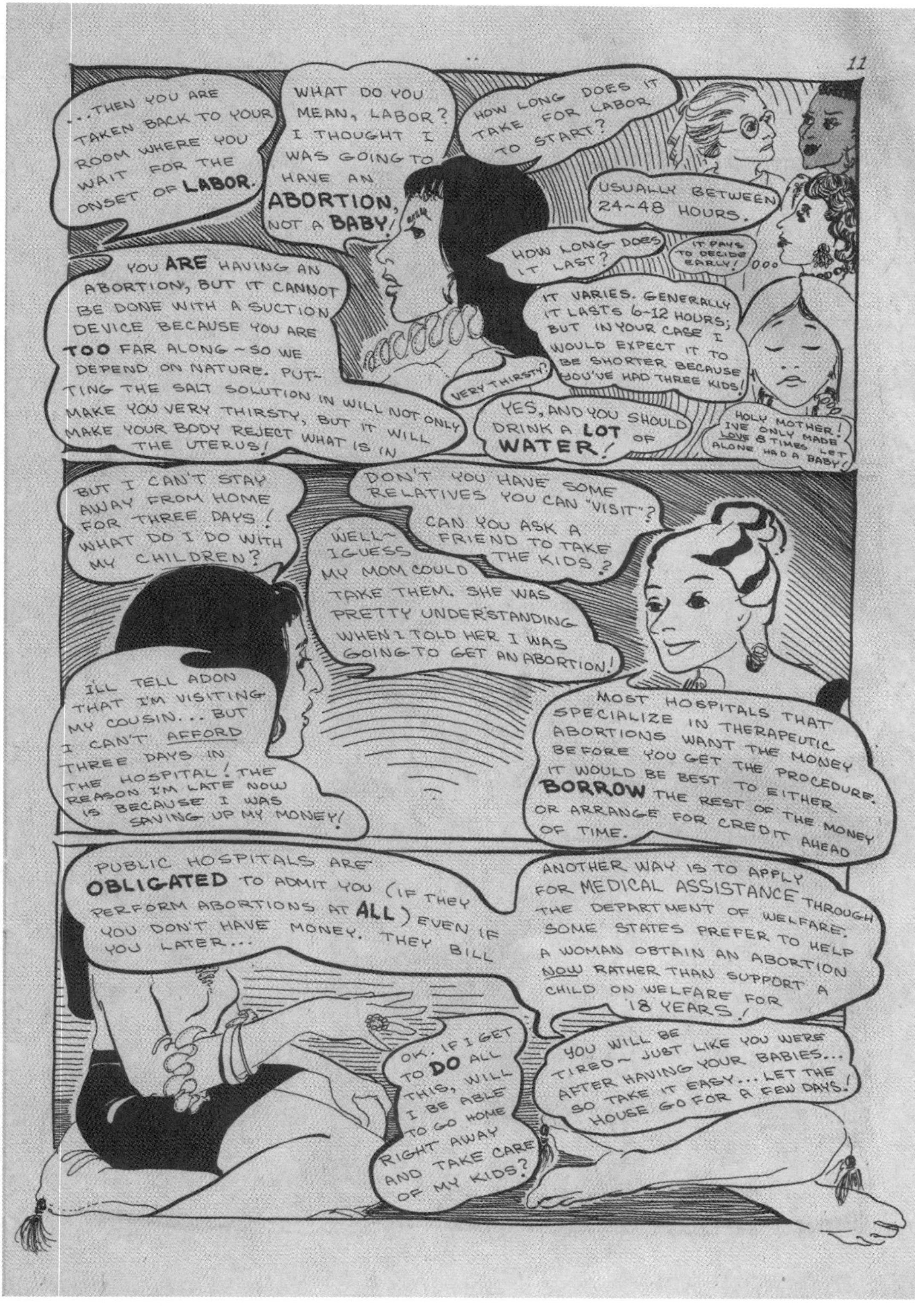
11
...THEN YOU ARE TAKEN BACK TO YOUR ROOM WHERE YOU WAIT FOR THE ONSET OF **LABOR**.
WHAT DO YOU MEAN, LABOR? I THOUGHT I WAS GOING TO HAVE AN **ABORTION**, NOT A **BABY**!
HOW LONG DOES IT TAKE FOR LABOR TO START?
USUALLY BETWEEN 24~48 HOURS.
HOW LONG DOES IT LAST?
IT PAYS TO DECIDE EARLY!
YOU **ARE** HAVING AN ABORTION, BUT IT CANNOT BE DONE WITH A SUCTION DEVICE BECAUSE YOU ARE **TOO** FAR ALONG ~ SO WE DEPEND ON NATURE. PUTTING THE SALT SOLUTION IN WILL NOT ONLY MAKE YOU VERY THIRSTY, BUT IT WILL MAKE YOUR BODY REJECT WHAT IS IN THE UTERUS!
IT VARIES. GENERALLY IT LASTS 6~12 HOURS; BUT IN YOUR CASE I WOULD EXPECT IT TO BE SHORTER BECAUSE YOU'VE HAD THREE KIDS!
VERY THIRSTY?
YES, AND YOU SHOULD DRINK A **LOT** OF **WATER**!
HOLY MOTHER! I'VE ONLY MADE LOVE 8 TIMES LET ALONE HAD A BABY!
BUT I CAN'T STAY AWAY FROM HOME FOR THREE DAYS! WHAT DO I DO WITH MY CHILDREN?
DON'T YOU HAVE SOME RELATIVES YOU CAN "VISIT"?
CAN YOU ASK A FRIEND TO TAKE THE KIDS?
WELL~ I GUESS MY MOM COULD TAKE THEM. SHE WAS PRETTY UNDERSTANDING WHEN I TOLD HER I WAS GOING TO GET AN ABORTION!
I'LL TELL ADON THAT I'M VISITING MY COUSIN... BUT I CAN'T AFFORD THREE DAYS IN THE HOSPITAL! THE REASON I'M LATE NOW IS BECAUSE I WAS SAVING UP MY MONEY!
MOST HOSPITALS THAT SPECIALIZE IN THERAPEUTIC ABORTIONS WANT THE MONEY BEFORE YOU GET THE PROCEDURE. IT WOULD BE BEST TO EITHER **BORROW** THE REST OF THE MONEY OR ARRANGE FOR CREDIT AHEAD OF TIME.
PUBLIC HOSPITALS ARE **OBLIGATED** TO ADMIT YOU (IF THEY PERFORM ABORTIONS AT **ALL**) EVEN IF YOU DON'T HAVE MONEY. THEY BILL YOU LATER...
ANOTHER WAY IS TO APPLY FOR MEDICAL ASSISTANCE THROUGH THE DEPARTMENT OF WELFARE. SOME STATES PREFER TO HELP A WOMAN OBTAIN AN ABORTION NOW RATHER THAN SUPPORT A CHILD ON WELFARE FOR 18 YEARS!
OK. IF I GET TO **DO** ALL THIS, WILL I BE ABLE TO GO HOME RIGHT AWAY AND TAKE CARE OF MY KIDS?
YOU WILL BE TIRED~ JUST LIKE YOU WERE AFTER HAVING YOUR BABIES... SO TAKE IT EASY... LET THE HOUSE GO FOR A FEW DAYS!

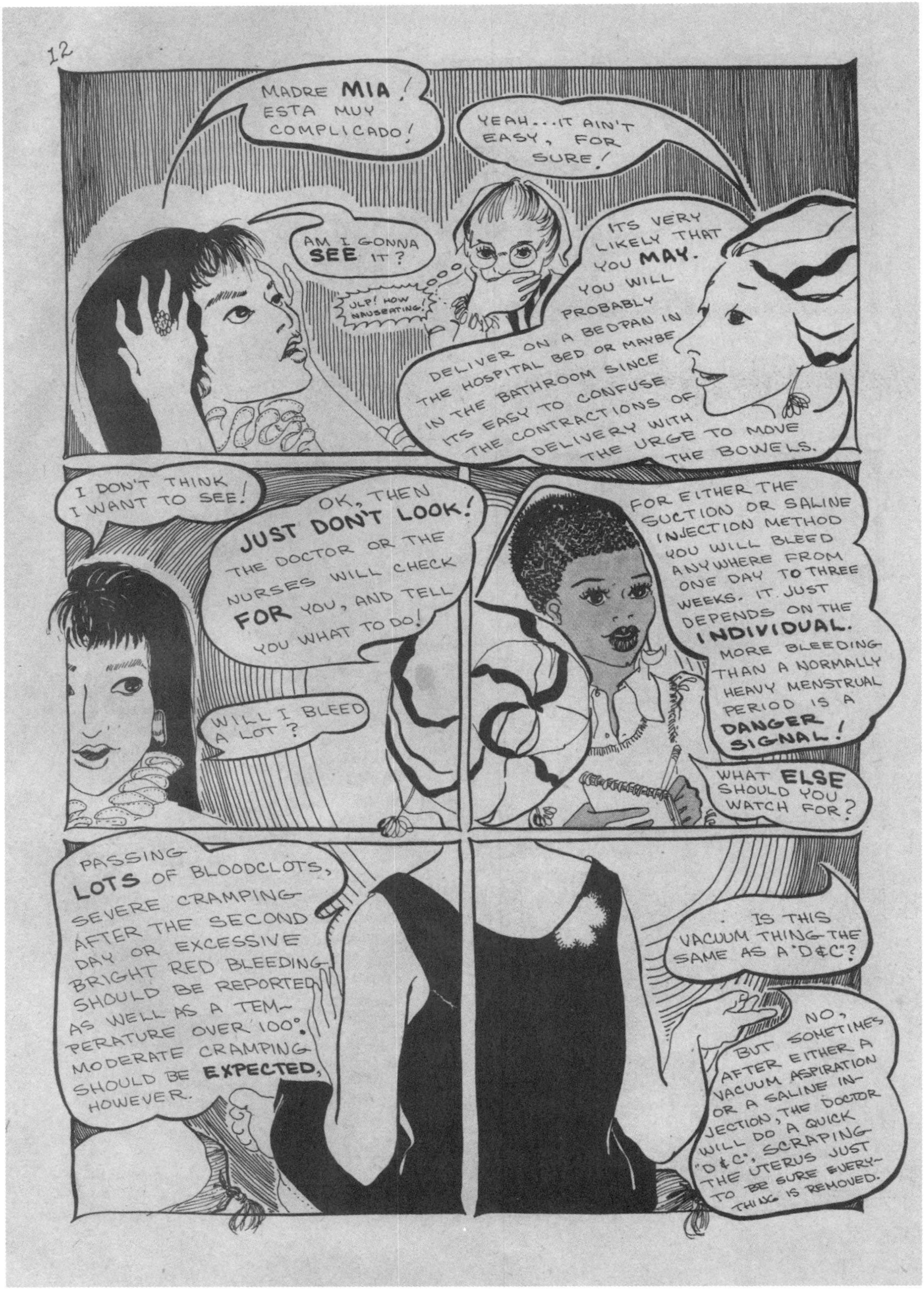
12
MADRE MIA! ESTA MUY COMPLICADO!
YEAH...IT AIN'T EASY, FOR SURE!
AM I GONNA SEE IT?
ULP! HOW NAUSEATING!
ITS VERY LIKELY THAT YOU MAY. YOU WILL PROBABLY DELIVER ON A BEDPAN IN THE HOSPITAL BED OR MAYBE IN THE BATHROOM SINCE ITS EASY TO CONFUSE THE CONTRACTIONS OF DELIVERY WITH THE URGE TO MOVE THE BOWELS.
I DON'T THINK I WANT TO SEE!
OK, THEN JUST DON'T LOOK! THE DOCTOR OR THE NURSES WILL CHECK FOR YOU, AND TELL YOU WHAT TO DO!
WILL I BLEED A LOT?
FOR EITHER THE SUCTION OR SALINE INJECTION METHOD YOU WILL BLEED ANYWHERE FROM ONE DAY TO THREE WEEKS. IT JUST DEPENDS ON THE INDIVIDUAL. MORE BLEEDING THAN A NORMALLY HEAVY MENSTRUAL PERIOD IS A DANGER SIGNAL!
WHAT ELSE SHOULD YOU WATCH FOR?
PASSING LOTS OF BLOODCLOTS, SEVERE CRAMPING AFTER THE SECOND DAY OR EXCESSIVE BRIGHT RED BLEEDING SHOULD BE REPORTED AS WELL AS A TEMPERATURE OVER 100°. MODERATE CRAMPING SHOULD BE EXPECTED, HOWEVER.
IS THIS VACUUM THING THE SAME AS A "D&C"?
NO, BUT SOMETIMES AFTER EITHER A VACUUM ASPIRATION OR A SALINE INJECTION, THE DOCTOR WILL DO A QUICK "D&C", SCRAPING THE UTERUS JUST TO BE SURE EVERYTHING IS REMOVED.

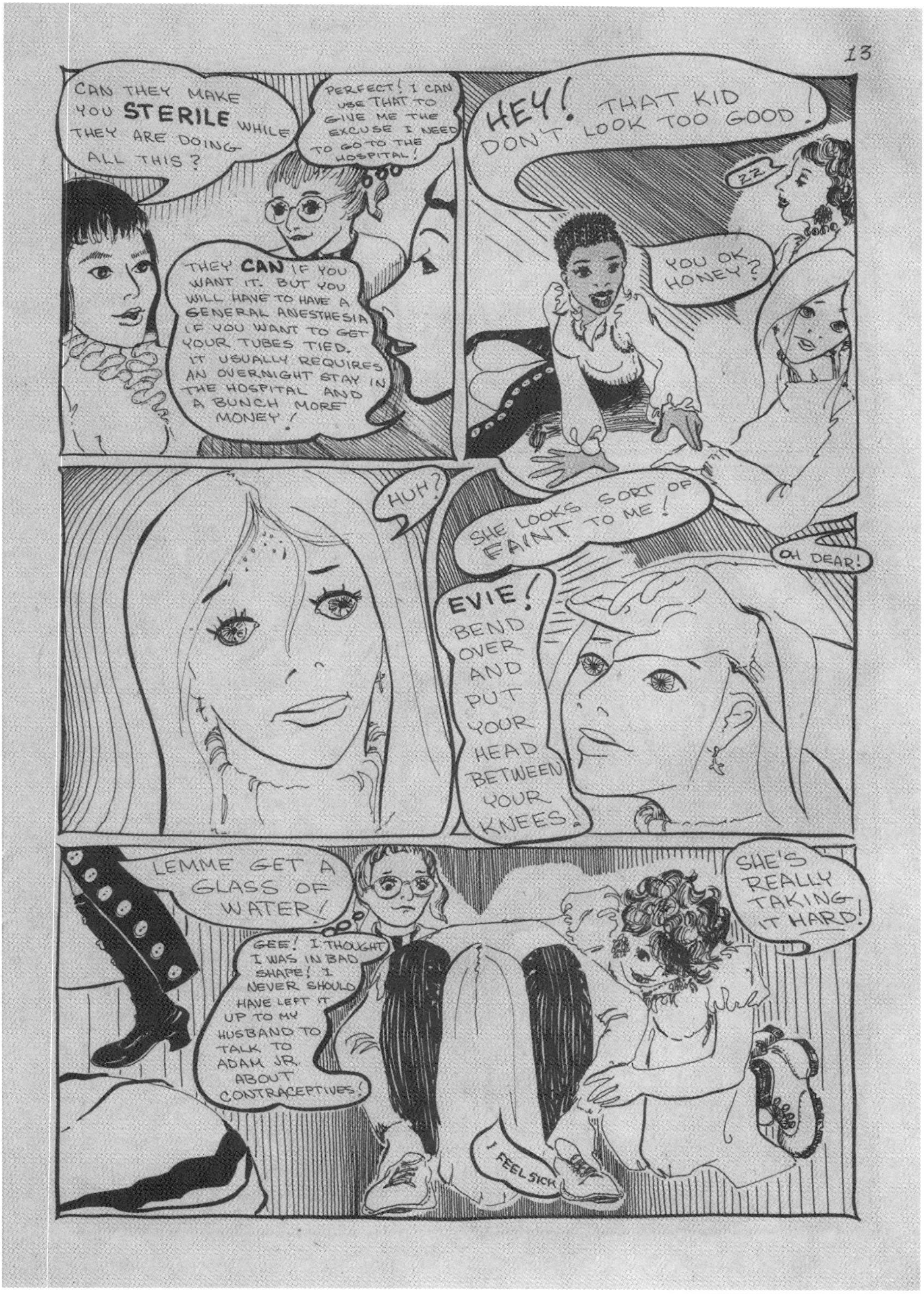
13
CAN THEY MAKE YOU STERILE WHILE THEY ARE DOING ALL THIS?
PERFECT! I CAN USE THAT TO GIVE ME THE EXCUSE I NEED TO GO TO THE HOSPITAL!
THEY CAN IF YOU WANT IT. BUT YOU WILL HAVE TO HAVE A GENERAL ANESTHESIA IF YOU WANT TO GET YOUR TUBES TIED. IT USUALLY REQUIRES AN OVERNIGHT STAY IN THE HOSPITAL AND A BUNCH MORE MONEY!
HEY! THAT KID DON'T LOOK TOO GOOD!
ZZ
YOU OK HONEY?
HUH?
SHE LOOKS SORT OF FAINT TO ME!
OH DEAR!
EVIE! BEND OVER AND PUT YOUR HEAD BETWEEN YOUR KNEES!
LEMME GET A GLASS OF WATER!
GEE! I THOUGHT I WAS IN BAD SHAPE! I NEVER SHOULD HAVE LEFT IT UP TO MY HUSBAND TO TALK TO ADAM JR. ABOUT CONTRACEPTIVES!
SHE'S REALLY TAKING IT HARD!
I FEEL SICK

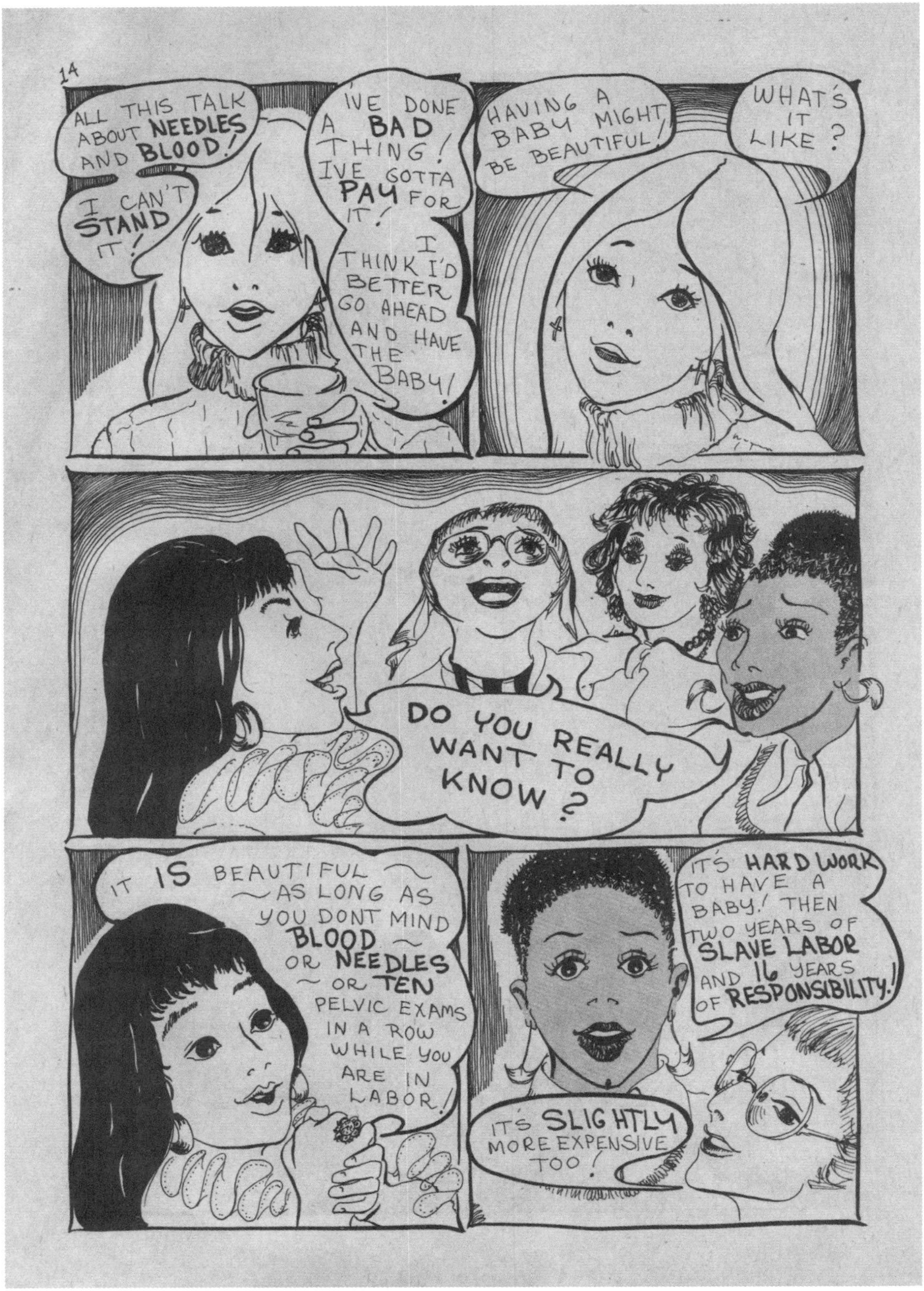
14
ALL THIS TALK ABOUT NEEDLES AND BLOOD!
I CAN'T STAND IT!
I'VE DONE A BAD THING! I'VE GOTTA PAY FOR IT!
I THINK I'D BETTER GO AHEAD AND HAVE THE BABY!
HAVING A BABY MIGHT BE BEAUTIFUL!
WHAT'S IT LIKE?
DO YOU REALLY WANT TO KNOW?
IT IS BEAUTIFUL ~ AS LONG AS YOU DONT MIND BLOOD ~ OR NEEDLES ~ OR TEN PELVIC EXAMS IN A ROW WHILE YOU ARE IN LABOR!
IT'S HARD WORK TO HAVE A BABY! THEN TWO YEARS OF SLAVE LABOR AND 16 YEARS OF RESPONSIBILITY!
IT'S SLIGHTLY MORE EXPENSIVE TOO!

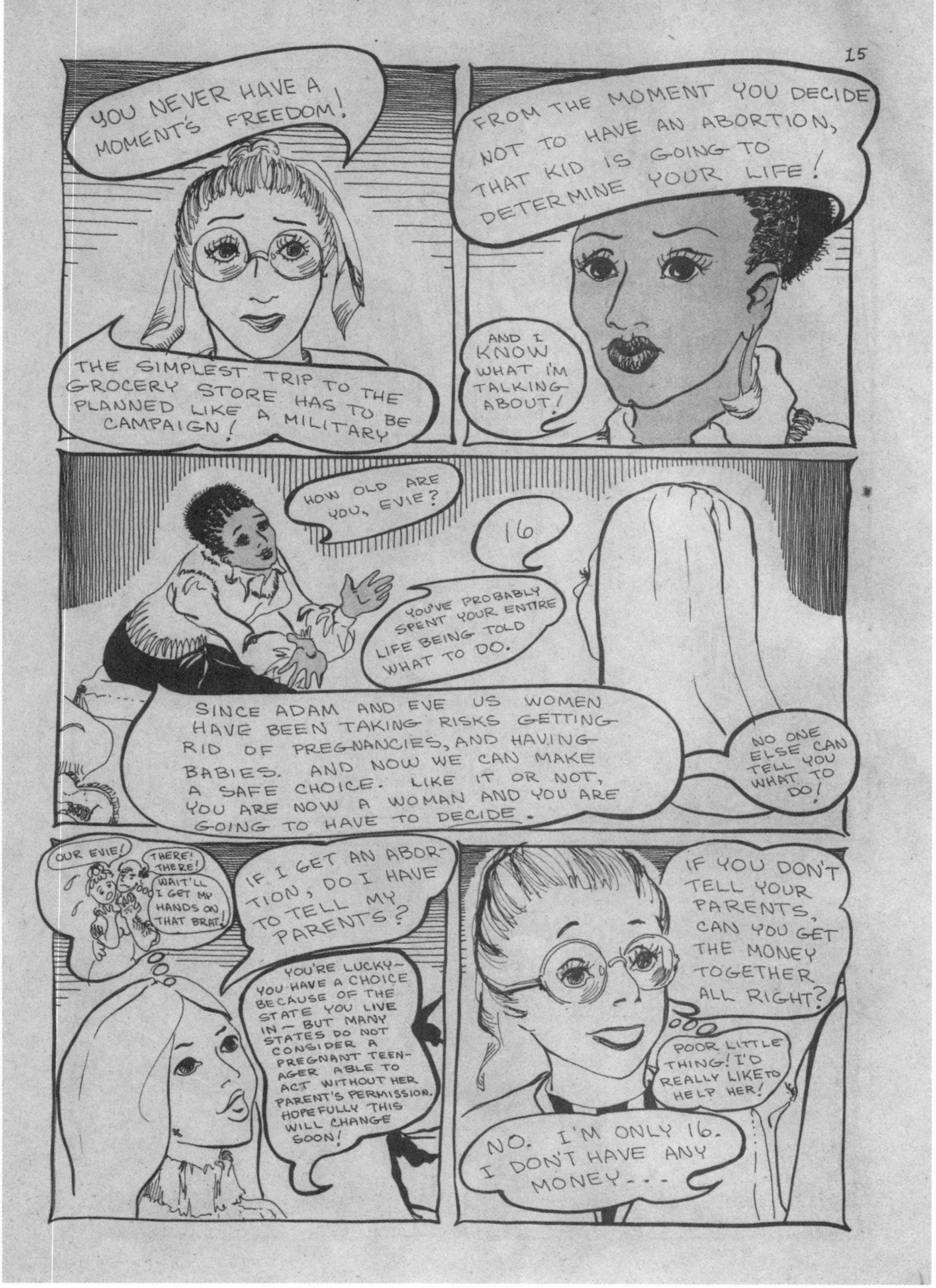
15
YOU NEVER HAVE A MOMENT'S FREEDOM!
THE SIMPLEST TRIP TO THE GROCERY STORE HAS TO BE PLANNED LIKE A MILITARY CAMPAIGN!
FROM THE MOMENT YOU DECIDE NOT TO HAVE AN ABORTION, THAT KID IS GOING TO DETERMINE YOUR LIFE!
AND I KNOW WHAT I'M TALKING ABOUT!
HOW OLD ARE YOU, EVIE?
16
YOU'VE PROBABLY SPENT YOUR ENTIRE LIFE BEING TOLD WHAT TO DO.
SINCE ADAM AND EVE US WOMEN HAVE BEEN TAKING RISKS GETTING RID OF PREGNANCIES, AND HAVING BABIES. AND NOW WE CAN MAKE A SAFE CHOICE. LIKE IT OR NOT, YOU ARE NOW A WOMAN AND YOU ARE GOING TO HAVE TO DECIDE.
NO ONE ELSE CAN TELL YOU WHAT TO DO!
OUR EVIE!
THERE! THERE!
WAIT'LL I GET MY HANDS ON THAT BRAT!
IF I GET AN ABORTION, DO I HAVE TO TELL MY PARENTS?
YOU'RE LUCKY~ YOU HAVE A CHOICE BECAUSE OF THE STATE YOU LIVE IN~ BUT MANY STATES DO NOT CONSIDER A PREGNANT TEEN-AGER ABLE TO ACT WITHOUT HER PARENT'S PERMISSION. HOPEFULLY THIS WILL CHANGE SOON!
IF YOU DON'T TELL YOUR PARENTS, CAN YOU GET THE MONEY TOGETHER ALL RIGHT?
POOR LITTLE THING! I'D REALLY LIKE TO HELP HER!
NO. I'M ONLY 16. I DON'T HAVE ANY MONEY...

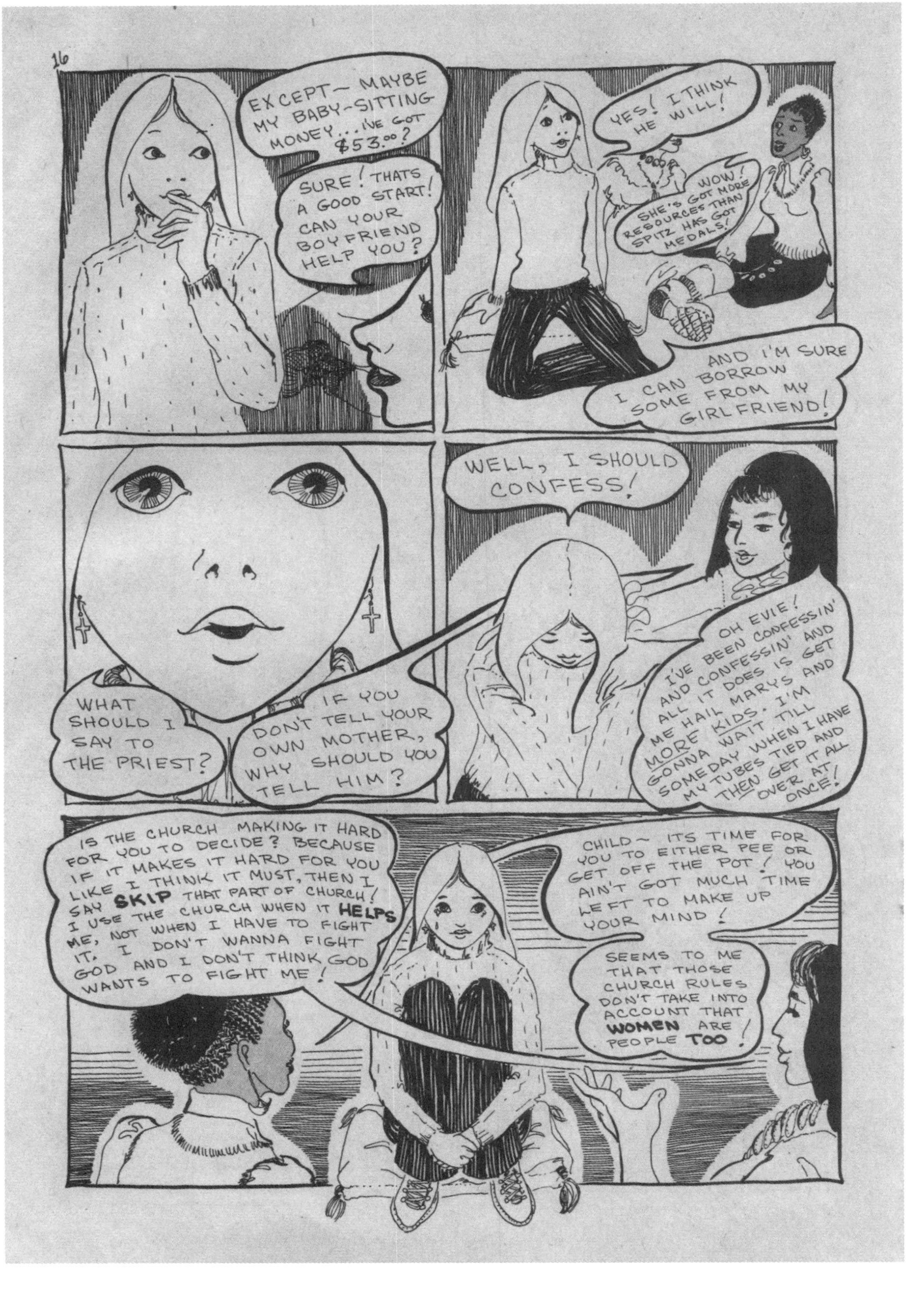
16
EXCEPT— MAYBE MY BABY-SITTING MONEY... I'VE GOT $53.00?
SURE! THATS A GOOD START! CAN YOUR BOYFRIEND HELP YOU?
YES! I THINK HE WILL!
WOW! SHE'S GOT MORE RESOURCES THAN SPITZ HAS GOT MEDALS!
AND I'M SURE I CAN BORROW SOME FROM MY GIRLFRIEND!
WHAT SHOULD I SAY TO THE PRIEST?
IF YOU DON'T TELL YOUR OWN MOTHER, WHY SHOULD YOU TELL HIM?
WELL, I SHOULD CONFESS!
OH EVIE! I'VE BEEN CONFESSIN' AND CONFESSIN' AND ALL IT DOES IS GET ME HAIL MARYS AND MORE KIDS. I'M GONNA WAIT TILL SOMEDAY WHEN I HAVE MY TUBES TIED AND THEN GET IT ALL OVER AT ONCE!
IS THE CHURCH MAKING IT HARD FOR YOU TO DECIDE? BECAUSE IF IT MAKES IT HARD FOR YOU LIKE I THINK IT MUST, THEN I SAY SKIP THAT PART OF CHURCH! I USE THE CHURCH WHEN IT HELPS ME, NOT WHEN I HAVE TO FIGHT IT. I DON'T WANNA FIGHT GOD AND I DON'T THINK GOD WANTS TO FIGHT ME!
CHILD~ ITS TIME FOR YOU TO EITHER PEE OR GET OFF THE POT! YOU AIN'T GOT MUCH TIME LEFT TO MAKE UP YOUR MIND!
SEEMS TO ME THAT THOSE CHURCH RULES DON'T TAKE INTO ACCOUNT THAT WOMEN ARE PEOPLE TOO!

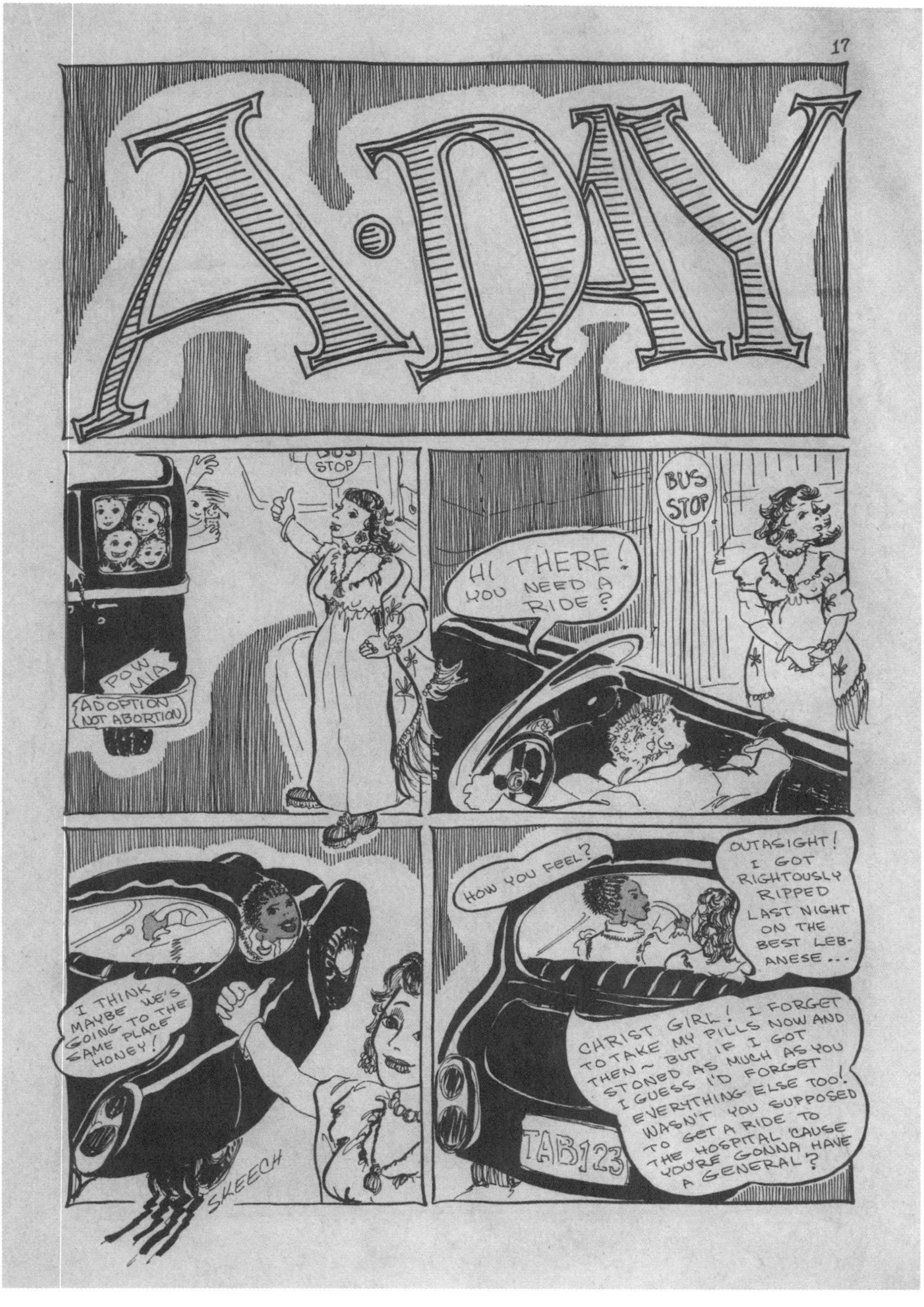
17
A-DAY
BUS STOP
POW MIA
ADOPTION NOT ABORTION
BUS STOP
HI THERE! YOU NEED A RIDE?
I THINK MAYBE WE'S GOING TO THE SAME PLACE HONEY!
SKEECH
HOW YOU FEEL?
OUTASIGHT! I GOT RIGHTOUSLY RIPPED LAST NIGHT ON THE BEST LEB-ANESE...
CHRIST GIRL! I FORGET TO TAKE MY PILLS NOW AND THEN~ BUT IF I GOT STONED AS MUCH AS YOU I GUESS I'D FORGET EVERYTHING ELSE TOO! WASN'T YOU SUPPOSED TO GET A RIDE TO THE HOSPITAL 'CAUSE YOU'RE GONNA HAVE A GENERAL?
TAB123

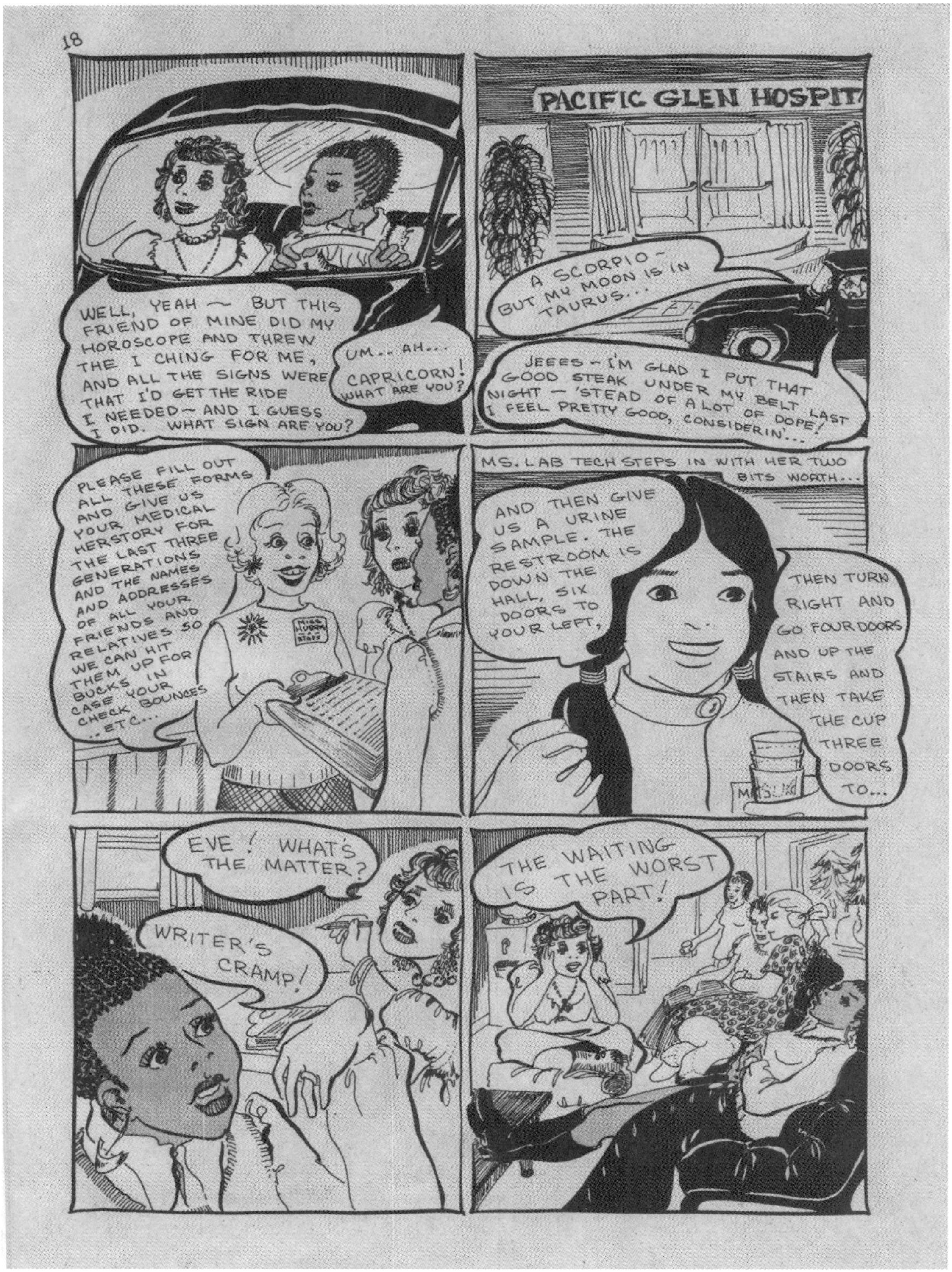
18
WELL, YEAH — BUT THIS FRIEND OF MINE DID MY HOROSCOPE AND THREW THE I CHING FOR ME, AND ALL THE SIGNS WERE THAT I'D GET THE RIDE I NEEDED— AND I GUESS I DID. WHAT SIGN ARE YOU?
UM.. AH... CAPRICORN! WHAT ARE YOU?
PACIFIC GLEN HOSPIT
A SCORPIO— BUT MY MOON IS IN TAURUS...
JEEES — I'M GLAD I PUT THAT GOOD STEAK UNDER MY BELT LAST NIGHT — 'STEAD OF A LOT OF DOPE! I FEEL PRETTY GOOD, CONSIDERIN'...
PLEASE FILL OUT ALL THESE FORMS AND GIVE US YOUR MEDICAL HERSTORY FOR THE LAST THREE GENERATIONS AND THE NAMES AND ADDRESSES OF ALL YOUR FRIENDS AND RELATIVES SO WE CAN HIT THEM UP FOR BUCKS IN CASE YOUR CHECK BOUNCES ..ETC...
MS. LAB TECH STEPS IN WITH HER TWO BITS WORTH...
AND THEN GIVE US A URINE SAMPLE. THE RESTROOM IS DOWN THE HALL, SIX DOORS TO YOUR LEFT,
THEN TURN RIGHT AND GO FOUR DOORS AND UP THE STAIRS AND THEN TAKE THE CUP THREE DOORS TO...
EVE! WHAT'S THE MATTER?
WRITER'S CRAMP!
THE WAITING IS THE WORST PART!

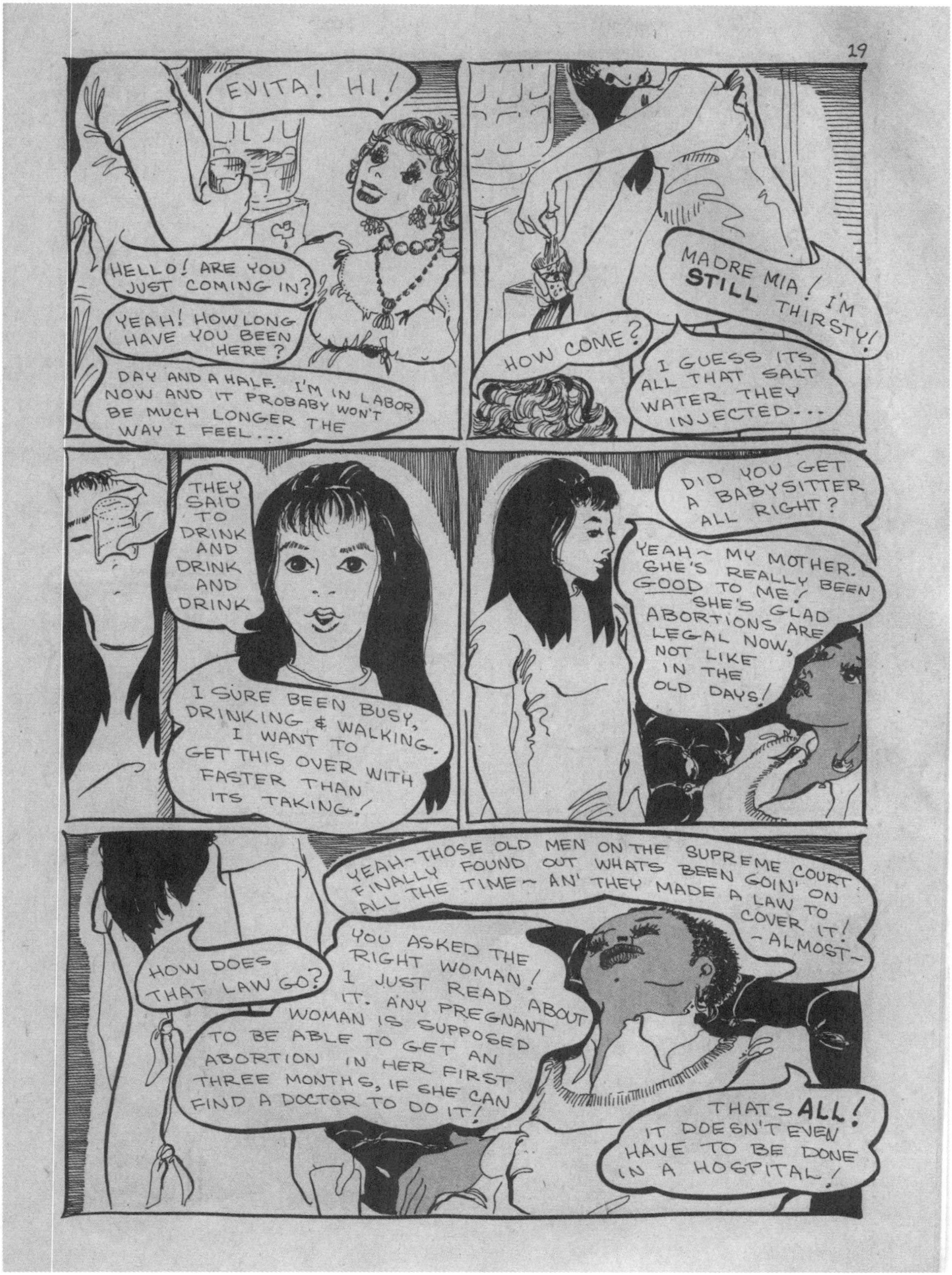
19
EVITA! HI!
HELLO! ARE YOU JUST COMING IN?
YEAH! HOW LONG HAVE YOU BEEN HERE?
DAY AND A HALF. I'M IN LABOR NOW AND IT PROBABY WON'T BE MUCH LONGER THE WAY I FEEL...
MADRE MIA! I'M STILL THIRSTY!
HOW COME?
I GUESS ITS ALL THAT SALT WATER THEY INJECTED...
THEY SAID TO DRINK AND DRINK AND DRINK
I SURE BEEN BUSY, DRINKING & WALKING. I WANT TO GET THIS OVER WITH FASTER THAN ITS TAKING!
DID YOU GET A BABYSITTER ALL RIGHT?
YEAH~ MY MOTHER. SHE'S REALLY BEEN GOOD TO ME! SHE'S GLAD ABORTIONS ARE LEGAL NOW, NOT LIKE IN THE OLD DAYS!
YEAH~THOSE OLD MEN ON THE SUPREME COURT FINALLY FOUND OUT WHATS BEEN GOIN' ON ALL THE TIME~ AN' THEY MADE A LAW TO COVER IT! ~ALMOST~
HOW DOES THAT LAW GO?
YOU ASKED THE RIGHT WOMAN! I JUST READ ABOUT IT. ANY PREGNANT WOMAN IS SUPPOSED TO BE ABLE TO GET AN ABORTION IN HER FIRST THREE MONTHS, IF SHE CAN FIND A DOCTOR TO DO IT!
THATS ALL! IT DOESN'T EVEN HAVE TO BE DONE IN A HOSPITAL!

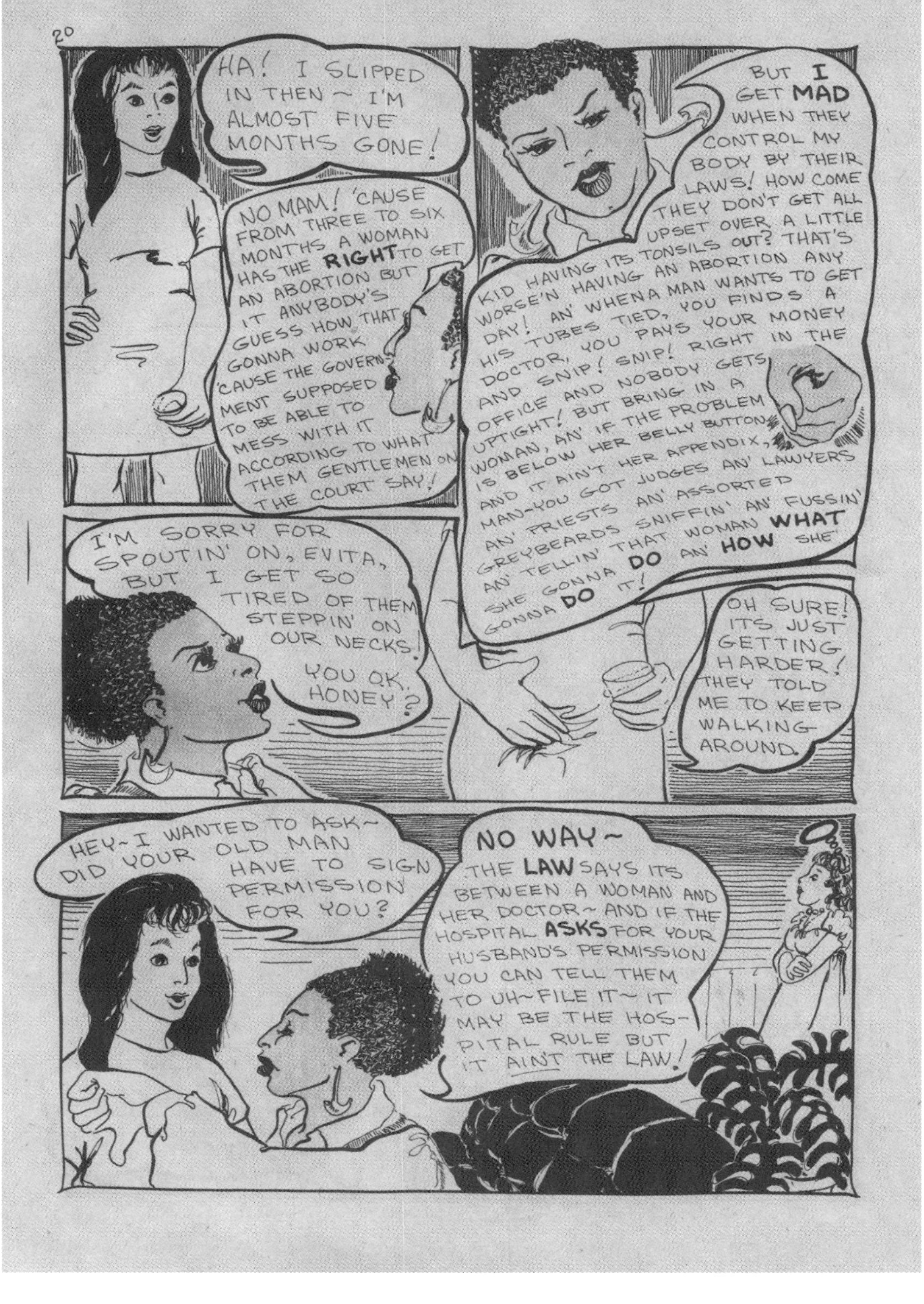
20
HA! I SLIPPED IN THEN ~ I'M ALMOST FIVE MONTHS GONE!
NO MAM! 'CAUSE FROM THREE TO SIX MONTHS A WOMAN HAS THE RIGHT TO GET AN ABORTION BUT IT ANYBODY'S GUESS HOW THAT GONNA WORK 'CAUSE THE GOVERNMENT SUPPOSED TO BE ABLE TO MESS WITH IT ACCORDING TO WHAT THEM GENTLEMEN ON THE COURT SAY!
BUT I GET MAD WHEN THEY CONTROL MY BODY BY THEIR LAWS! HOW COME THEY DON'T GET ALL UPSET OVER A LITTLE KID HAVING ITS TONSILS OUT? THAT'S WORSE'N HAVING AN ABORTION ANY DAY! AN' WHEN A MAN WANTS TO GET HIS TUBES TIED, YOU FINDS A DOCTOR, YOU PAYS YOUR MONEY AND SNIP! SNIP! RIGHT IN THE OFFICE AND NOBODY GETS UPTIGHT! BUT BRING IN A WOMAN, AN' IF THE PROBLEM IS BELOW HER BELLY BUTTON, AND IT AIN'T HER APPENDIX, MAN~YOU GOT JUDGES AN' LAWYERS AN' PRIESTS AN' ASSORTED GREYBEARDS SNIFFIN' AN' FUSSIN' AN' TELLIN' THAT WOMAN WHAT SHE GONNA DO AN' HOW SHE GONNA DO IT!
I'M SORRY FOR SPOUTIN' ON, EVITA, BUT I GET SO TIRED OF THEM STEPPIN' ON OUR NECKS! YOU OK, HONEY?
OH SURE! ITS JUST GETTING HARDER! THEY TOLD ME TO KEEP WALKING AROUND.
HEY~I WANTED TO ASK~ DID YOUR OLD MAN HAVE TO SIGN PERMISSION FOR YOU?
NO WAY~ THE LAW SAYS ITS BETWEEN A WOMAN AND HER DOCTOR~ AND IF THE HOSPITAL ASKS FOR YOUR HUSBAND'S PERMISSION YOU CAN TELL THEM TO UH~FILE IT~ IT MAY BE THE HOSPITAL RULE BUT IT AIN'T THE LAW!

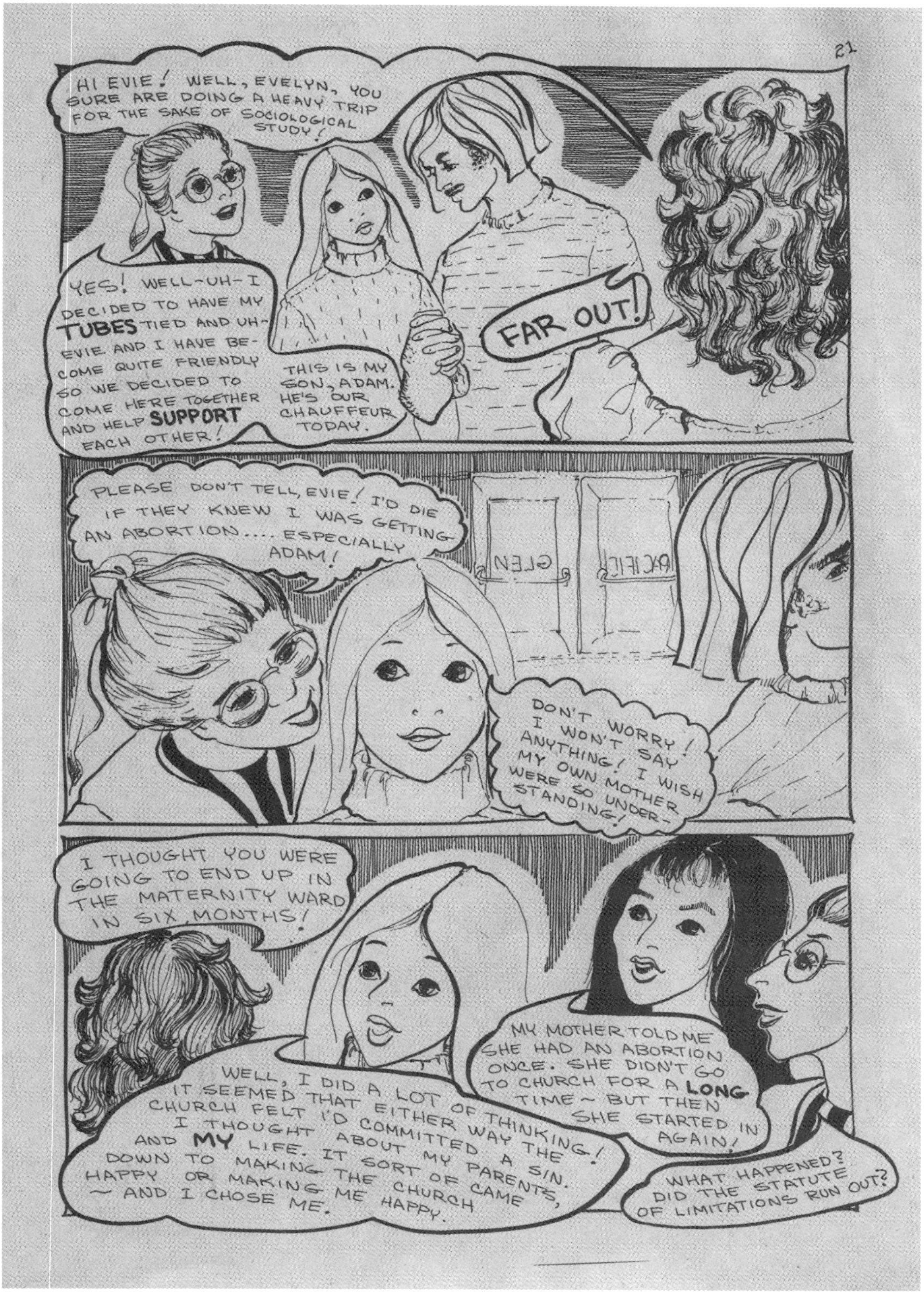
21
HI EVIE! WELL, EVELYN, YOU SURE ARE DOING A HEAVY TRIP FOR THE SAKE OF SOCIOLOGICAL STUDY!
YES! WELL-UH-I DECIDED TO HAVE MY TUBES TIED AND UH- EVIE AND I HAVE BECOME QUITE FRIENDLY SO WE DECIDED TO COME HERE TOGETHER AND HELP SUPPORT EACH OTHER!
THIS IS MY SON, ADAM. HE'S OUR CHAUFFEUR TODAY.
FAR OUT!
PLEASE DON'T TELL, EVIE! I'D DIE IF THEY KNEW I WAS GETTING AN ABORTION.... ESPECIALLY ADAM!
DON'T WORRY! I WON'T SAY ANYTHING! I WISH MY OWN MOTHER WERE SO UNDERSTANDING!
I THOUGHT YOU WERE GOING TO END UP IN THE MATERNITY WARD IN SIX MONTHS!
WELL, I DID A LOT OF THINKING! IT SEEMED THAT EITHER WAY THE CHURCH FELT I'D COMMITTED A SIN. I THOUGHT ABOUT MY PARENTS, AND MY LIFE. IT SORT OF CAME DOWN TO MAKING THE CHURCH HAPPY OR MAKING ME HAPPY. ~ AND I CHOSE ME.
MY MOTHER TOLD ME SHE HAD AN ABORTION ONCE. SHE DIDN'T GO TO CHURCH FOR A LONG TIME ~ BUT THEN SHE STARTED IN AGAIN!
WHAT HAPPENED? DID THE STATUTE OF LIMITATIONS RUN OUT?

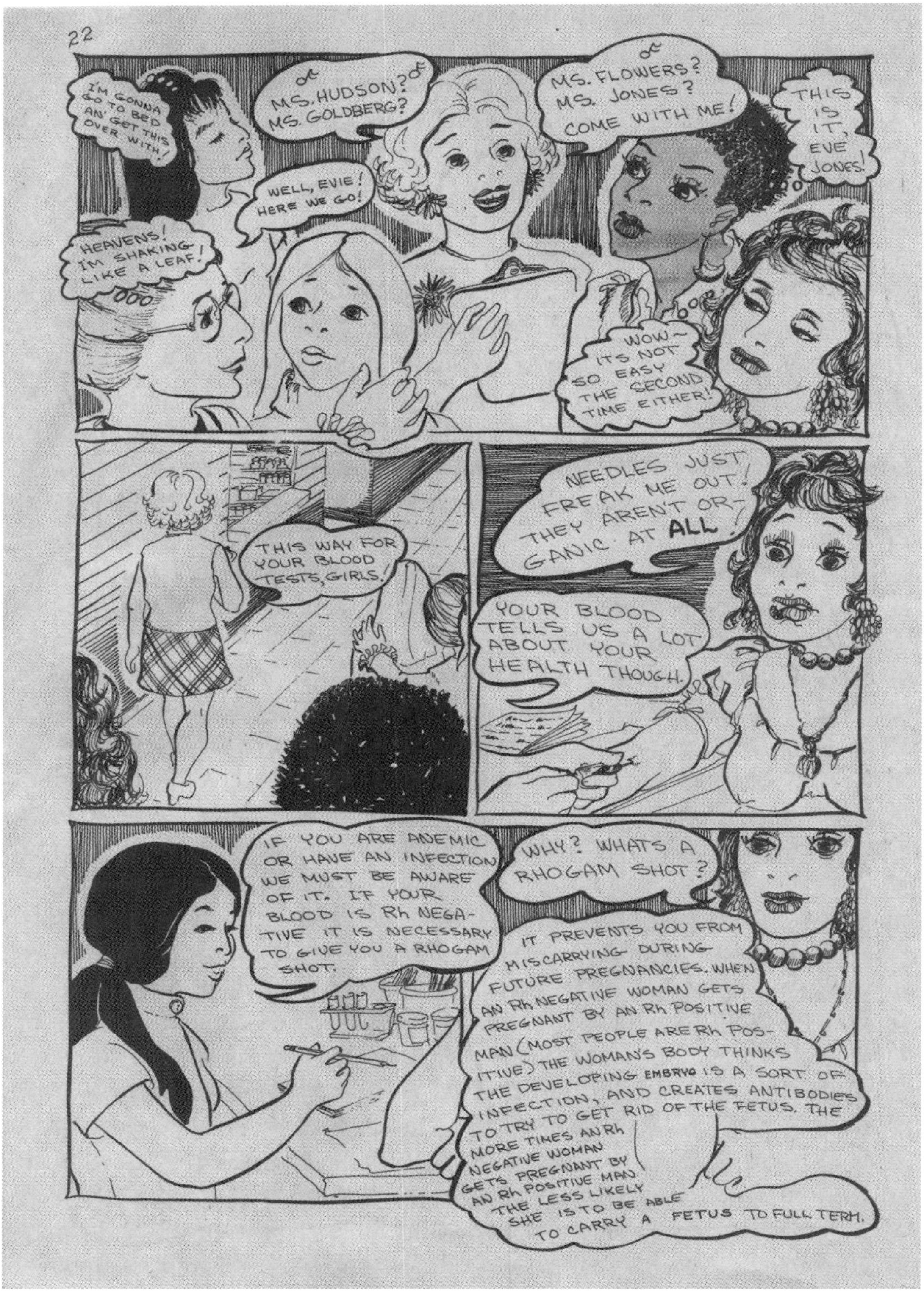
22
I'M GONNA GO TO BED AN' GET THIS OVER WITH!
MS. HUDSON? or MS. GOLDBERG? or
MS. FLOWERS? or MS. JONES? COME WITH ME!
THIS IS IT, EVE JONES!
WELL, EVIE! HERE WE GO!
HEAVENS! I'M SHAKING LIKE A LEAF!
WOW~ ITS NOT SO EASY THE SECOND TIME EITHER!
THIS WAY FOR YOUR BLOOD TESTS, GIRLS!
NEEDLES JUST FREAK ME OUT! THEY AREN'T OR-GANIC AT ALL!
YOUR BLOOD TELLS US A LOT ABOUT YOUR HEALTH THOUGH.
IF YOU ARE ANEMIC OR HAVE AN INFECTION WE MUST BE AWARE OF IT. IF YOUR BLOOD IS Rh NEGA-TIVE IT IS NECESSARY TO GIVE YOU A RHOGAM SHOT.
WHY? WHATS A RHOGAM SHOT?
IT PREVENTS YOU FROM MISCARRYING DURING FUTURE PREGNANCIES. WHEN AN Rh NEGATIVE WOMAN GETS PREGNANT BY AN Rh POSITIVE MAN (MOST PEOPLE ARE Rh POS-ITIVE) THE WOMAN'S BODY THINKS THE DEVELOPING EMBRYO IS A SORT OF INFECTION, AND CREATES ANTIBODIES TO TRY TO GET RID OF THE FETUS. THE MORE TIMES AN Rh NEGATIVE WOMAN GETS PREGNANT BY AN Rh POSITIVE MAN THE LESS LIKELY SHE IS TO BE ABLE TO CARRY A FETUS TO FULL TERM.

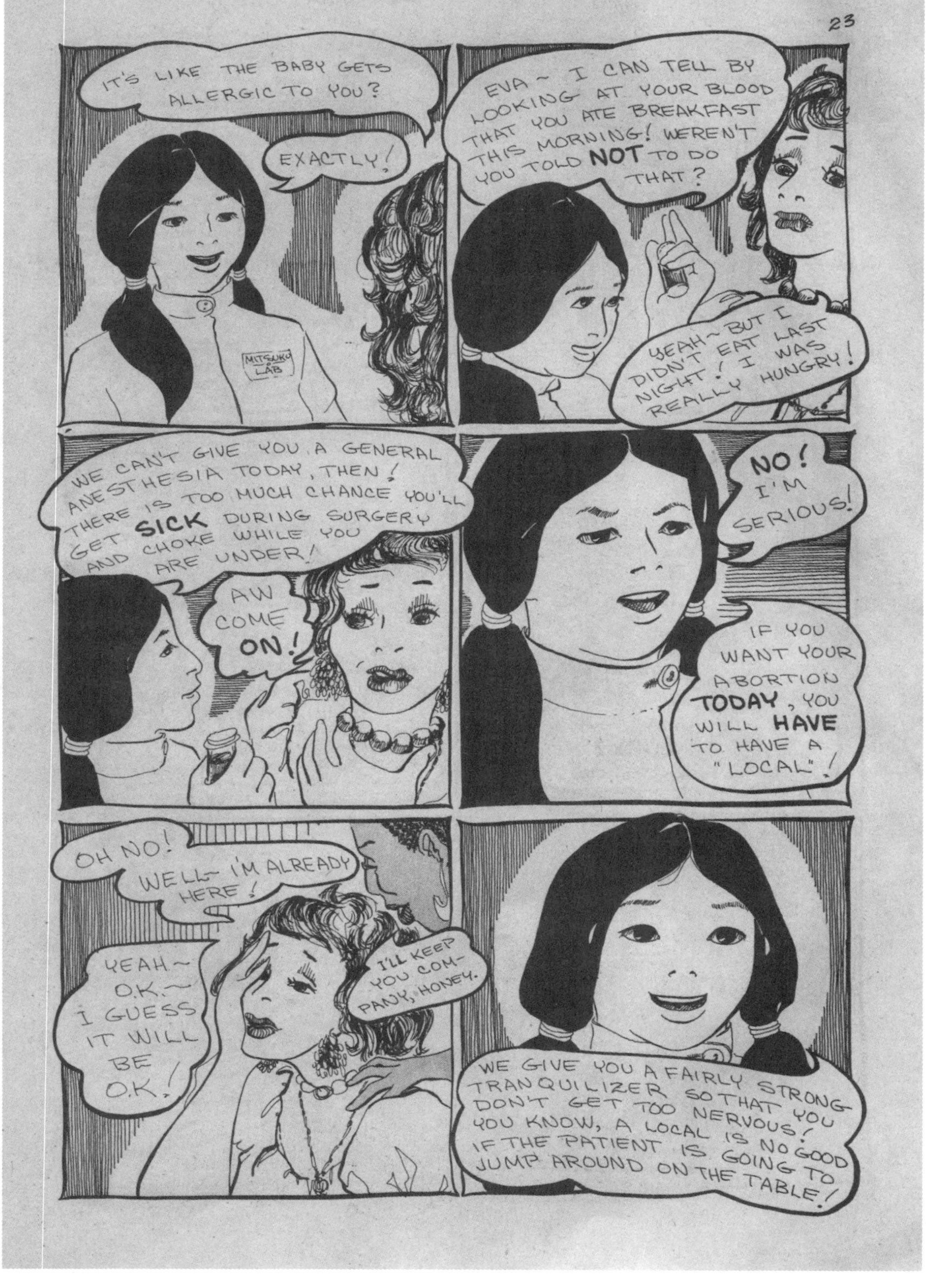
23
IT'S LIKE THE BABY GETS ALLERGIC TO YOU?
EXACTLY!
MITSUKO LAB
EVA~ I CAN TELL BY LOOKING AT YOUR BLOOD THAT YOU ATE BREAKFAST THIS MORNING! WEREN'T YOU TOLD NOT TO DO THAT?
YEAH~ BUT I DIDN'T EAT LAST NIGHT! I WAS REALLY HUNGRY!
WE CAN'T GIVE YOU A GENERAL ANESTHESIA TODAY, THEN! THERE IS TOO MUCH CHANCE YOU'LL GET SICK DURING SURGERY AND CHOKE WHILE YOU ARE UNDER!
AW COME ON!
NO! I'M SERIOUS!
IF YOU WANT YOUR ABORTION TODAY, YOU WILL HAVE TO HAVE A "LOCAL"!
OH NO! WELL~ I'M ALREADY HERE!
YEAH~ O.K.~ I GUESS IT WILL BE O.K.!
I'LL KEEP YOU COMPANY, HONEY.
WE GIVE YOU A FAIRLY STRONG TRANQUILIZER SO THAT YOU DON'T GET TOO NERVOUS! YOU KNOW, A LOCAL IS NO GOOD IF THE PATIENT IS GOING TO JUMP AROUND ON THE TABLE!

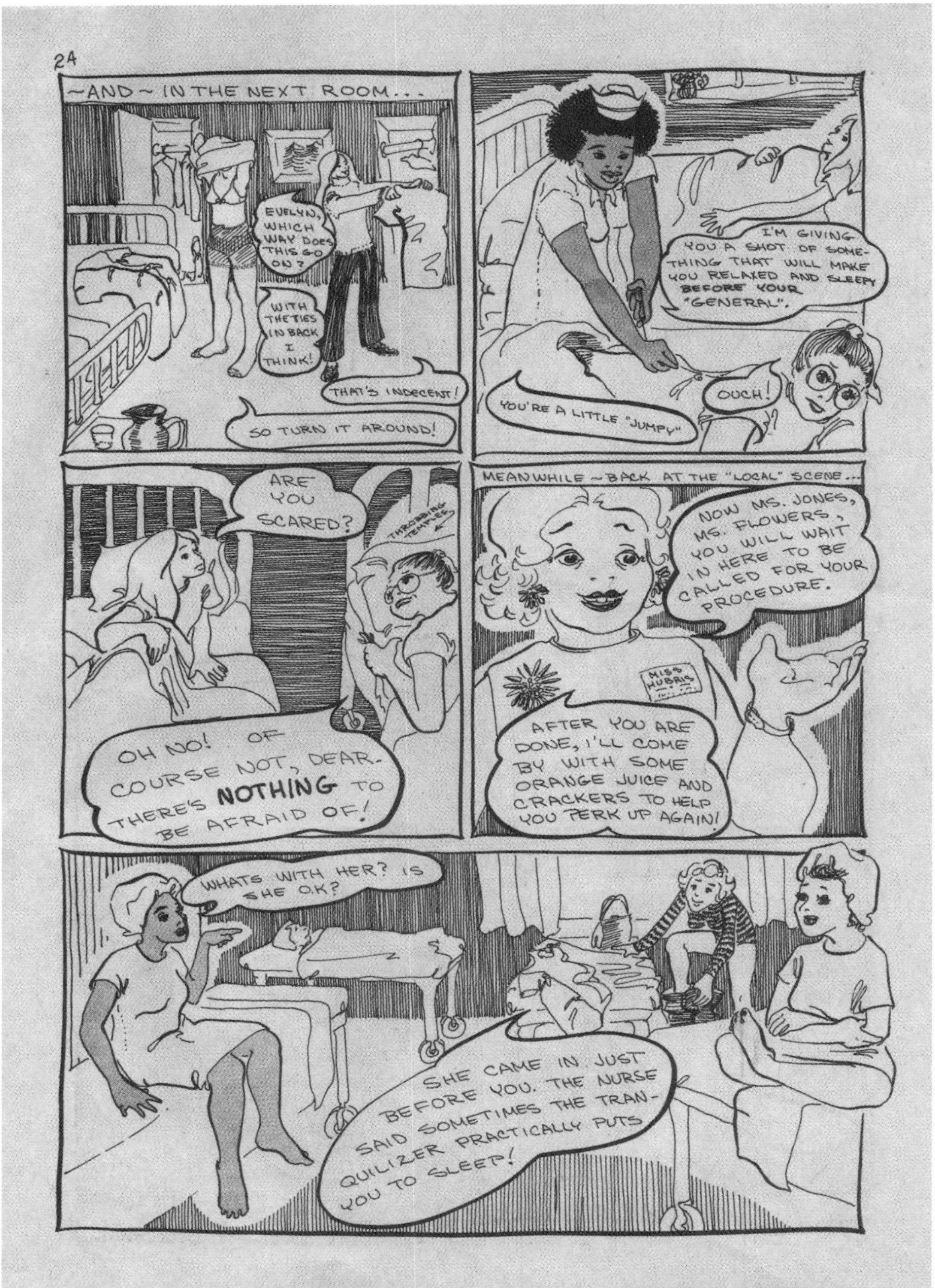
24
~AND~ IN THE NEXT ROOM...
EVELYN, WHICH WAY DOES THIS GO ON?
WITH THE TIES IN BACK I THINK!
THAT'S INDECENT!
SO TURN IT AROUND!
I'M GIVING YOU A SHOT OF SOME-THING THAT WILL MAKE YOU RELAXED AND SLEEPY BEFORE YOUR "GENERAL".
OUCH!
YOU'RE A LITTLE "JUMPY"
ARE YOU SCARED?
THROBBING TEMPLES
OH NO! OF COURSE NOT, DEAR. THERE'S NOTHING TO BE AFRAID OF!
MEANWHILE ~ BACK AT THE "LOCAL" SCENE...
NOW MS. JONES, MS. FLOWERS, YOU WILL WAIT IN HERE TO BE CALLED FOR YOUR PROCEDURE.
MISS HUBRIS
AFTER YOU ARE DONE, I'LL COME BY WITH SOME ORANGE JUICE AND CRACKERS TO HELP YOU PERK UP AGAIN!
WHATS WITH HER? IS SHE O.K?
SHE CAME IN JUST BEFORE YOU. THE NURSE SAID SOMETIMES THE TRAN-QUILIZER PRACTICALLY PUTS YOU TO SLEEP!

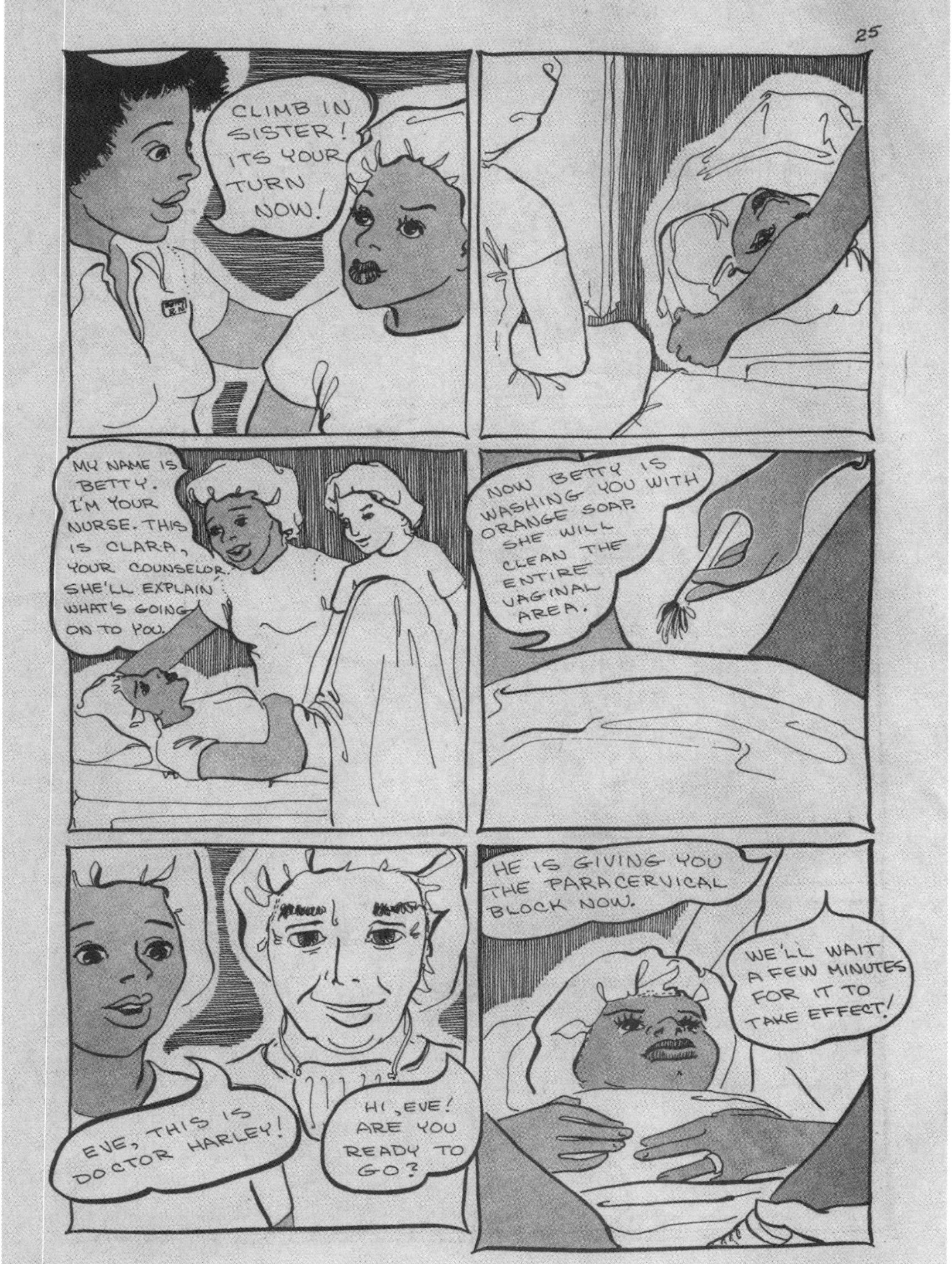
25
CLIMB IN SISTER! ITS YOUR TURN NOW!
MY NAME IS BETTY. I'M YOUR NURSE. THIS IS CLARA, YOUR COUNSELOR. SHE'LL EXPLAIN WHAT'S GOING ON TO YOU.
NOW BETTY IS WASHING YOU WITH ORANGE SOAP. SHE WILL CLEAN THE ENTIRE VAGINAL AREA.
EVE, THIS IS DOCTOR HARLEY!
HI, EVE! ARE YOU READY TO GO?
HE IS GIVING YOU THE PARACERVICAL BLOCK NOW.
WE'LL WAIT A FEW MINUTES FOR IT TO TAKE EFFECT!

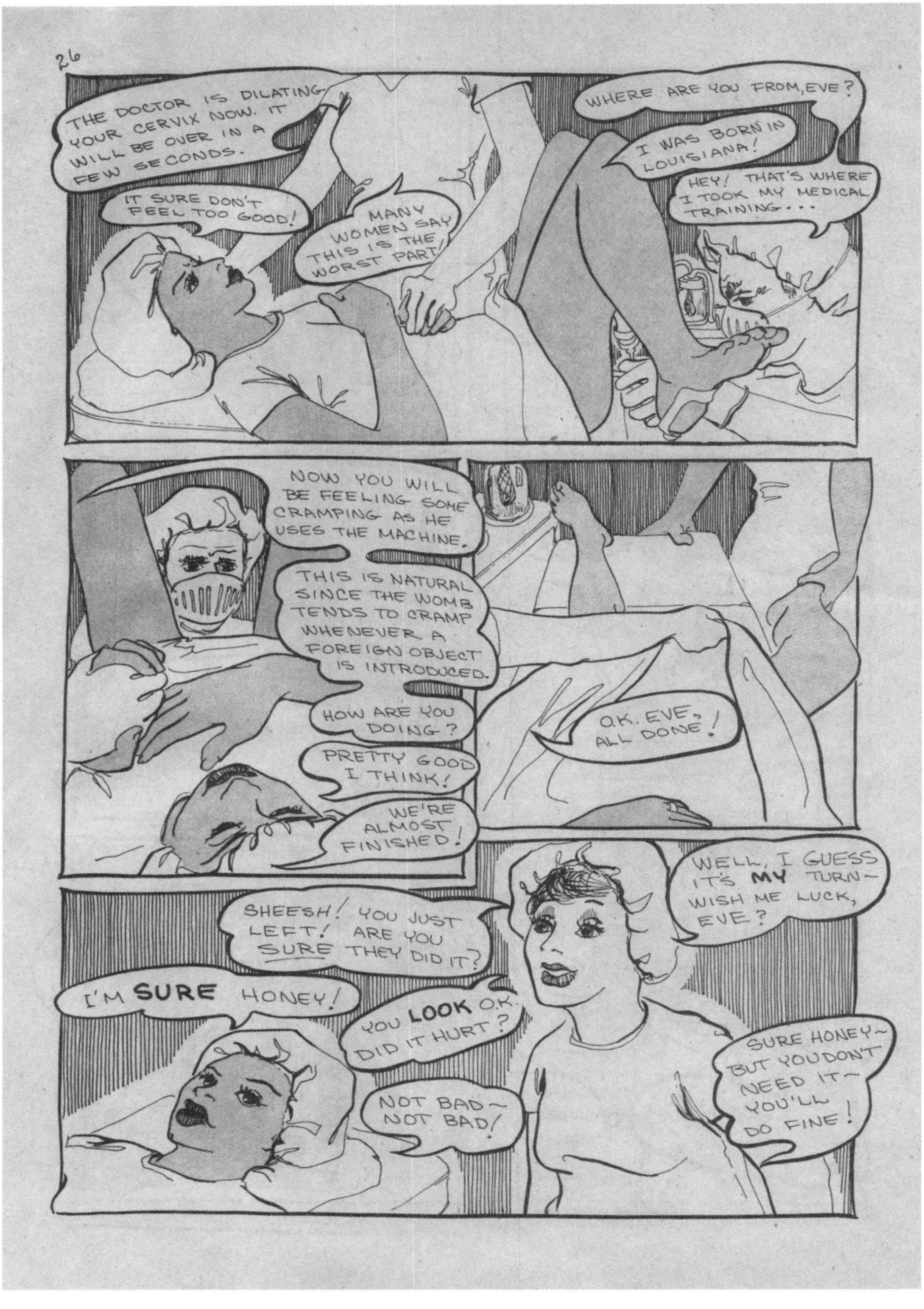
26
THE DOCTOR IS DILATING YOUR CERVIX NOW. IT WILL BE OVER IN A FEW SECONDS.
IT SURE DON'T FEEL TOO GOOD!
MANY WOMEN SAY THIS IS THE WORST PART!
WHERE ARE YOU FROM, EVE?
I WAS BORN IN LOUISIANA!
HEY! THAT'S WHERE I TOOK MY MEDICAL TRAINING...
NOW YOU WILL BE FEELING SOME CRAMPING AS HE USES THE MACHINE.
THIS IS NATURAL SINCE THE WOMB TENDS TO CRAMP WHENEVER A FOREIGN OBJECT IS INTRODUCED.
HOW ARE YOU DOING?
PRETTY GOOD I THINK!
WE'RE ALMOST FINISHED!
O.K. EVE, ALL DONE!
SHEESH! YOU JUST LEFT! ARE YOU SURE THEY DID IT?
I'M SURE HONEY!
WELL, I GUESS IT'S MY TURN– WISH ME LUCK, EVE?
YOU LOOK O.K. DID IT HURT?
NOT BAD– NOT BAD!
SURE HONEY– BUT YOU DON'T NEED IT– YOU'LL DO FINE!

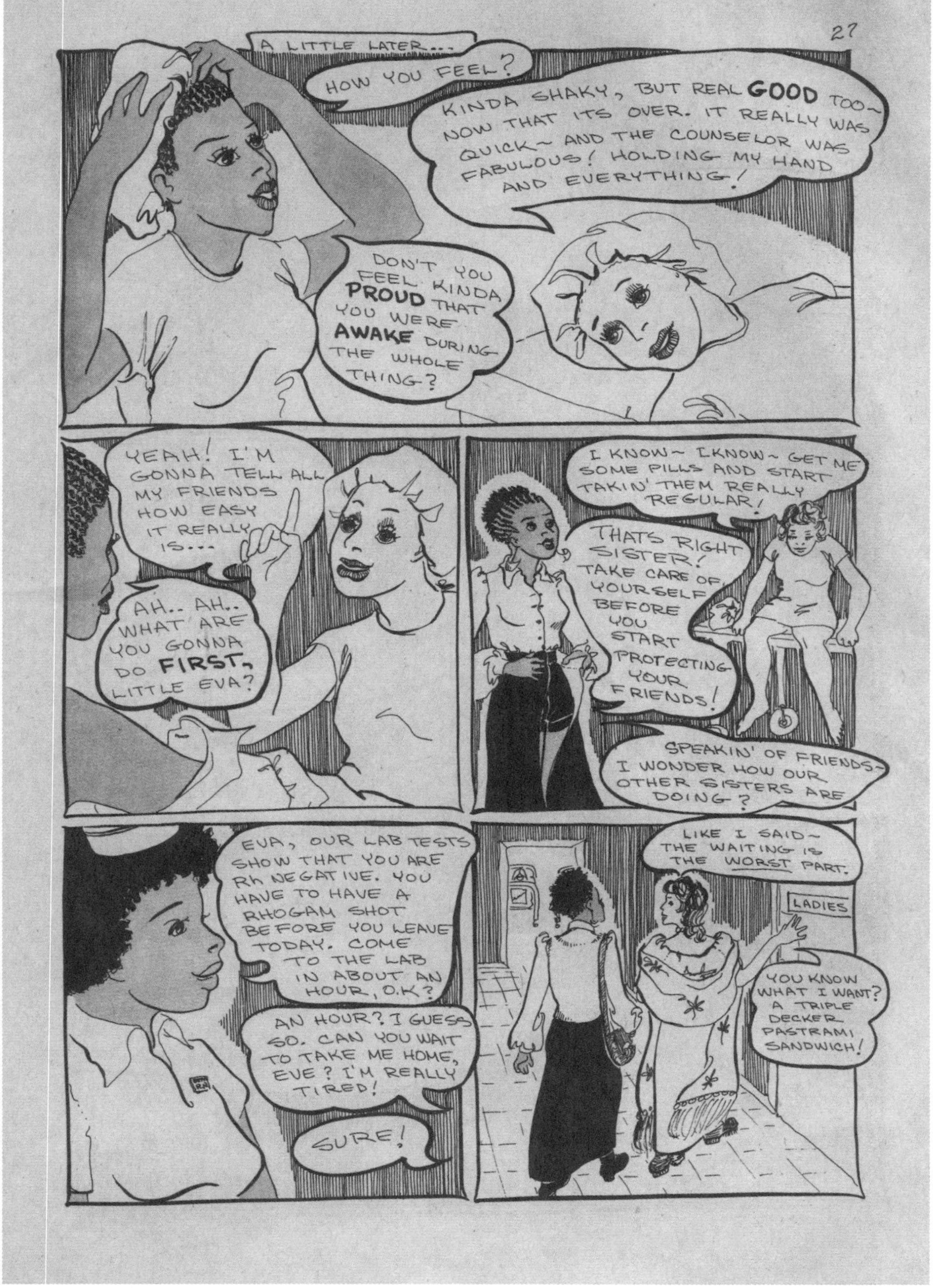
27
A LITTLE LATER...
HOW YOU FEEL?
KINDA SHAKY, BUT REAL GOOD TOO~ NOW THAT ITS OVER. IT REALLY WAS QUICK~ AND THE COUNSELOR WAS FABULOUS! HOLDING MY HAND AND EVERYTHING!
DON'T YOU FEEL KINDA PROUD THAT YOU WERE AWAKE DURING THE WHOLE THING?
YEAH! I'M GONNA TELL ALL MY FRIENDS HOW EASY IT REALLY IS...
AH.. AH.. WHAT ARE YOU GONNA DO FIRST, LITTLE EVA?
I KNOW~ I KNOW~ GET ME SOME PILLS AND START TAKIN' THEM REALLY REGULAR!
THAT'S RIGHT SISTER! TAKE CARE OF YOURSELF BEFORE YOU START PROTECTING YOUR FRIENDS!
SPEAKIN' OF FRIENDS~ I WONDER HOW OUR OTHER SISTERS ARE DOING?
EVA, OUR LAB TESTS SHOW THAT YOU ARE Rh NEGATIVE. YOU HAVE TO HAVE A RHOGAM SHOT BEFORE YOU LEAVE TODAY. COME TO THE LAB IN ABOUT AN HOUR, O.K?
AN HOUR? I GUESS SO. CAN YOU WAIT TO TAKE ME HOME, EVE? I'M REALLY TIRED!
SURE!
LIKE I SAID~ THE WAITING IS THE WORST PART.
LADIES
YOU KNOW WHAT I WANT? A TRIPLE DECKER PASTRAMI SANDWICH!

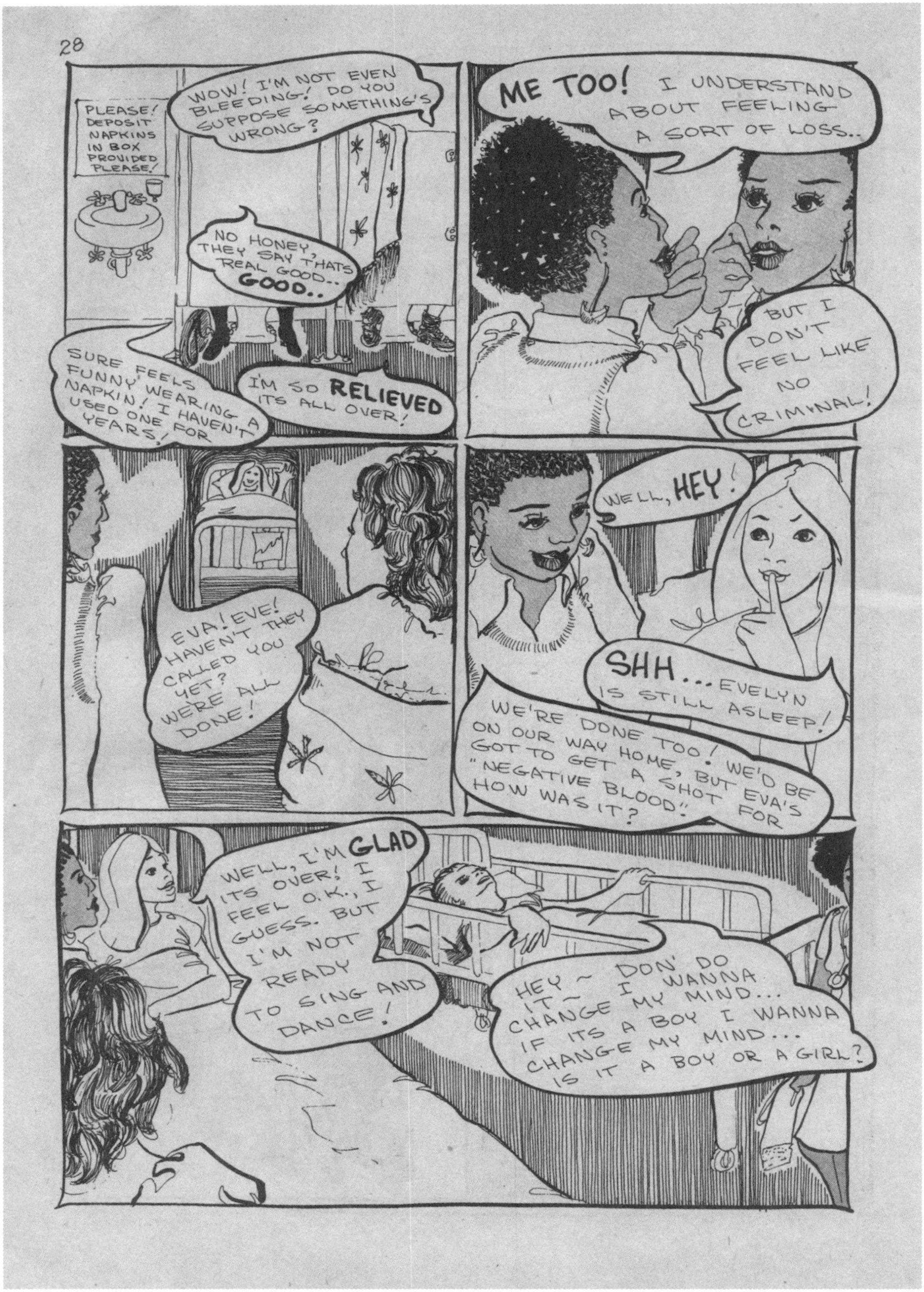
28
PLEASE! DEPOSIT NAPKINS IN BOX PROVIDED PLEASE!
WOW! I'M NOT EVEN BLEEDING! DO YOU SUPPOSE SOMETHING'S WRONG?
NO HONEY, THEY SAY THATS REAL GOOD... GOOD..
SURE FEELS FUNNY WEARING A NAPKIN! I HAVEN'T USED ONE FOR YEARS!
I'M SO RELIEVED ITS ALL OVER!
ME TOO! I UNDERSTAND ABOUT FEELING A SORT OF LOSS..
BUT I DON'T FEEL LIKE NO CRIMINAL!
EVA! EVE! HAVEN'T THEY CALLED YOU YET? WE'RE ALL DONE!
WELL, HEY!
SHH... EVELYN IS STILL ASLEEP!
WE'RE DONE TOO! WE'D BE ON OUR WAY HOME, BUT EVA'S GOT TO GET A SHOT FOR "NEGATIVE BLOOD"! HOW WAS IT?
WELL, I'M GLAD ITS OVER! I FEEL O.K., I GUESS. BUT I'M NOT READY TO SING AND DANCE!
HEY ~ DON' DO IT ~ I WANNA CHANGE MY MIND... IF ITS A BOY I WANNA CHANGE MY MIND... IS IT A BOY OR A GIRL?

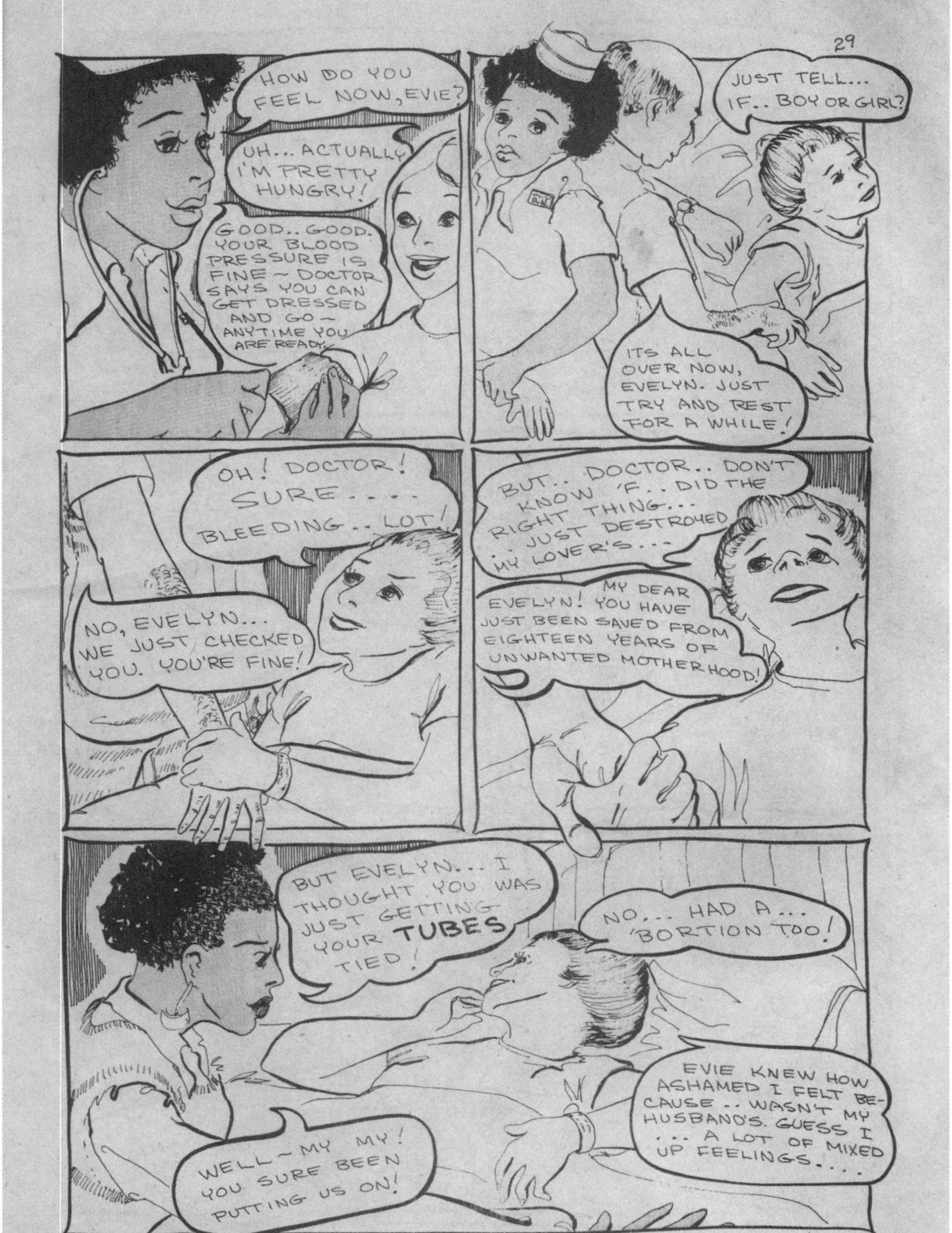
29
HOW DO YOU FEEL NOW, EVIE?
UH... ACTUALLY I'M PRETTY HUNGRY!
GOOD.. GOOD. YOUR BLOOD PRESSURE IS FINE ~ DOCTOR SAYS YOU CAN GET DRESSED AND GO ~ ANYTIME YOU ARE READY.
JUST TELL... IF.. BOY OR GIRL?
ITS ALL OVER NOW, EVELYN. JUST TRY AND REST FOR A WHILE!
OH! DOCTOR! SURE.... BLEEDING.. LOT!
NO, EVELYN... WE JUST CHECKED YOU. YOU'RE FINE!
BUT.. DOCTOR.. DON'T KNOW 'F.. DID THE RIGHT THING... ..JUST DESTROYED MY LOVER'S...
MY DEAR EVELYN! YOU HAVE JUST BEEN SAVED FROM EIGHTEEN YEARS OF UNWANTED MOTHERHOOD!
BUT EVELYN... I THOUGHT YOU WAS JUST GETTING YOUR TUBES TIED!
NO,.. HAD A... 'BORTION TOO!
WELL ~ MY MY! YOU SURE BEEN PUTTING US ON!
EVIE KNEW HOW ASHAMED I FELT BE-CAUSE .. WASN'T MY HUSBAND'S. GUESS I ... A LOT OF MIXED UP FEELINGS...

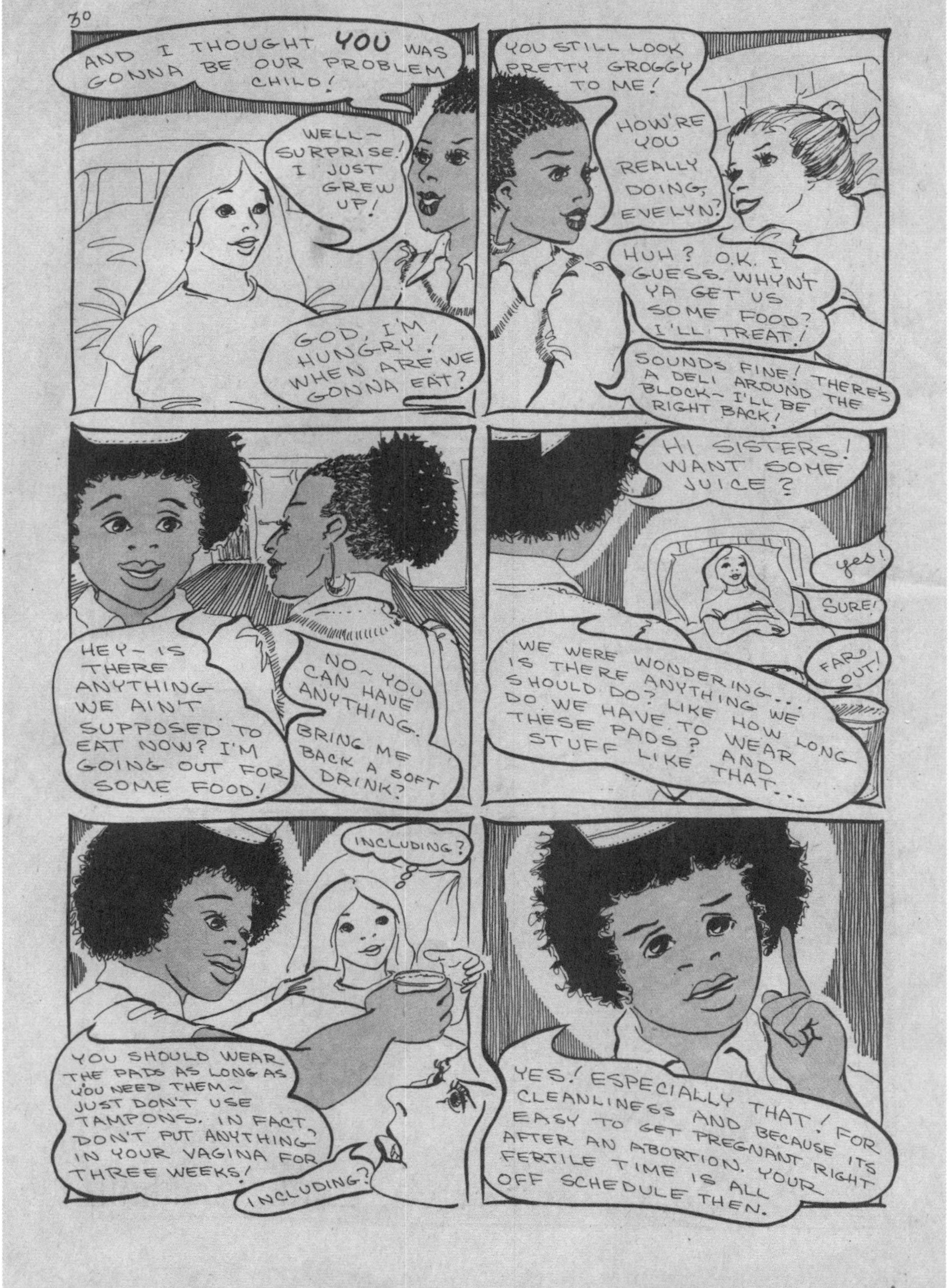
30
AND I THOUGHT YOU WAS GONNA BE OUR PROBLEM CHILD!
WELL~ SURPRISE! I JUST GREW UP!
GOD, I'M HUNGRY! WHEN ARE WE GONNA EAT?
YOU STILL LOOK PRETTY GROGGY TO ME!
HOW'RE YOU REALLY DOING, EVELYN?
HUH? O.K. I GUESS. WHYN'T YA GET US SOME FOOD? I'LL TREAT!
SOUNDS FINE! THERE'S A DELI AROUND THE BLOCK~ I'LL BE RIGHT BACK!
HEY~ IS THERE ANYTHING WE AIN'T SUPPOSED TO EAT NOW? I'M GOING OUT FOR SOME FOOD!
NO~ YOU CAN HAVE ANYTHING.
BRING ME BACK A SOFT DRINK?
HI SISTERS! WANT SOME JUICE?
yes!
SURE!
FAR OUT!
WE WERE WONDERING... IS THERE ANYTHING WE SHOULD DO? LIKE HOW LONG DO WE HAVE TO WEAR THESE PADS? AND STUFF LIKE THAT...
INCLUDING?
YOU SHOULD WEAR THE PADS AS LONG AS YOU NEED THEM~ JUST DON'T USE TAMPONS. IN FACT, DON'T PUT ANYTHING IN YOUR VAGINA FOR THREE WEEKS!
INCLUDING?
YES! ESPECIALLY THAT! FOR CLEANLINESS AND BECAUSE ITS EASY TO GET PREGNANT RIGHT AFTER AN ABORTION. YOUR FERTILE TIME IS ALL OFF SCHEDULE THEN.

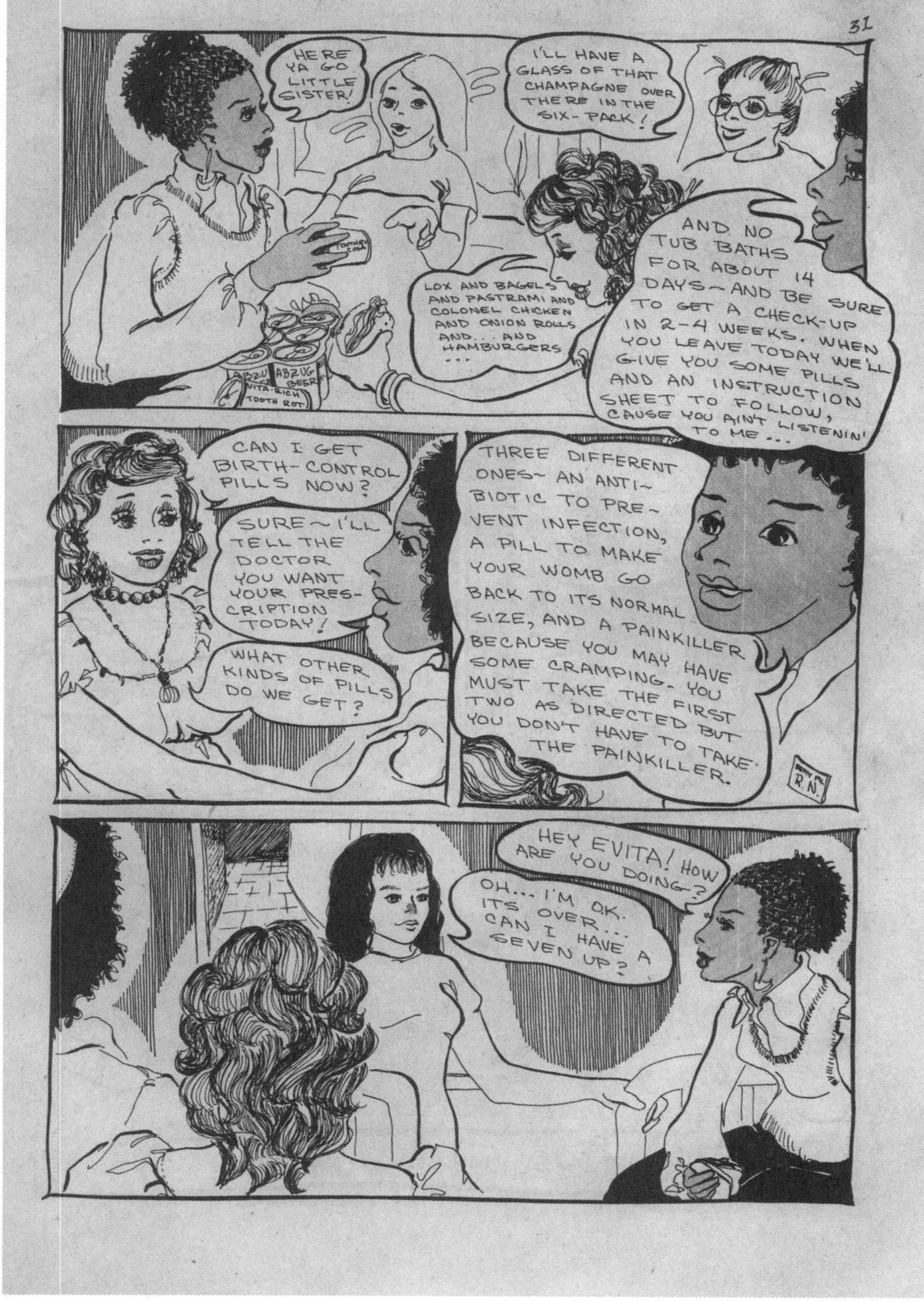
31
HERE YA GO LITTLE SISTER!
I'LL HAVE A GLASS OF THAT CHAMPAGNE OVER THERE IN THE SIX-PACK!
LOX AND BAGELS AND PASTRAMI AND COLONEL CHICKEN AND ONION ROLLS AND... AND HAMBURGERS ...
AND NO TUB BATHS FOR ABOUT 14 DAYS~ AND BE SURE TO GET A CHECK-UP IN 2-4 WEEKS. WHEN YOU LEAVE TODAY WE'LL GIVE YOU SOME PILLS AND AN INSTRUCTION SHEET TO FOLLOW, CAUSE YOU AIN'T LISTENIN' TO ME...
ABZUG BEER
VITA-RICH TOOTH ROT
CAN I GET BIRTH-CONTROL PILLS NOW?
SURE~ I'LL TELL THE DOCTOR YOU WANT YOUR PRES-CRIPTION TODAY!
WHAT OTHER KINDS OF PILLS DO WE GET?
THREE DIFFERENT ONES~ AN ANTI-BIOTIC TO PRE-VENT INFECTION, A PILL TO MAKE YOUR WOMB GO BACK TO ITS NORMAL SIZE, AND A PAINKILLER BECAUSE YOU MAY HAVE SOME CRAMPING. YOU MUST TAKE THE FIRST TWO AS DIRECTED BUT YOU DON'T HAVE TO TAKE THE PAINKILLER.
R.N.
HEY EVITA! HOW ARE YOU DOING?
OH... I'M O.K. ITS OVER... CAN I HAVE A SEVEN UP?

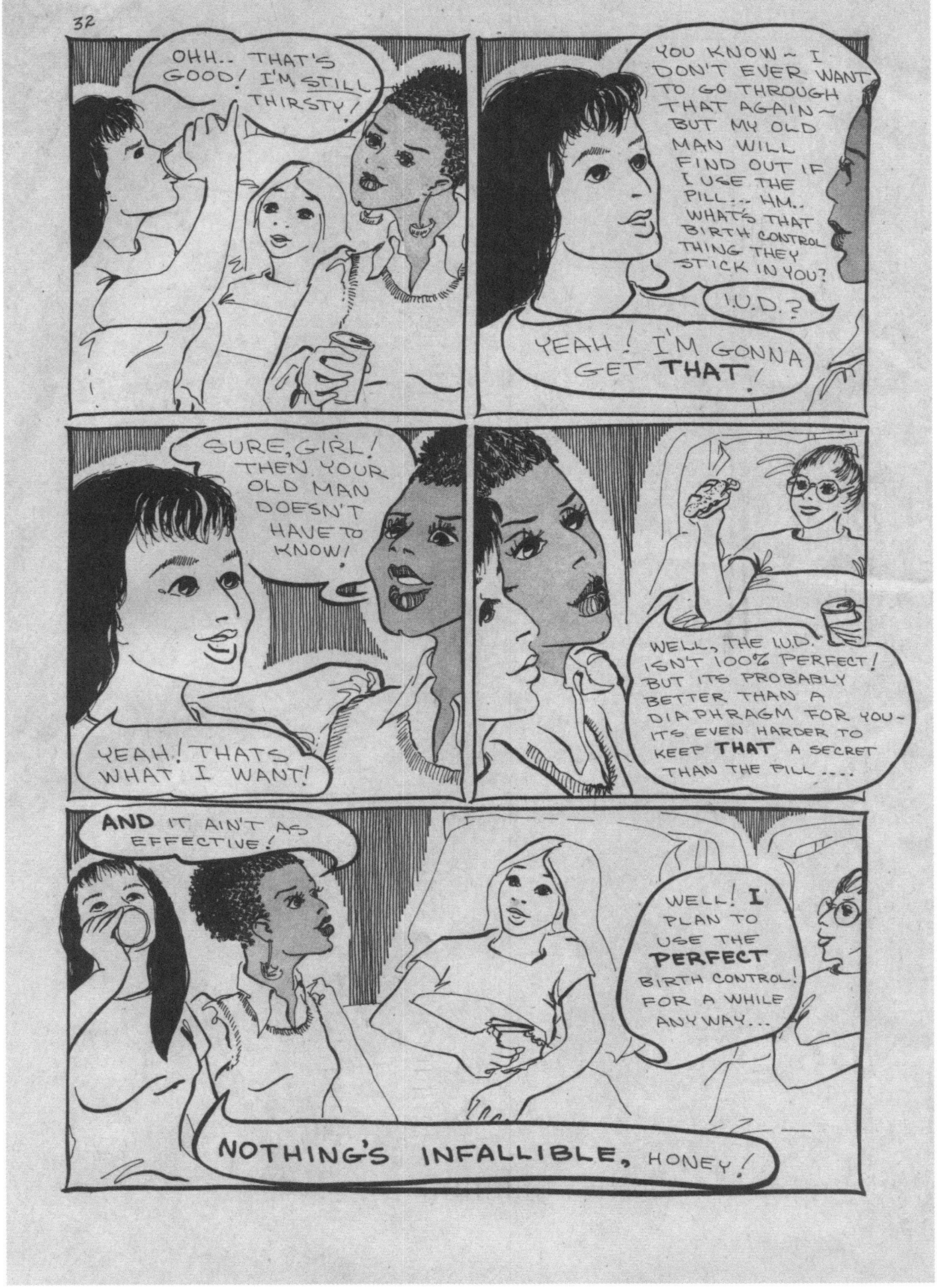
32
OHH.. THAT'S GOOD! I'M STILL THIRSTY!
YOU KNOW ~ I DON'T EVER WANT TO GO THROUGH THAT AGAIN ~ BUT MY OLD MAN WILL FIND OUT IF I USE THE PILL... HM.. WHAT'S THAT BIRTH CONTROL THING THEY STICK IN YOU?
I.U.D.?
YEAH! I'M GONNA GET THAT!
SURE, GIRL! THEN YOUR OLD MAN DOESN'T HAVE TO KNOW!
YEAH! THATS WHAT I WANT!
WELL, THE I.U.D. ISN'T 100% PERFECT! BUT ITS PROBABLY BETTER THAN A DIAPHRAGM FOR YOU- ITS EVEN HARDER TO KEEP THAT A SECRET THAN THE PILL....
AND IT AIN'T AS EFFECTIVE!
WELL! I PLAN TO USE THE PERFECT BIRTH CONTROL! FOR A WHILE ANYWAY...
NOTHING'S INFALLIBLE, HONEY!

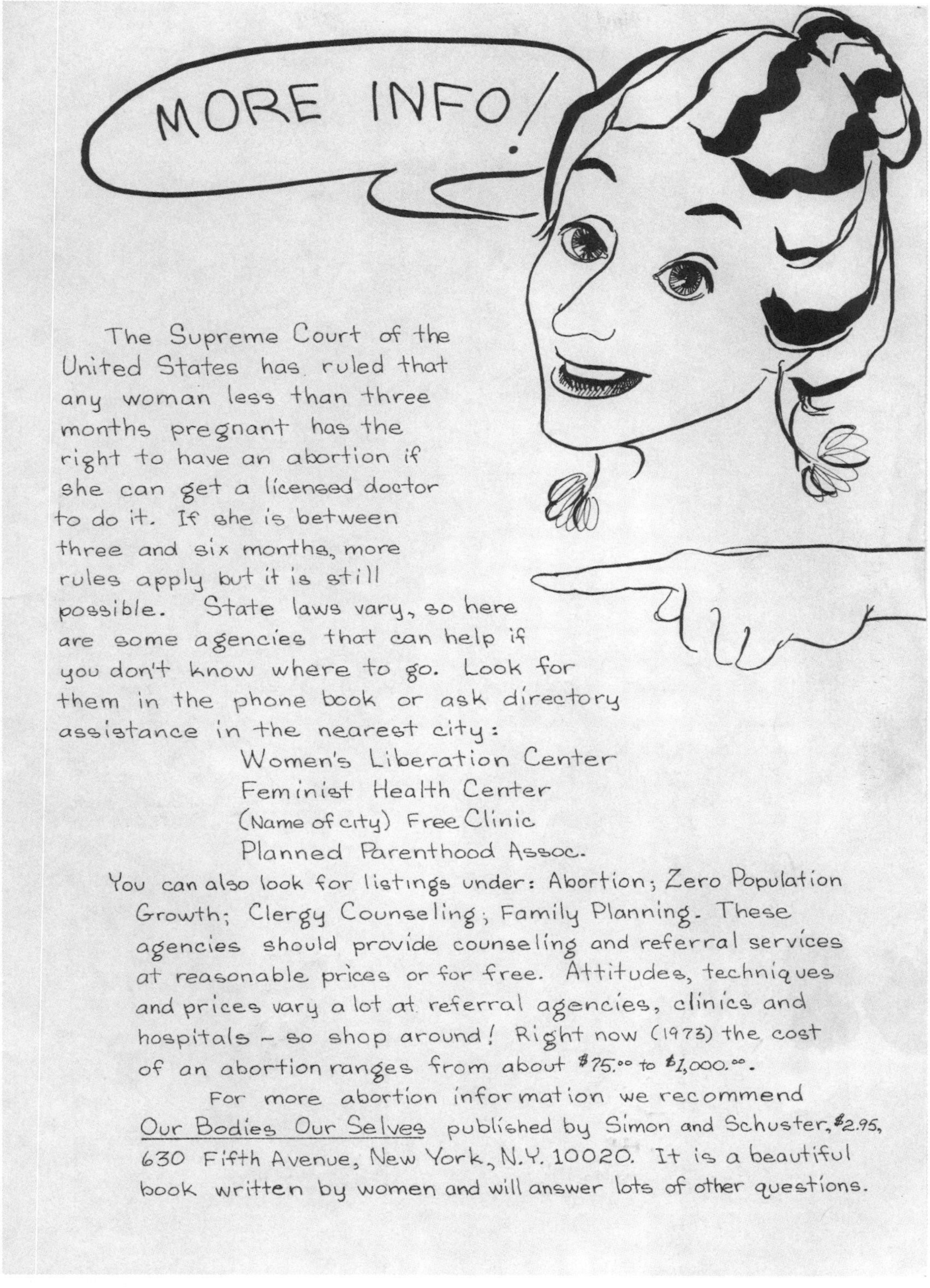
MORE INFO!
The Supreme Court of the United States has ruled that any woman less than three months pregnant has the right to have an abortion if she can get a licensed doctor to do it. If she is between three and six months, more rules apply but it is still possible. State laws vary, so here are some agencies that can help if you don't know where to go. Look for them in the phone book or ask directory assistance in the nearest city:
Women's Liberation Center
Feminist Health Center
(Name of city) Free Clinic
Planned Parenthood Assoc.
You can also look for listings under: Abortion; Zero Population Growth; Clergy Counseling; Family Planning. These agencies should provide counseling and referral services at reasonable prices or for free. Attitudes, techniques and prices vary a lot at referral agencies, clinics and hospitals - so shop around! Right now (1973) the cost of an abortion ranges from about $75.00 to $1,000.00.
For more abortion information we recommend Our Bodies Our Selves published by Simon and Schuster, $2.95, 630 Fifth Avenue, New York, N.Y. 10020. It is a beautiful book written by women and will answer lots of other questions.

EXCERPT FROM

Not Funny Ha-Ha

(2015)

Leah Hayes

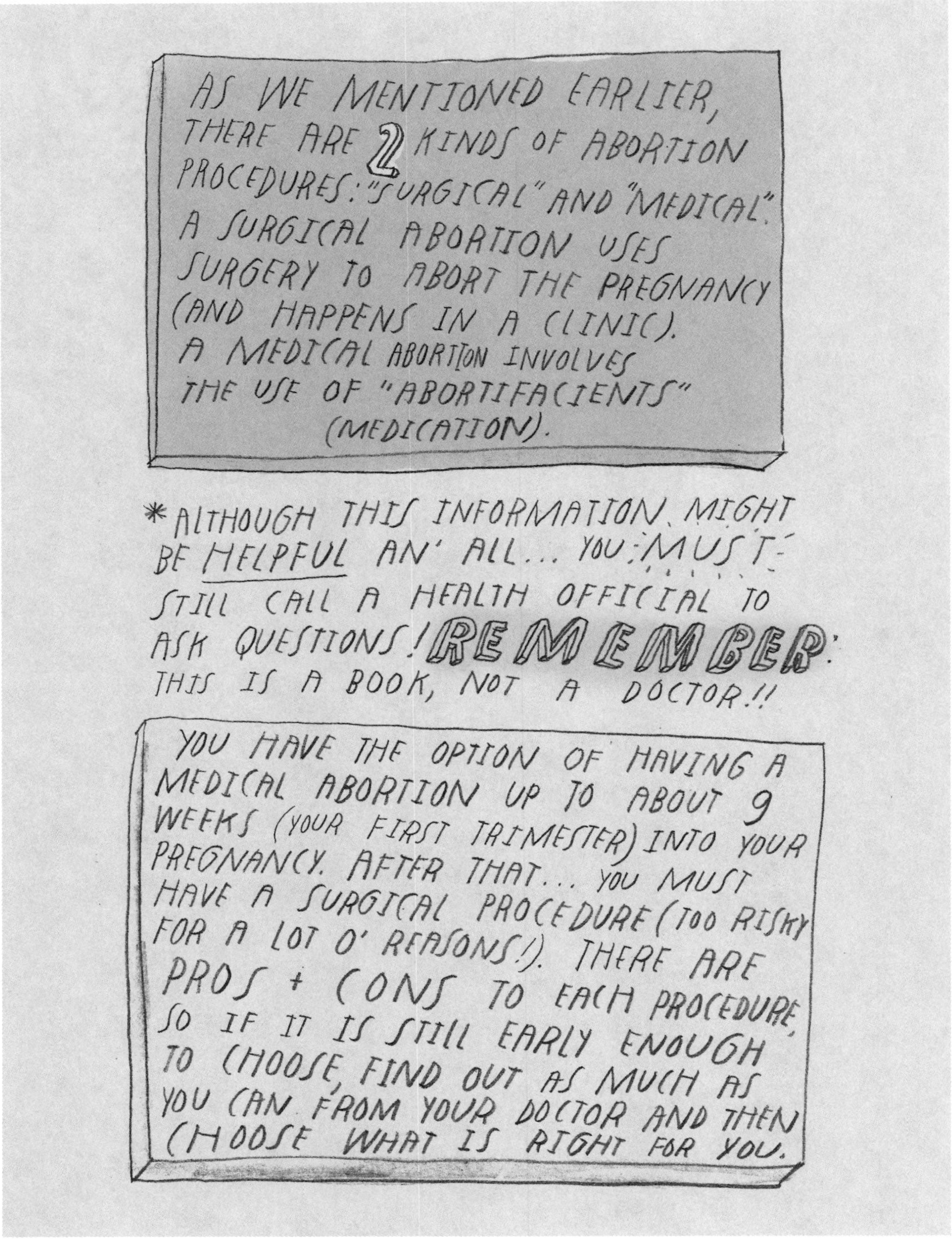

AS WE MENTIONED EARLIER, THERE ARE 2 KINDS OF ABORTION PROCEDURES: "SURGICAL" AND "MEDICAL". A SURGICAL ABORTION USES SURGERY TO ABORT THE PREGNANCY (AND HAPPENS IN A CLINIC). A MEDICAL ABORTION INVOLVES THE USE OF "ABORTIFACIENTS" (MEDICATION).

* ALTHOUGH THIS INFORMATION MIGHT BE HELPFUL AN' ALL... YOU MUST STILL CALL A HEALTH OFFICIAL TO ASK QUESTIONS! REMEMBER: THIS IS A BOOK, NOT A DOCTOR!!

YOU HAVE THE OPTION OF HAVING A MEDICAL ABORTION UP TO ABOUT 9 WEEKS (YOUR FIRST TRIMESTER) INTO YOUR PREGNANCY. AFTER THAT... YOU MUST HAVE A SURGICAL PROCEDURE (TOO RISKY FOR A LOT O' REASONS!). THERE ARE PROS + CONS TO EACH PROCEDURE, SO IF IT IS STILL EARLY ENOUGH TO CHOOSE, FIND OUT AS MUCH AS YOU CAN FROM YOUR DOCTOR AND THEN CHOOSE WHAT IS RIGHT FOR YOU.

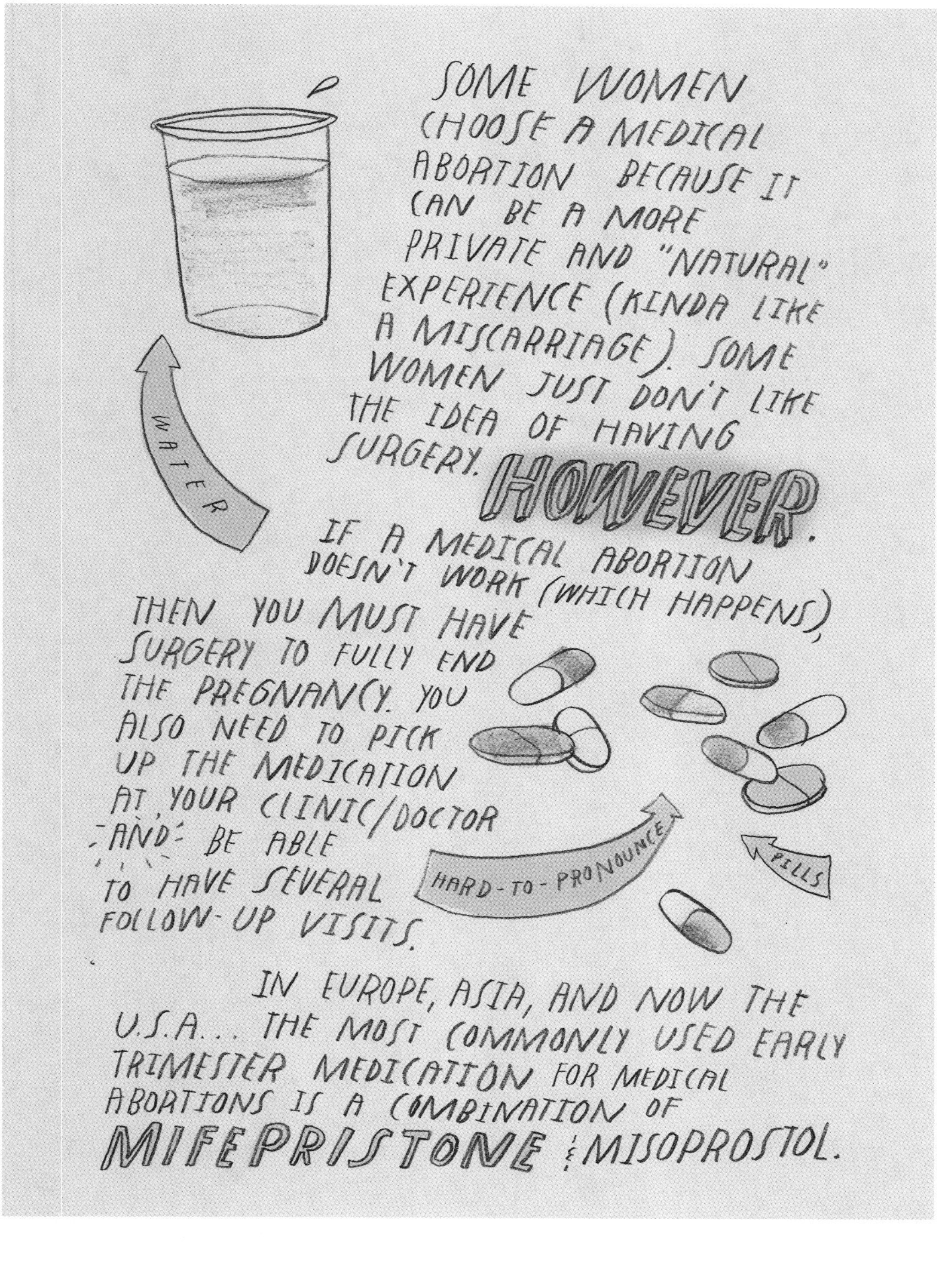
SOME WOMEN CHOOSE A MEDICAL ABORTION BECAUSE IT CAN BE A MORE PRIVATE AND "NATURAL" EXPERIENCE (KINDA LIKE A MISCARRIAGE). SOME WOMEN JUST DON'T LIKE THE IDEA OF HAVING SURGERY.
HOWEVER.
IF A MEDICAL ABORTION DOESN'T WORK (WHICH HAPPENS), THEN YOU MUST HAVE SURGERY TO FULLY END THE PREGNANCY. YOU ALSO NEED TO PICK UP THE MEDICATION AT YOUR CLINIC/DOCTOR AND BE ABLE TO HAVE SEVERAL FOLLOW-UP VISITS.
WATER
HARD-TO-PRONOUNCE
PILLS
IN EUROPE, ASIA, AND NOW THE U.S.A... THE MOST COMMONLY USED EARLY TRIMESTER MEDICATION FOR MEDICAL ABORTIONS IS A COMBINATION OF MIFEPRISTONE & MISOPROSTOL.

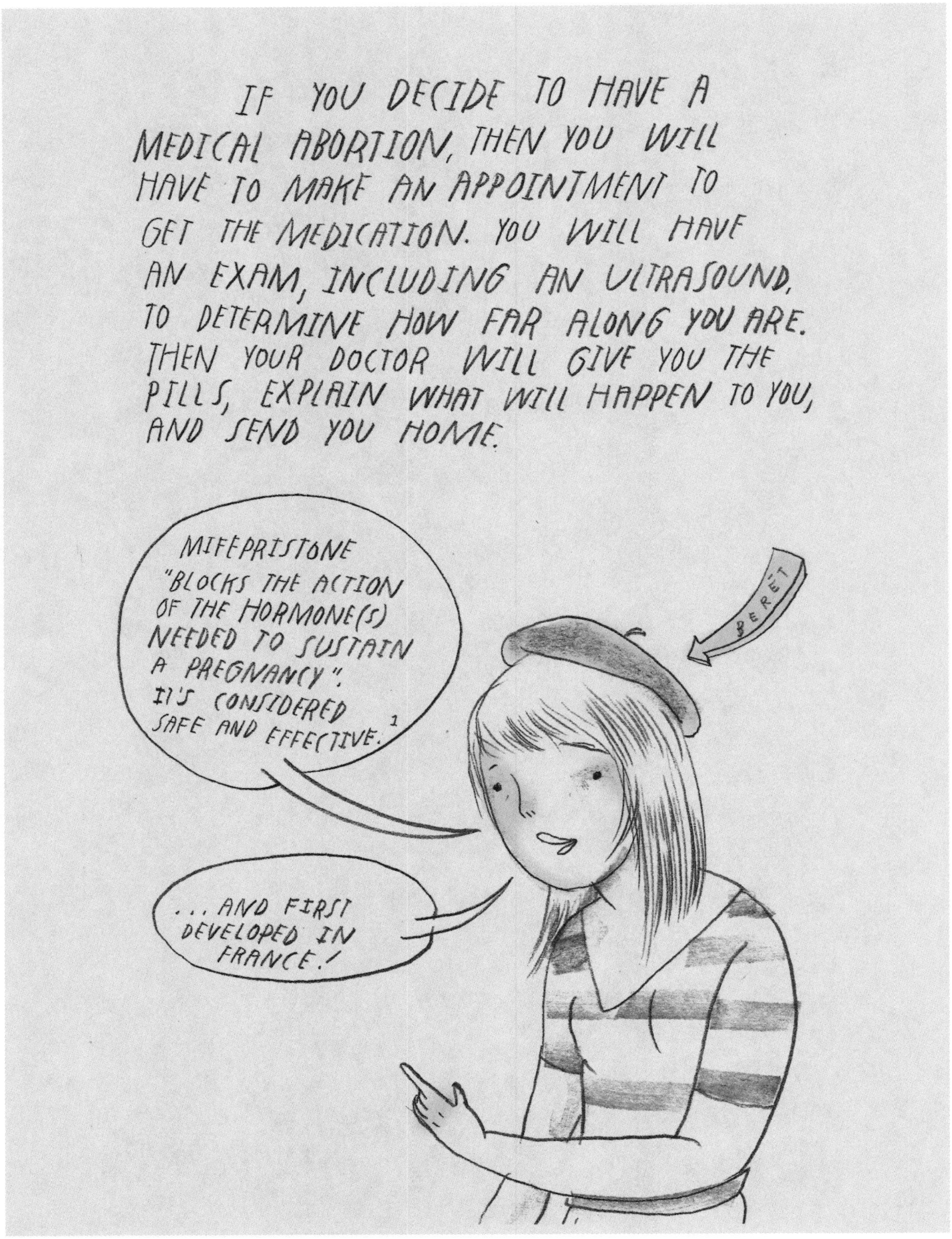
IF YOU DECIDE TO HAVE A MEDICAL ABORTION, THEN YOU WILL HAVE TO MAKE AN APPOINTMENT TO GET THE MEDICATION. YOU WILL HAVE AN EXAM, INCLUDING AN ULTRASOUND, TO DETERMINE HOW FAR ALONG YOU ARE. THEN YOUR DOCTOR WILL GIVE YOU THE PILLS, EXPLAIN WHAT WILL HAPPEN TO YOU, AND SEND YOU HOME.
MIFEPRISTONE "BLOCKS THE ACTION OF THE HORMONE(S) NEEDED TO SUSTAIN A PREGNANCY". IT'S CONSIDERED SAFE AND EFFECTIVE.[1]
BERET
...AND FIRST DEVELOPED IN FRANCE!

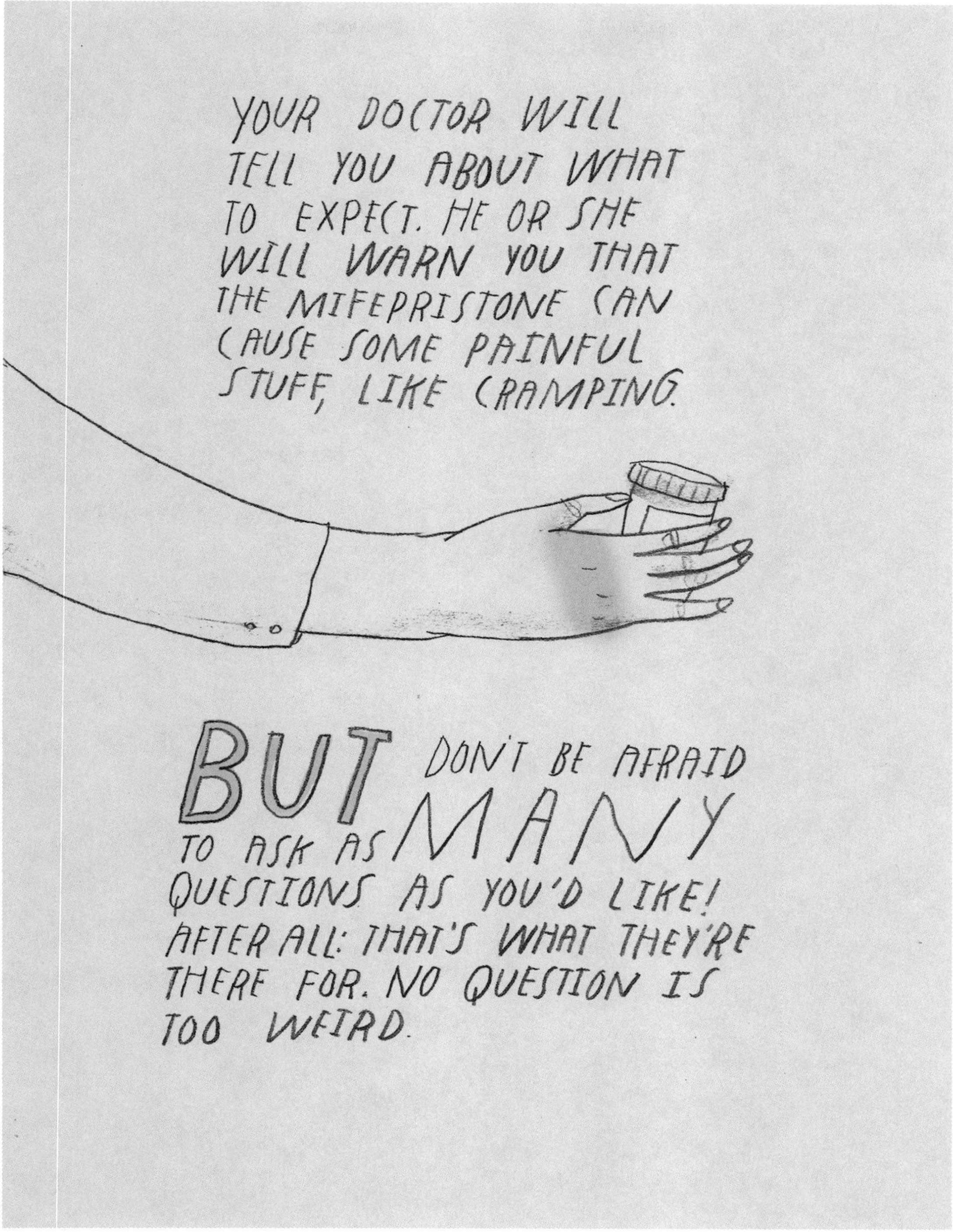

YOUR DOCTOR WILL
TELL YOU ABOUT WHAT
TO EXPECT. HE OR SHE
WILL WARN YOU THAT
THE MIFEPRISTONE CAN
CAUSE SOME PAINFUL
STUFF, LIKE CRAMPING.

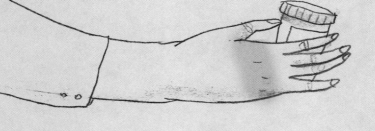

BUT DON'T BE AFRAID
TO ASK AS MANY
QUESTIONS AS YOU'D LIKE!
AFTER ALL: THAT'S WHAT THEY'RE
THERE FOR. NO QUESTION IS
TOO WEIRD.

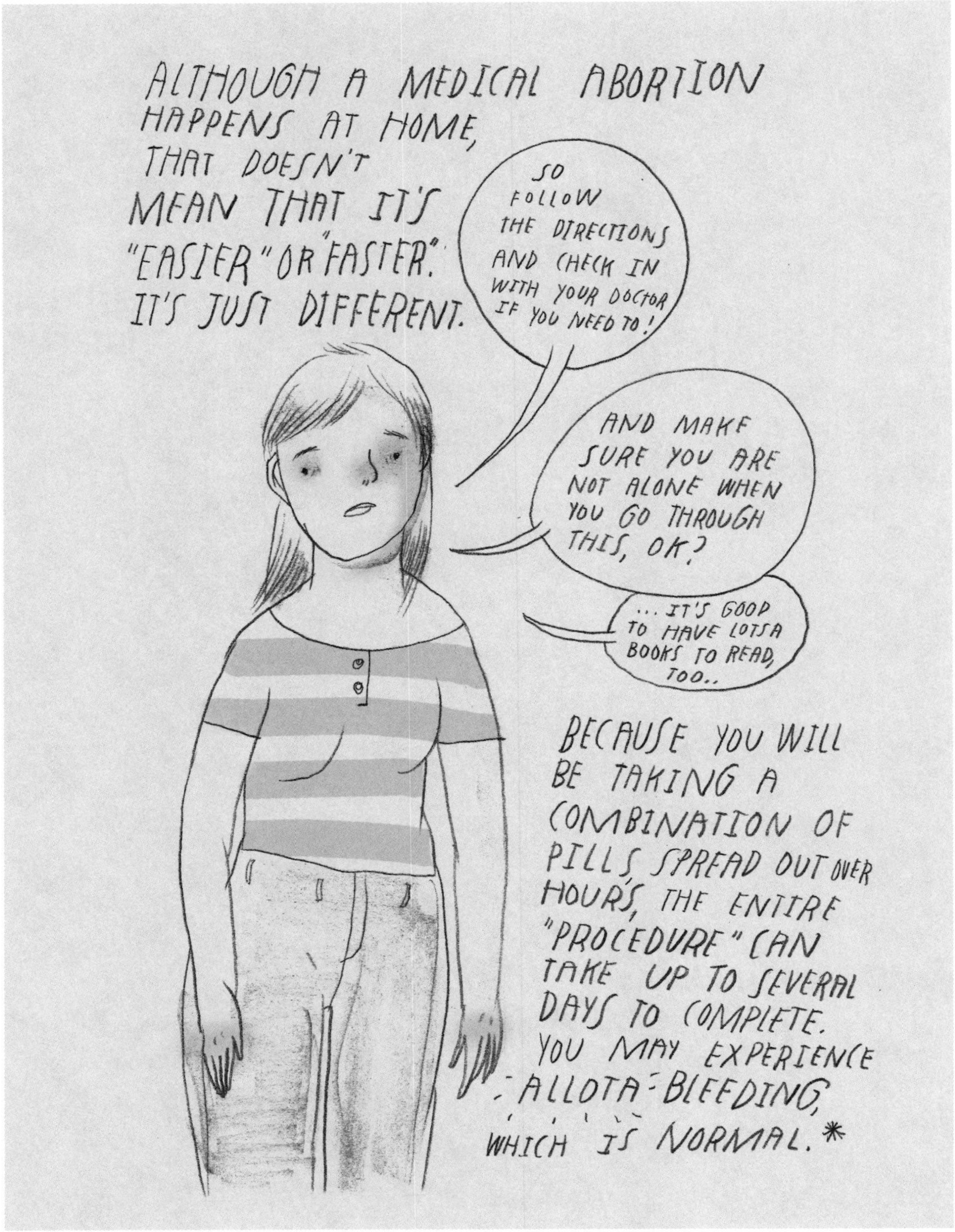
ALTHOUGH A MEDICAL ABORTION HAPPENS AT HOME, THAT DOESN'T MEAN THAT IT'S "EASIER" OR "FASTER". IT'S JUST DIFFERENT.
SO FOLLOW THE DIRECTIONS AND CHECK IN WITH YOUR DOCTOR IF YOU NEED TO!
AND MAKE SURE YOU ARE NOT ALONE WHEN YOU GO THROUGH THIS, OK?
... IT'S GOOD TO HAVE LOTSA BOOKS TO READ, TOO..
BECAUSE YOU WILL BE TAKING A COMBINATION OF PILLS SPREAD OUT OVER HOURS, THE ENTIRE "PROCEDURE" CAN TAKE UP TO SEVERAL DAYS TO COMPLETE. YOU MAY EXPERIENCE ALLOTA BLEEDING, WHICH IS NORMAL.*

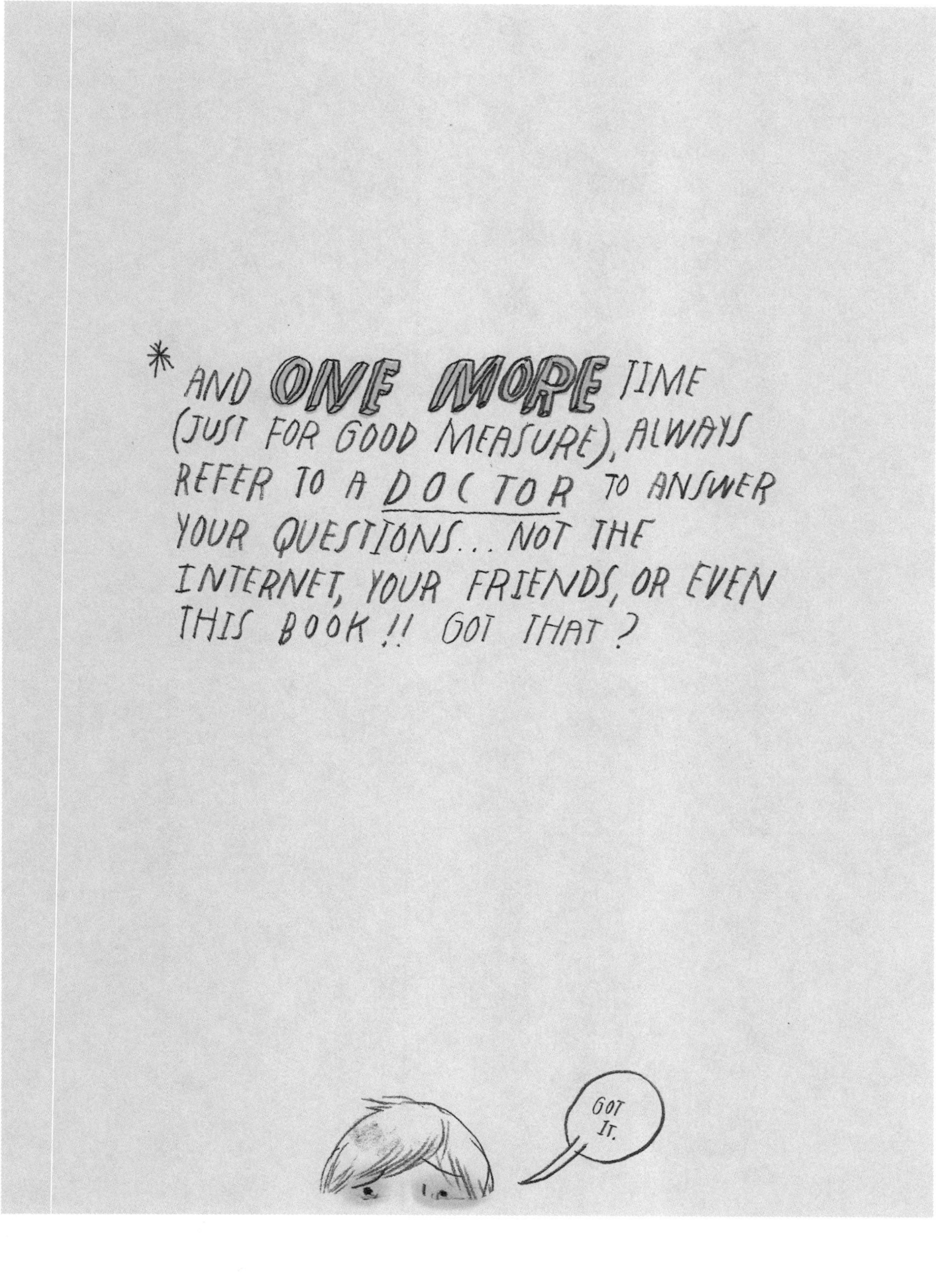
* AND ONE MORE TIME (JUST FOR GOOD MEASURE), ALWAYS REFER TO A DOCTOR TO ANSWER YOUR QUESTIONS... NOT THE INTERNET, YOUR FRIENDS, OR EVEN THIS BOOK!! GOT THAT?
GOT IT.

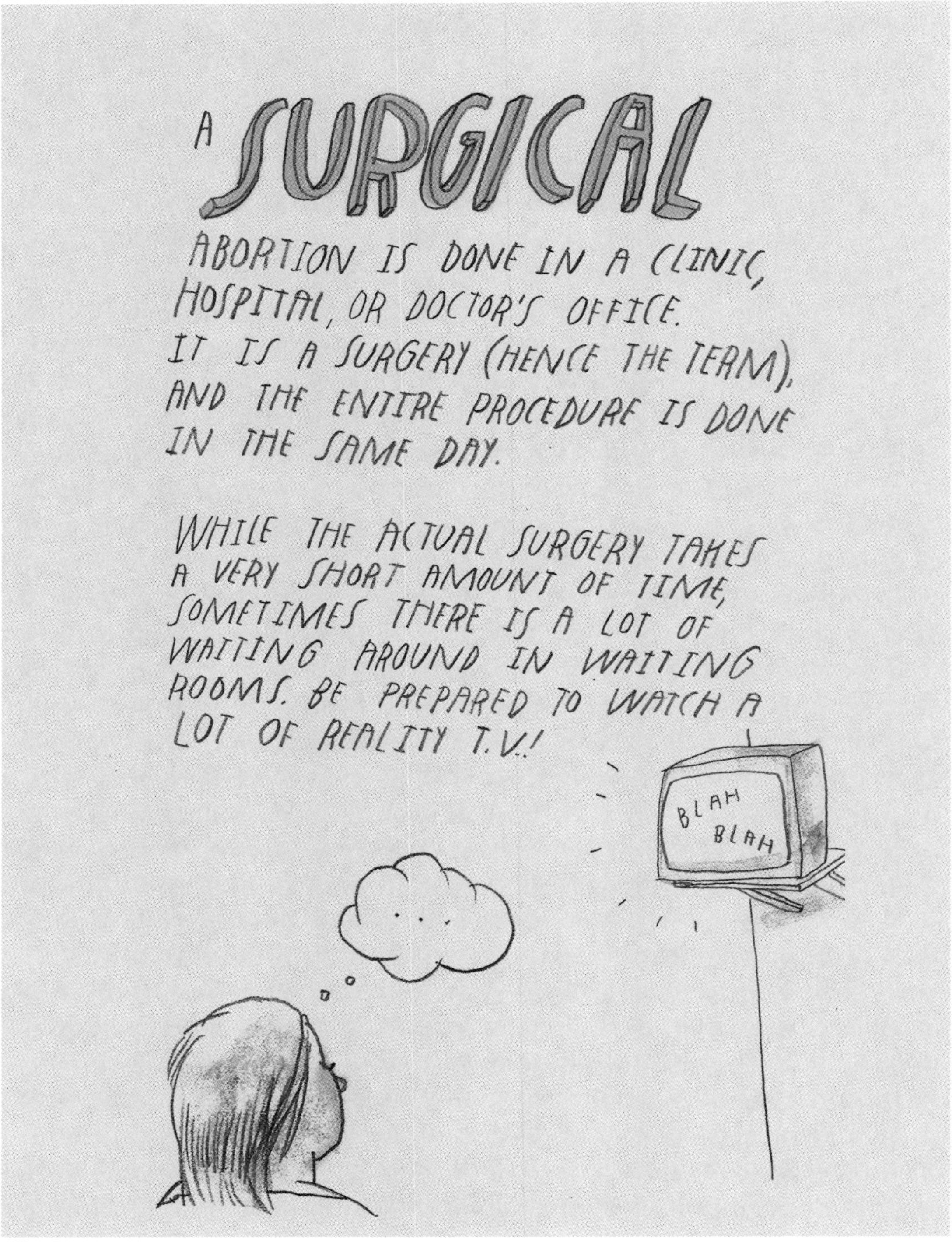
A SURGICAL
ABORTION IS DONE IN A CLINIC, HOSPITAL, OR DOCTOR'S OFFICE. IT IS A SURGERY (HENCE THE TERM), AND THE ENTIRE PROCEDURE IS DONE IN THE SAME DAY.
WHILE THE ACTUAL SURGERY TAKES A VERY SHORT AMOUNT OF TIME, SOMETIMES THERE IS A LOT OF WAITING AROUND IN WAITING ROOMS. BE PREPARED TO WATCH A LOT OF REALITY T.V.!
BLAH BLAH
. . .

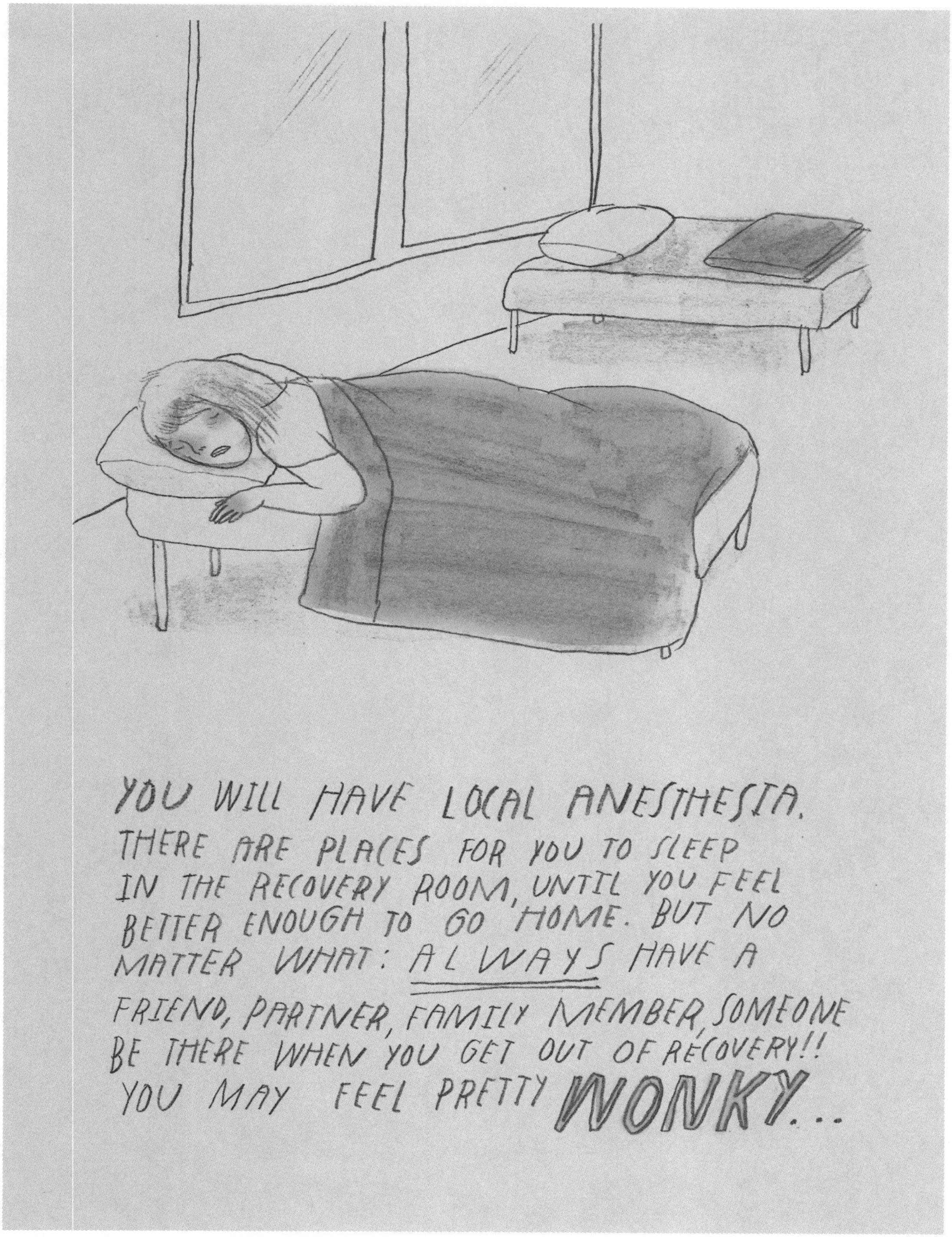
YOU WILL HAVE LOCAL ANESTHESIA.
THERE ARE PLACES FOR YOU TO SLEEP
IN THE RECOVERY ROOM, UNTIL YOU FEEL
BETTER ENOUGH TO GO HOME. BUT NO
MATTER WHAT: ALWAYS HAVE A
FRIEND, PARTNER, FAMILY MEMBER, SOMEONE
BE THERE WHEN YOU GET OUT OF RECOVERY!!
YOU MAY FEEL PRETTY WONKY...

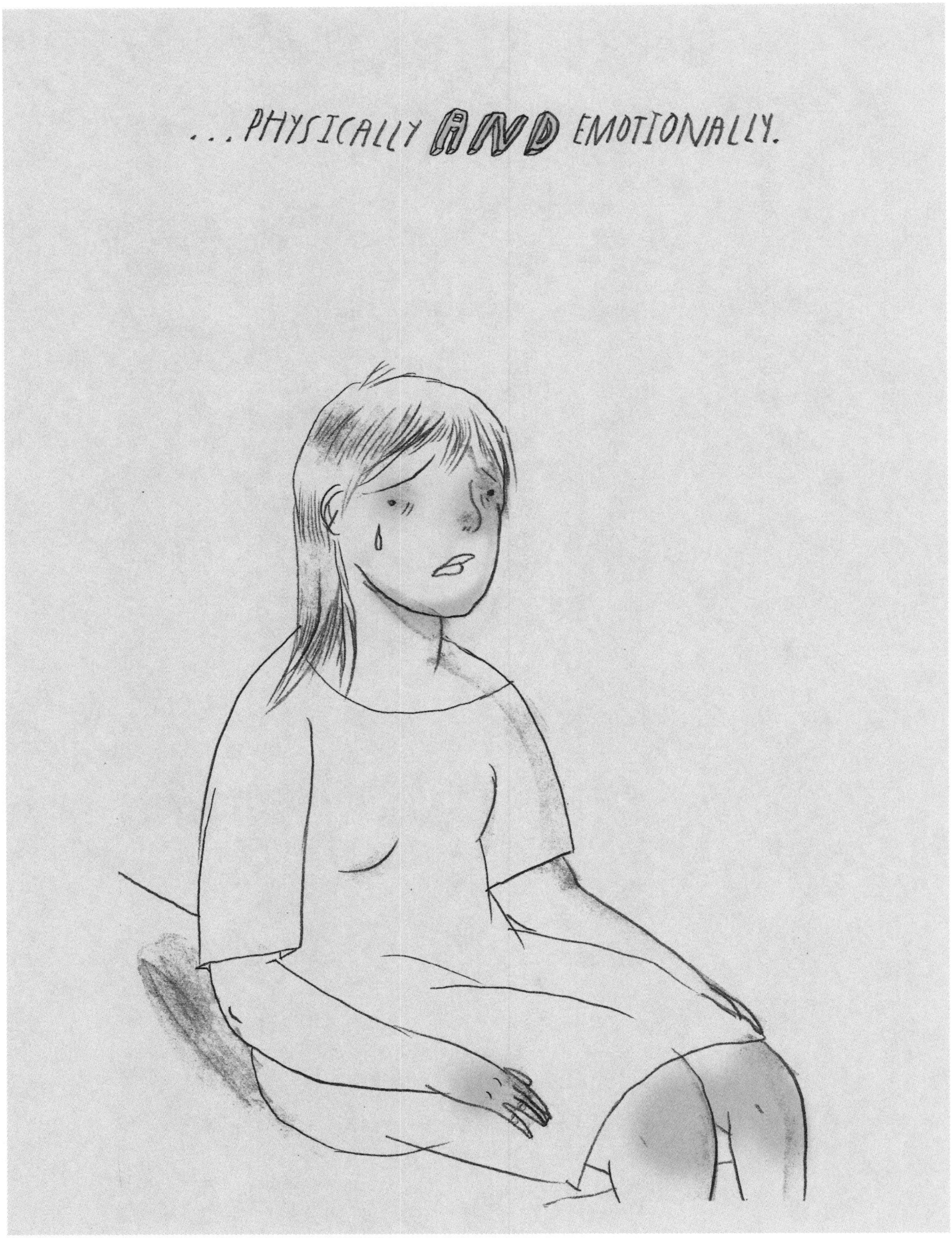
...PHYSICALLY AND EMOTIONALLY.

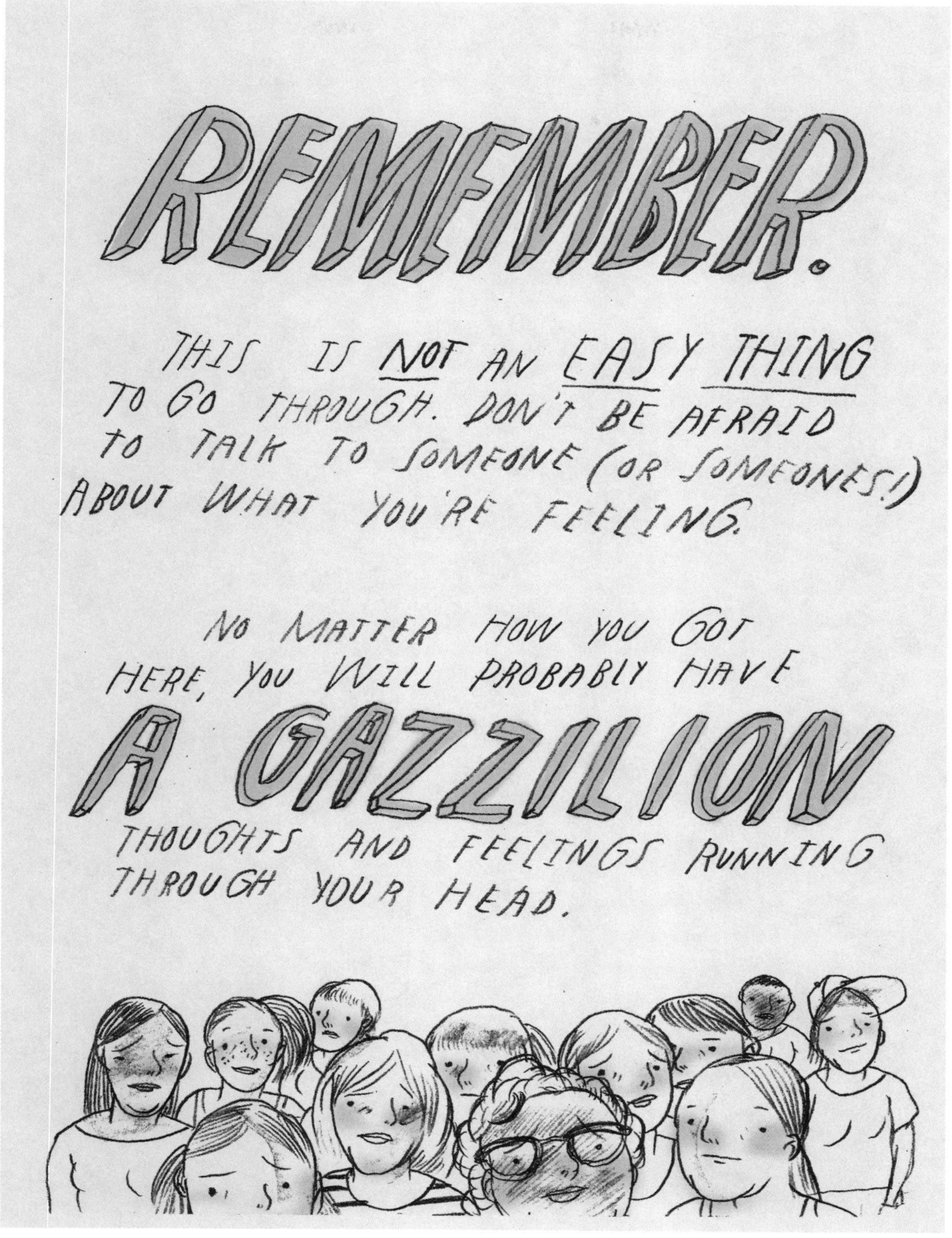
REMEMBER.
THIS IS NOT AN EASY THING TO GO THROUGH. DON'T BE AFRAID TO TALK TO SOMEONE (OR SOMEONES!) ABOUT WHAT YOU'RE FEELING.
NO MATTER HOW YOU GOT HERE, YOU WILL PROBABLY HAVE
A GAZZILION
THOUGHTS AND FEELINGS RUNNING THROUGH YOUR HEAD.

EXCERPTS FROM

Spooky Womb

(2012)

AND

X Utero

(2013)

Paula Knight

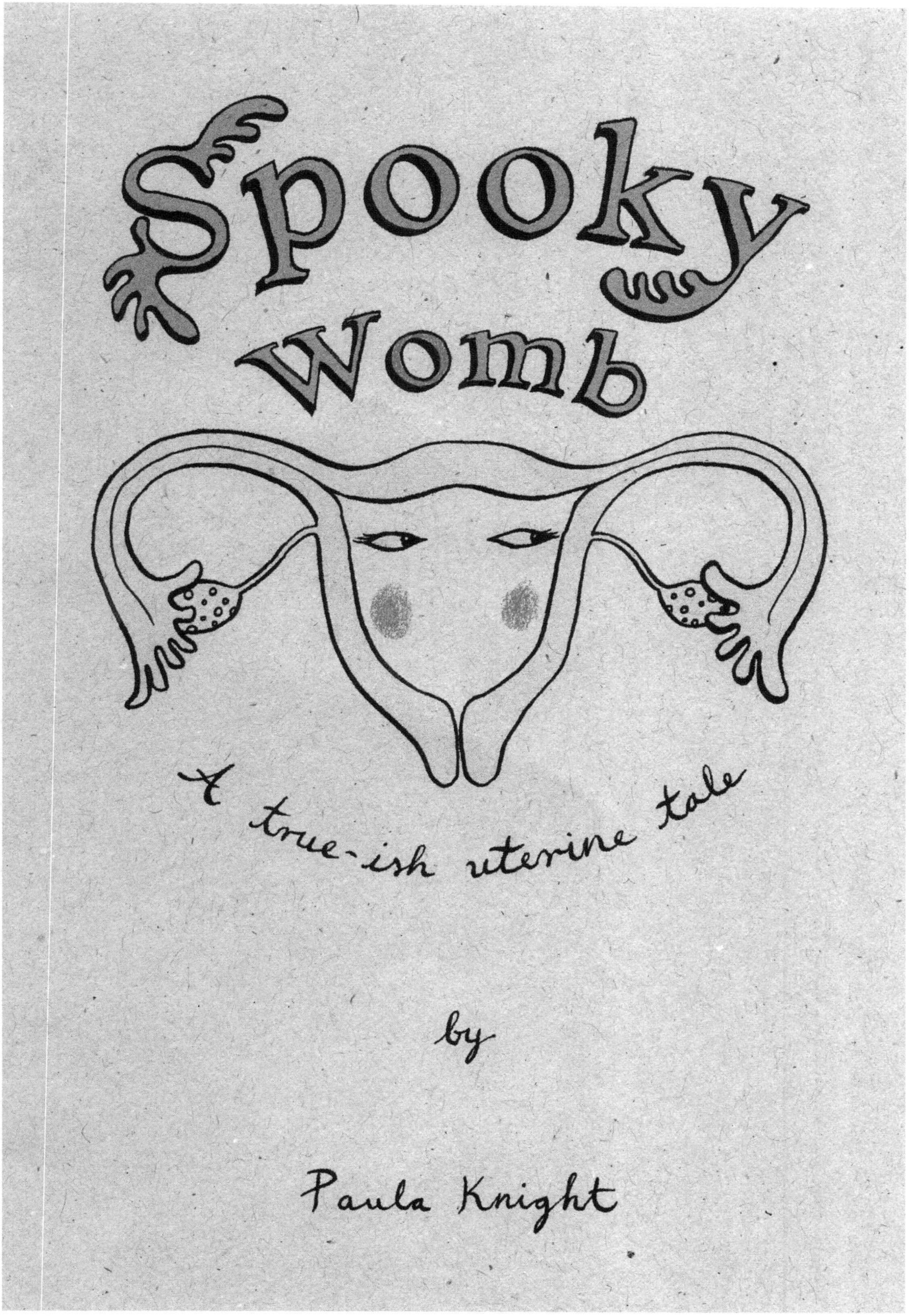
Spooky
Womb
A true-ish uterine tale
by
Paula Knight

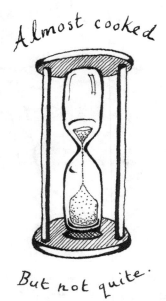

Almost cooked

But not quite.

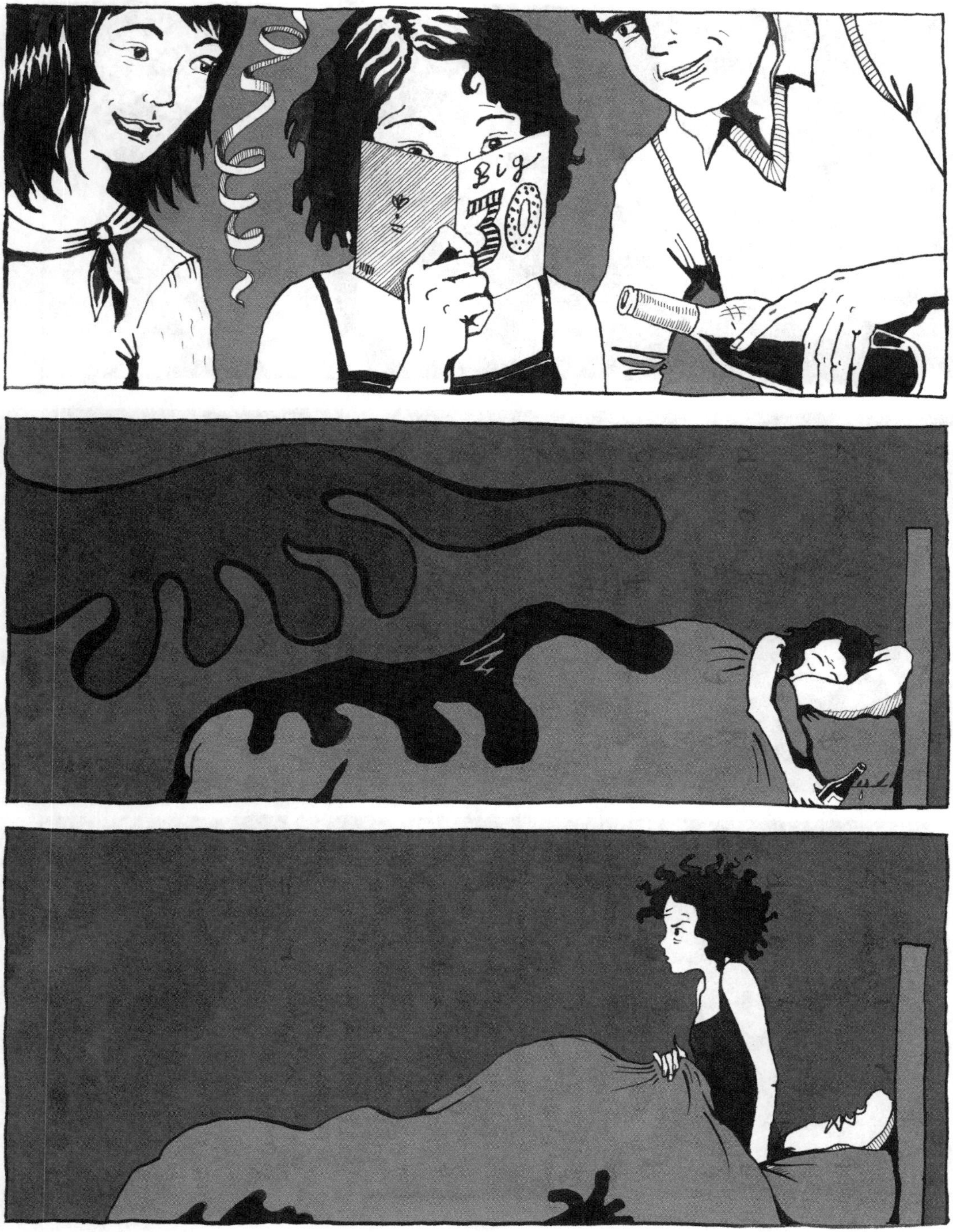
Big 30

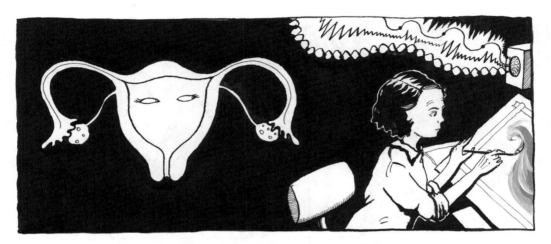

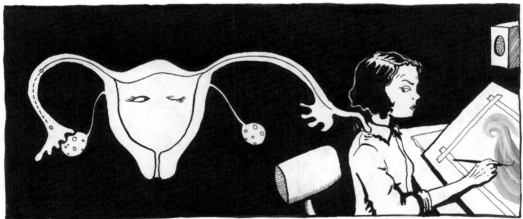

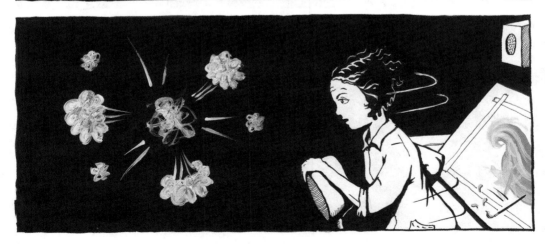

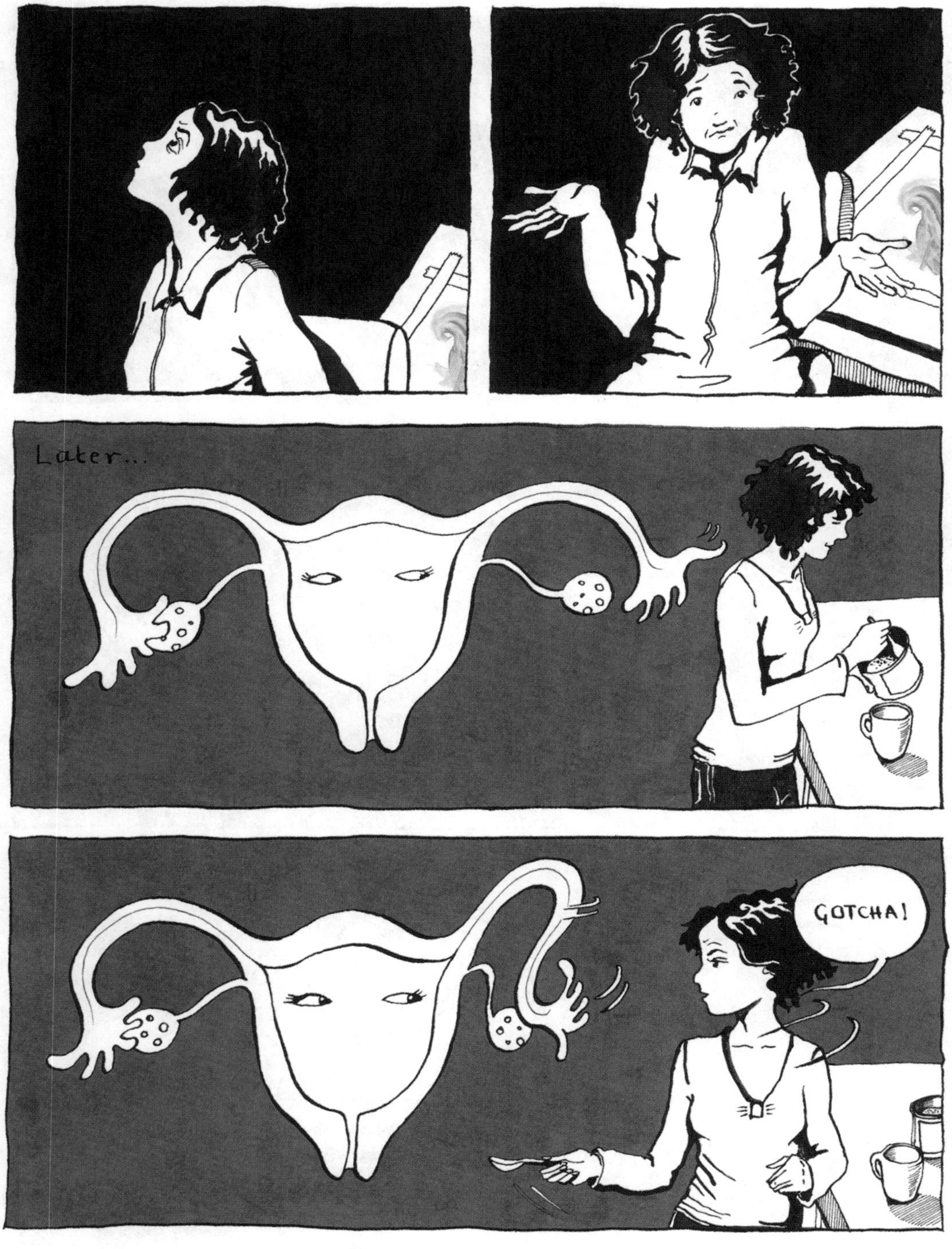
Later...
GOTCHA!

What do you want?
Creeping up on me like that!
Huh?
Oh! I get it!
Well, it's not just up to me you know!

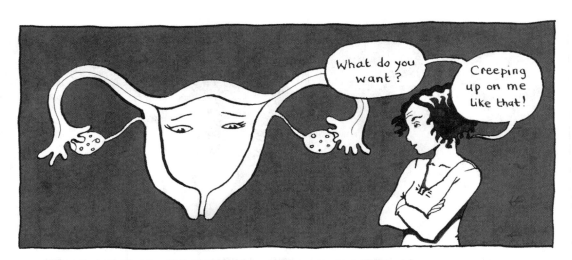

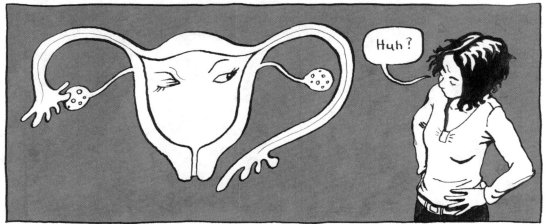

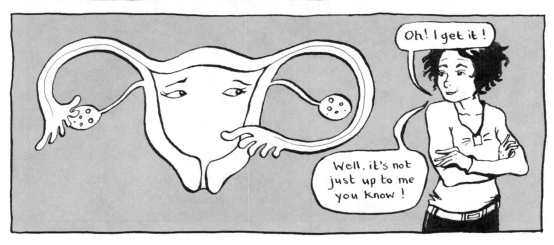

A couple of years later.
OK OK!
I'll see what I can do.
But you've got to stop being such a pest!

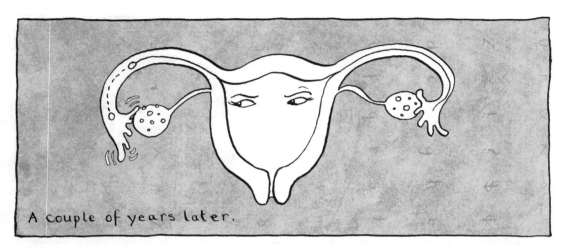

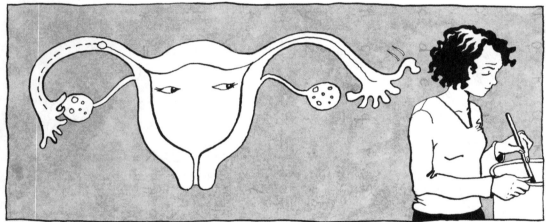

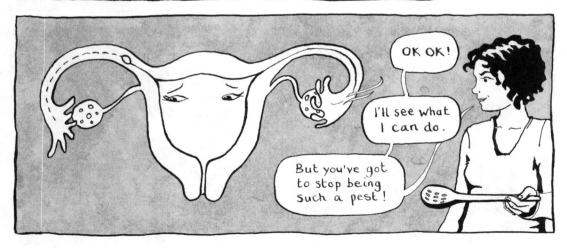

Wait for me!
You're going the wrong way.
Me first!
No! ME first!

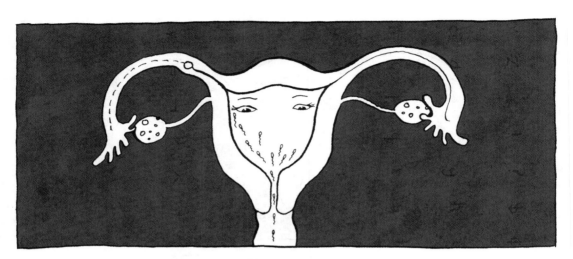

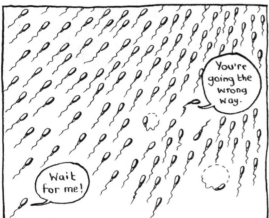

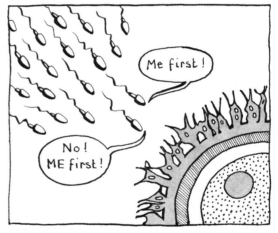

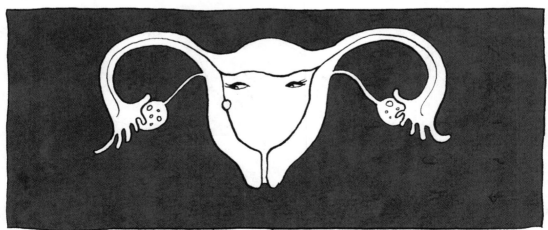

Oh wow!
I was wondering
Nice work!

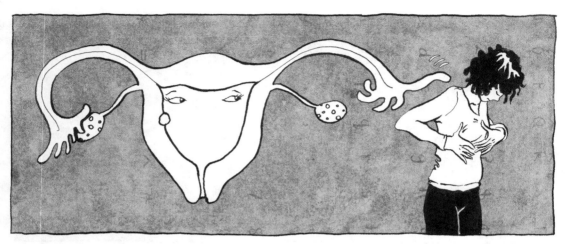

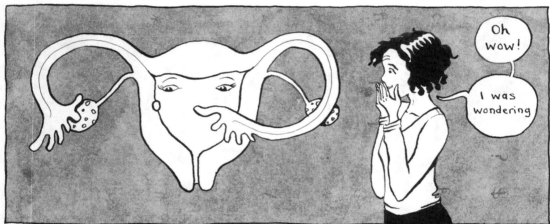

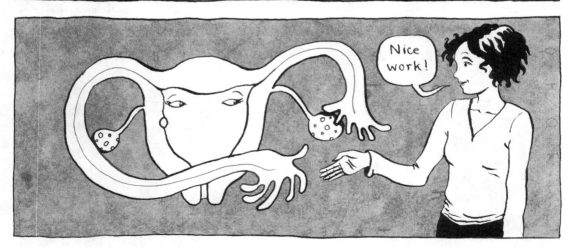

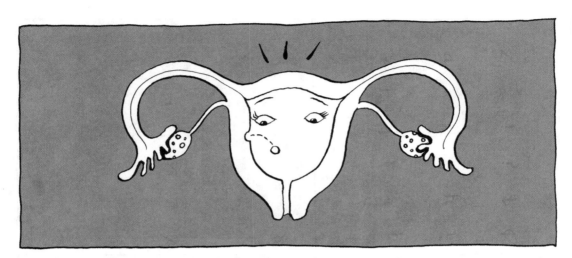

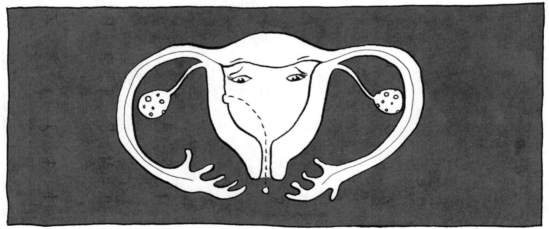

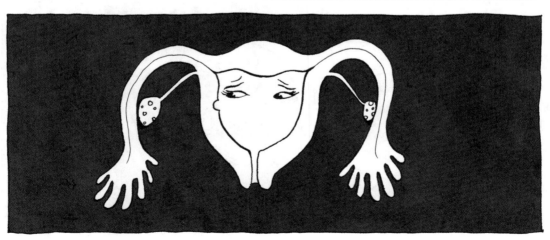

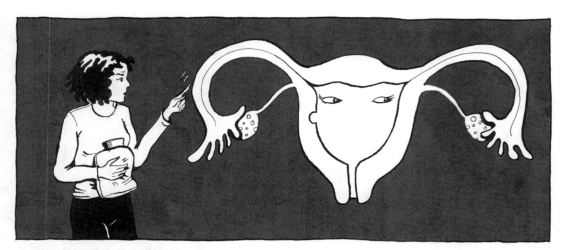

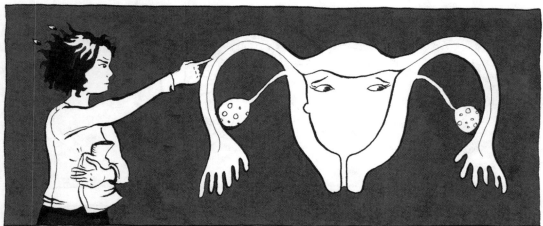

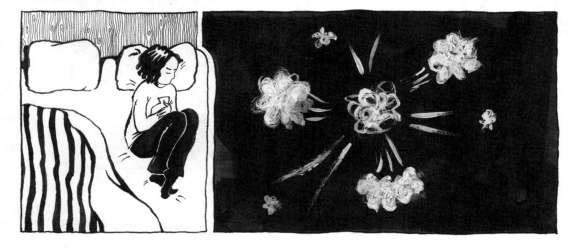

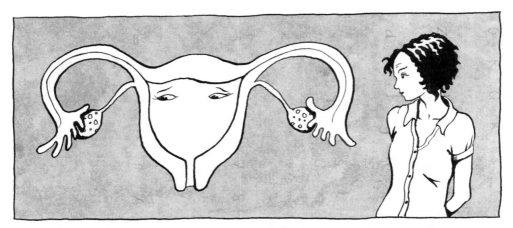

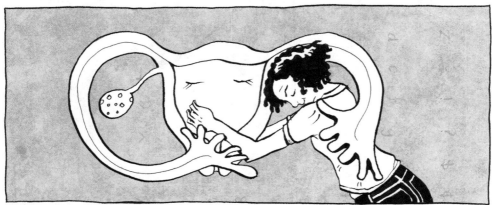

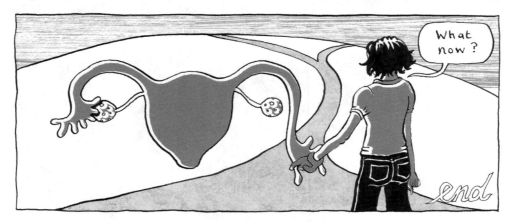

The answer to 'What now?' will become evident in my longer work, The Facts of Life.

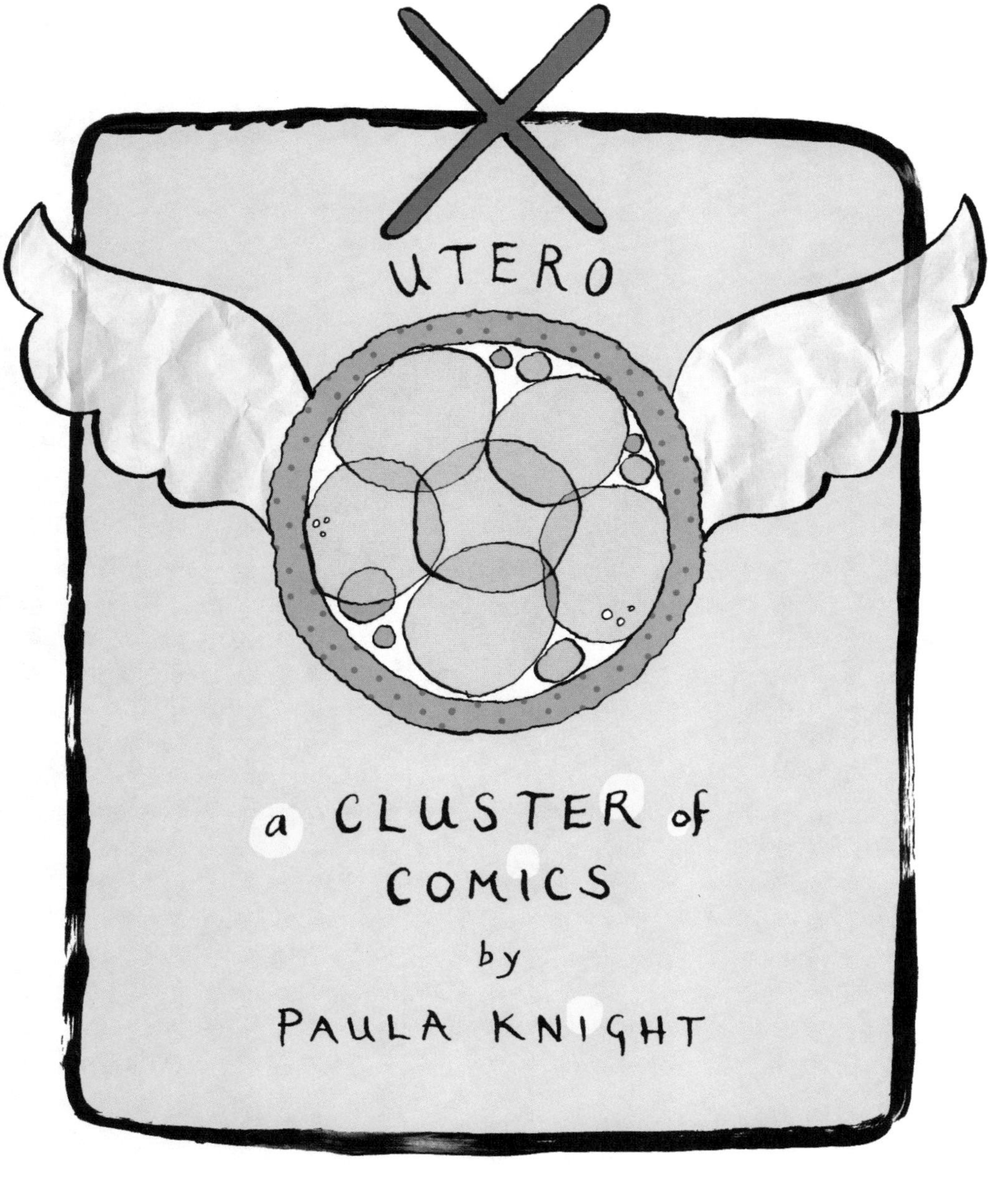
X
UTERO
a CLUSTER of
COMICS
by
PAULA KNIGHT

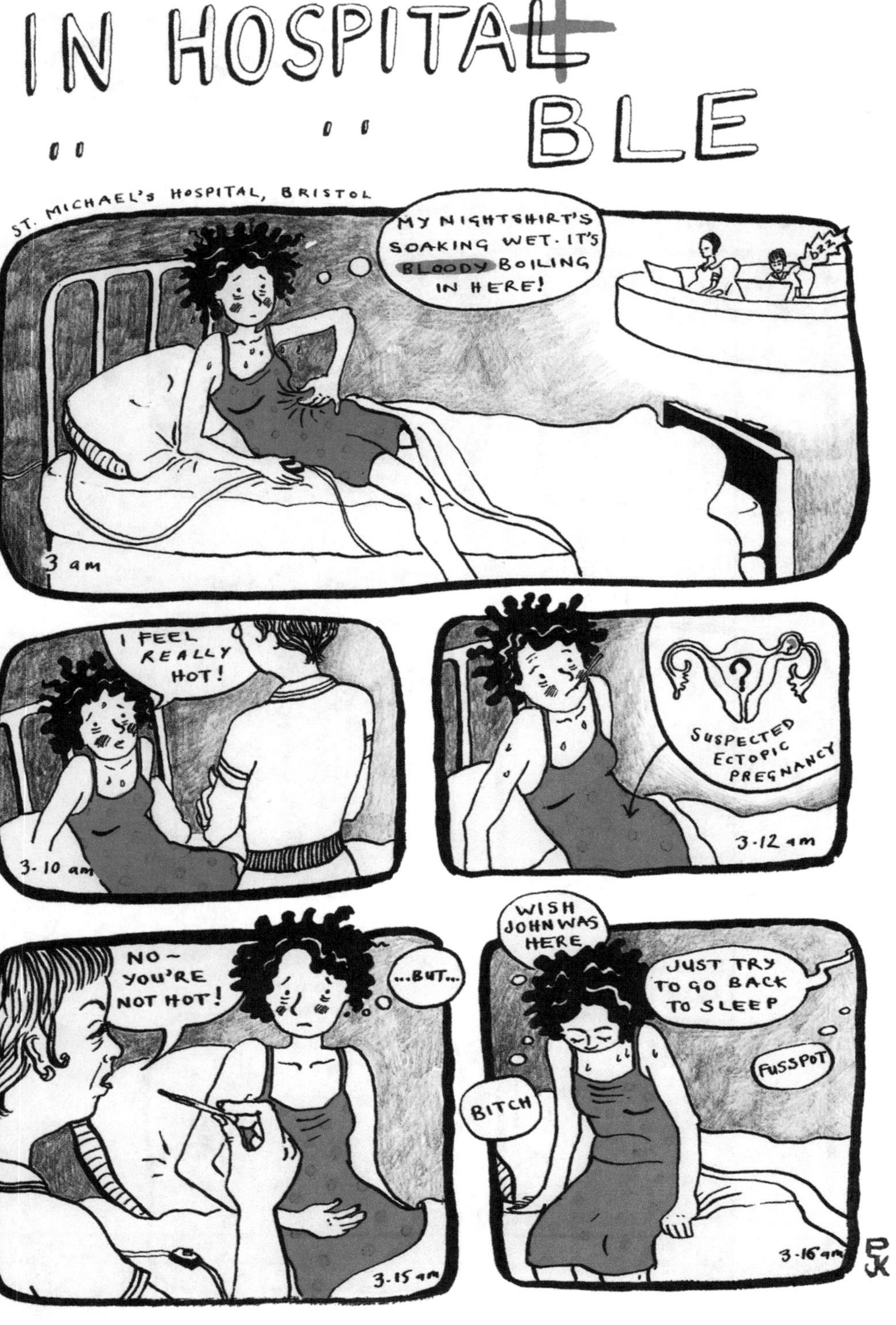
IN HOSPITAL
BLE
ST. MICHAEL'S HOSPITAL, BRISTOL
MY NIGHTSHIRT'S SOAKING WET. IT'S BLOODY BOILING IN HERE!
bzz
3 am
I FEEL REALLY HOT!
3-10 am
SUSPECTED ECTOPIC PREGNANCY
3-12 am
NO ~ YOU'RE NOT HOT!
...BUT...
3-15 am
WISH JOHN WAS HERE
JUST TRY TO GO BACK TO SLEEP
FUSSPOT
BITCH
3-16 am
PJK

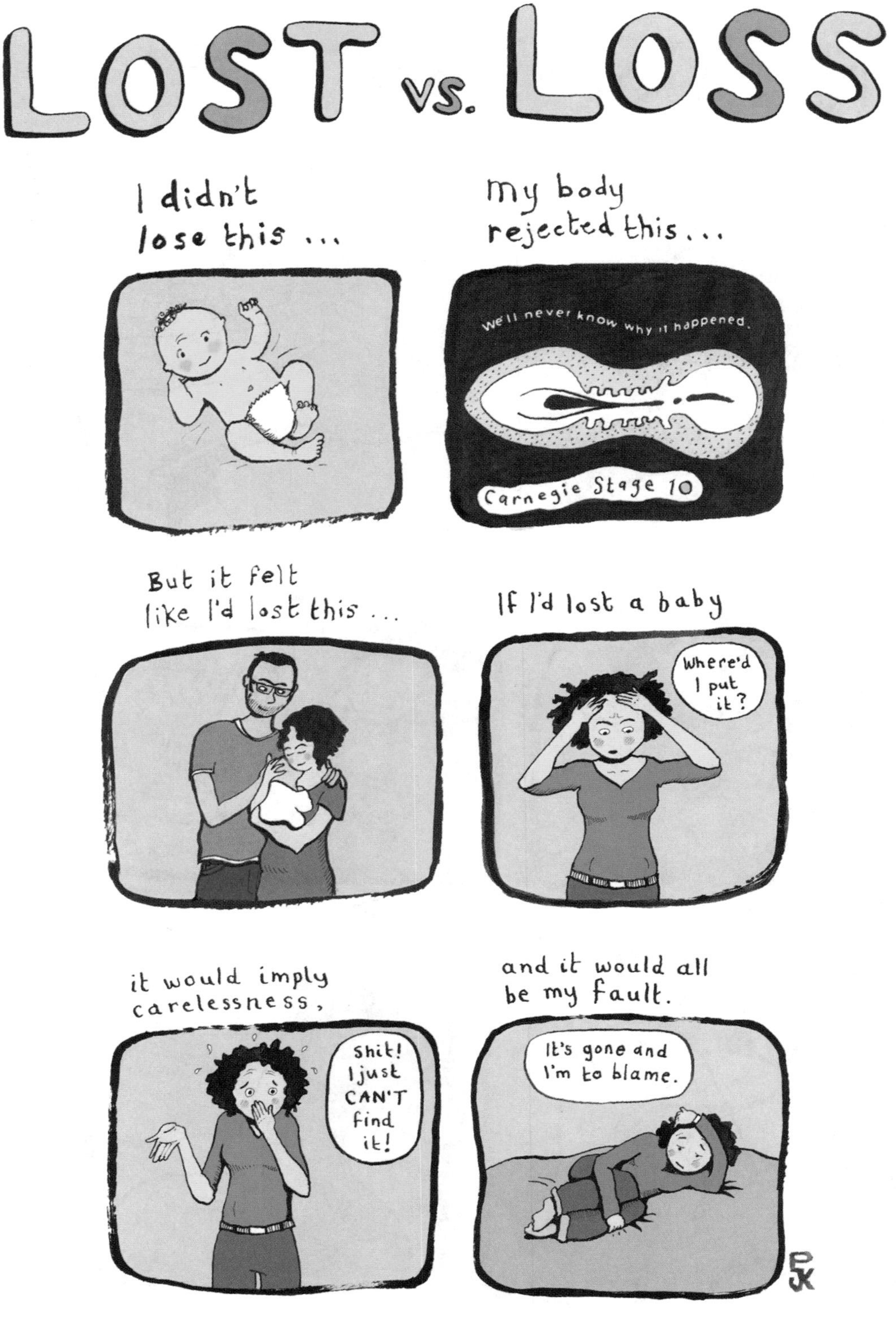
LOST vs. LOSS
I didn't lose this ...
My body rejected this ...
We'll never know why it happened.
Carnegie Stage 10
But it felt like I'd lost this ...
If I'd lost a baby
Where'd I put it?
it would imply carelessness,
Shit! I just CAN'T find it!
and it would all be my fault.
It's gone and I'm to blame.
PJK

"IT WASN'T MEANT TO BE"

I beg to differ!
DAY 14
We did this on purpose
UNPROTECTED because we meant it.
The sperm was quite intent on its path
and that particular sperm REALLY did mean it.
But it just went wrong,
as bodies are prone to do.

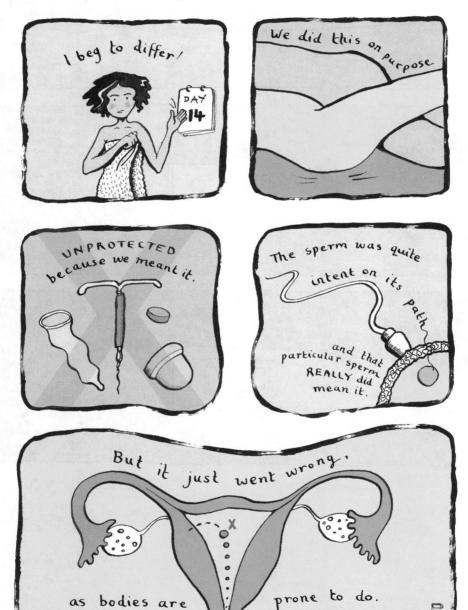

Once a
hCG FRI 140
collection
SUN 313
of lines,
THURS 400

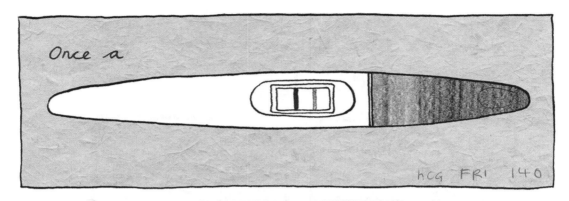

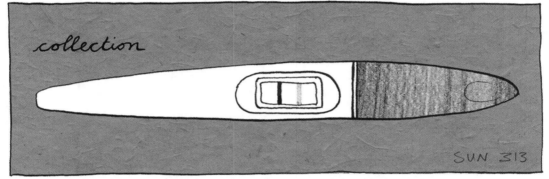

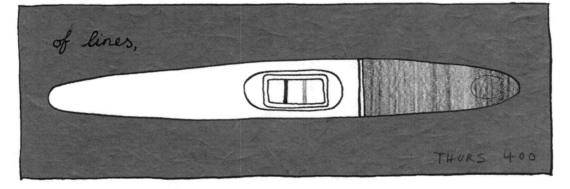

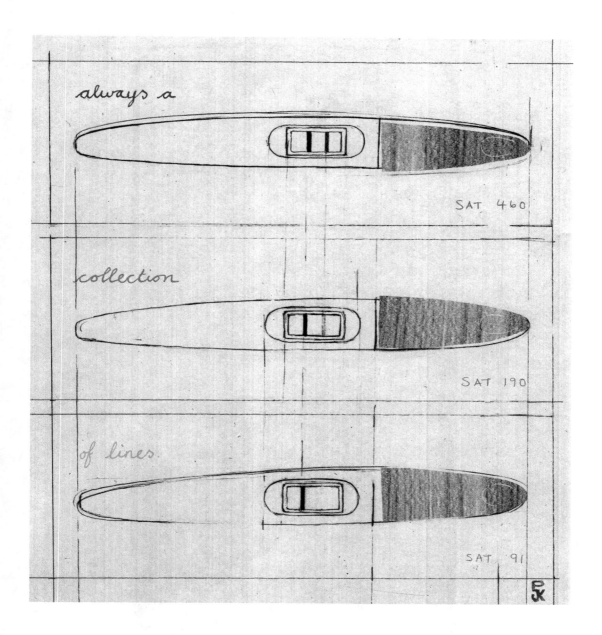

always a

SAT 460

collection

SAT 190

of lines.

SAT 91

FAILED
must
try
harder

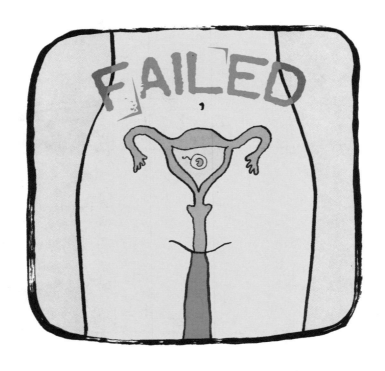

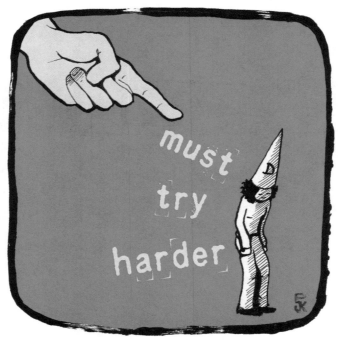

It was only a cluster of cells
But it was my cluster of cells!

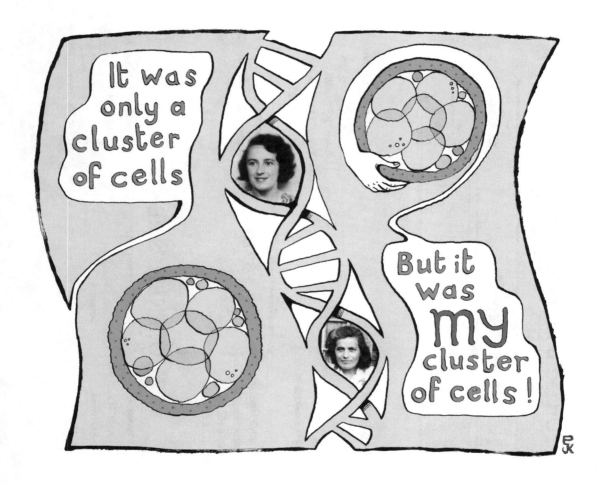

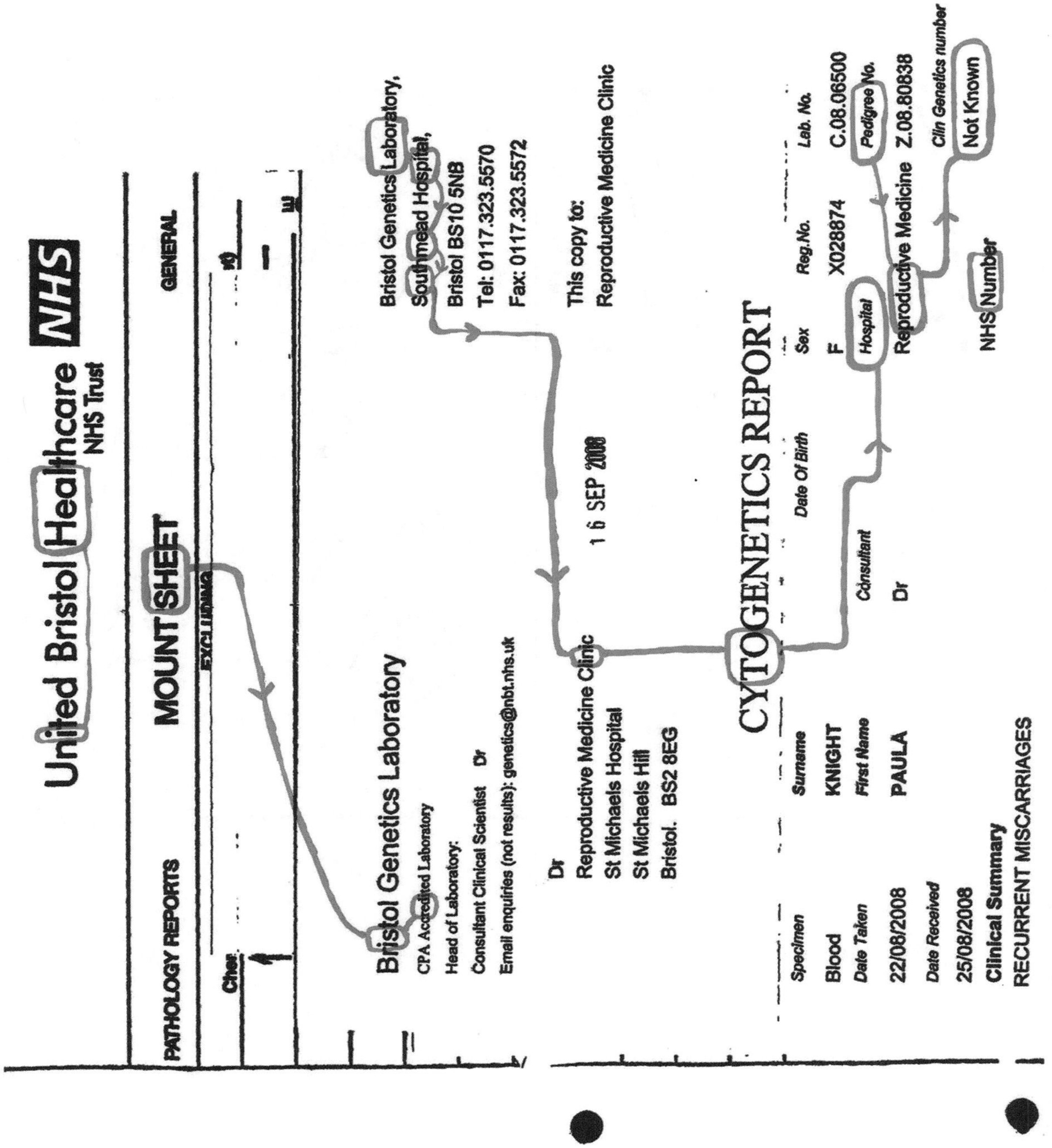

United Bristol Healthcare NHS Trust

NHS

PATHOLOGY REPORTS

MOUNT SHEET

GENERAL

EXCLUDING

Bristol Genetics Laboratory

CPA Accredited Laboratory

Head of Laboratory:

Consultant Clinical Scientist Dr

Email enquiries (not results): genetics@nbt.nhs.uk

Bristol Genetics Laboratory,
Southmead Hospital,
Bristol BS10 5NB
Tel: 0117.323.5570
Fax: 0117.323.5572

Dr
Reproductive Medicine Clinic
St Michaels Hospital
St Michaels Hill
Bristol. BS2 8EG

16 SEP 2008

This copy to:
Reproductive Medicine Clinic

CYTOGENETICS REPORT

Specimen	Surname	Date Of Birth	Sex	Reg.No.	Lab. No.
Blood	KNIGHT		F	X028874	C.08.06500
Date Taken	First Name	Consultant	Hospital		Pedigree No.
22/08/2008	PAULA	Dr	Reproductive Medicine		Z.08.80838
Date Received			NHS Number		Clin Genetics number
25/08/2008					Not Known

Clinical Summary
RECURRENT MISCARRIAGES

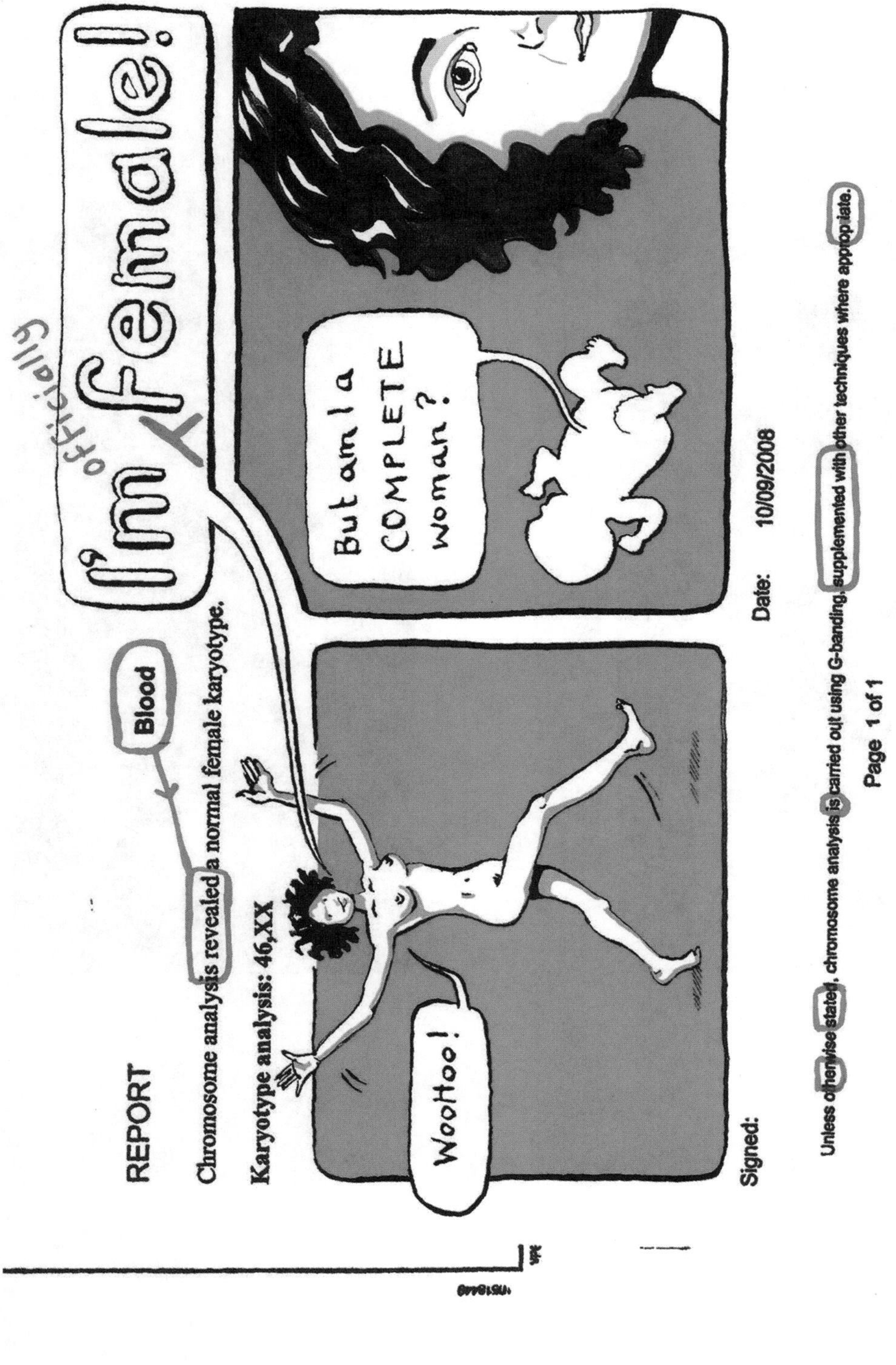
REPORT
Chromosome analysis revealed a normal female karyotype.
Karyotype analysis: 46,XX
Blood
I'm officially female!
WooHoo!
But am I a COMPLETE woman?
Signed:
Date: 10/09/2008
Unless otherwise stated, chromosome analysis is carried out using G-banding, supplemented with other techniques where appropriate.
Page 1 of 1

Childless or Childfree?

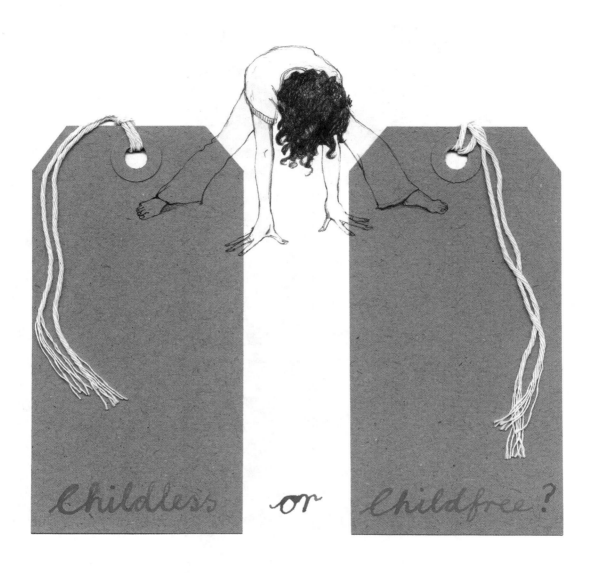

Neither
Just
Me

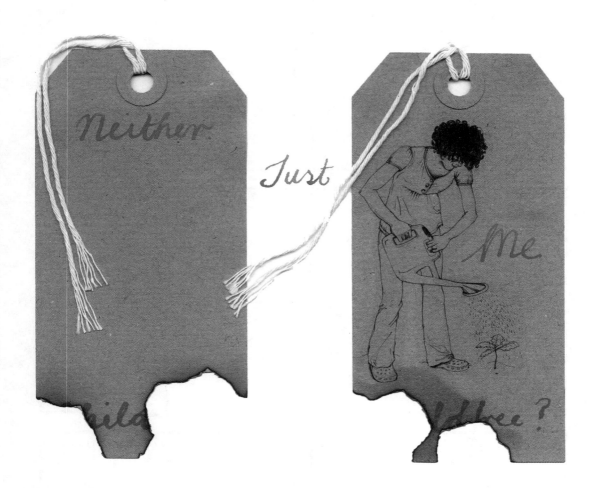

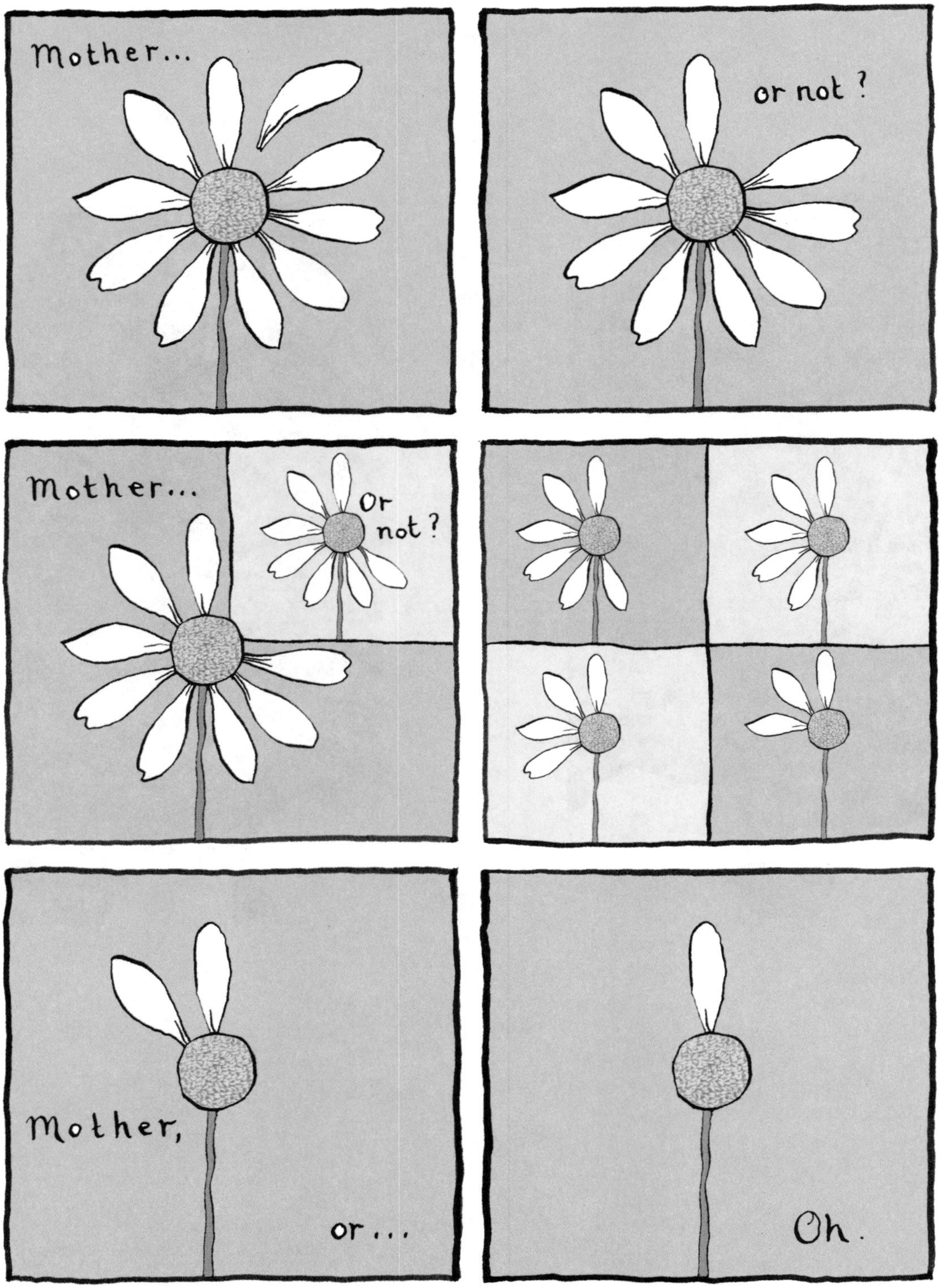
Mother...
or not ?
Mother...
Or not ?
Mother,
or...
Oh.

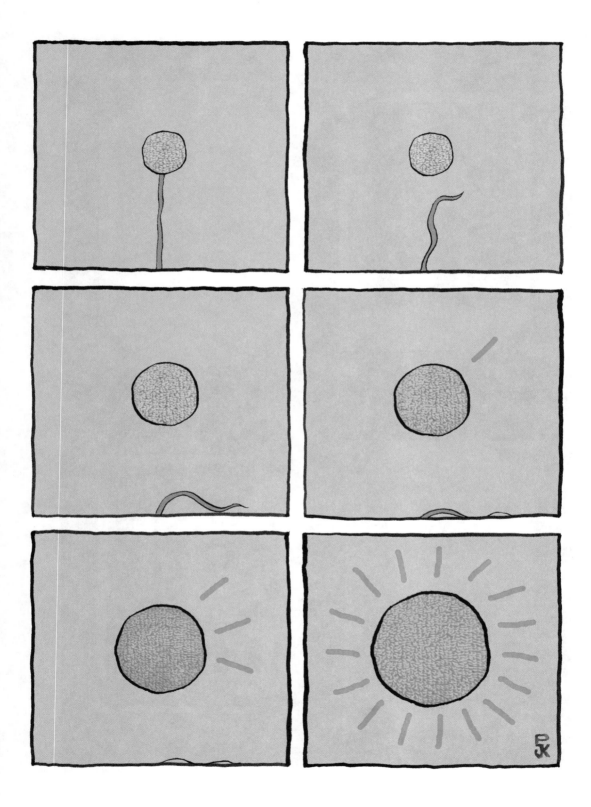

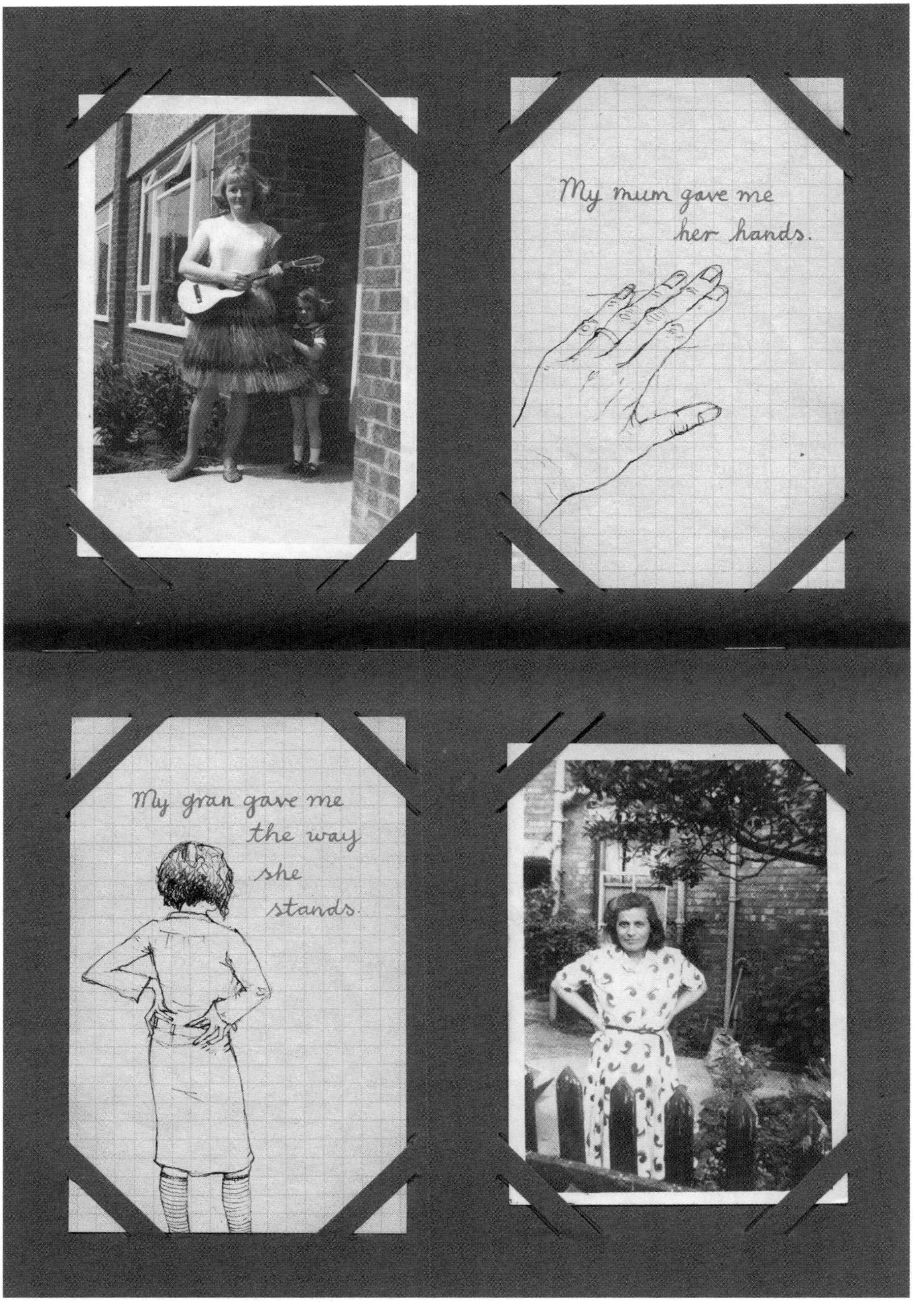
My mum gave me
her hands.
My gran gave me
the way
she
stands.

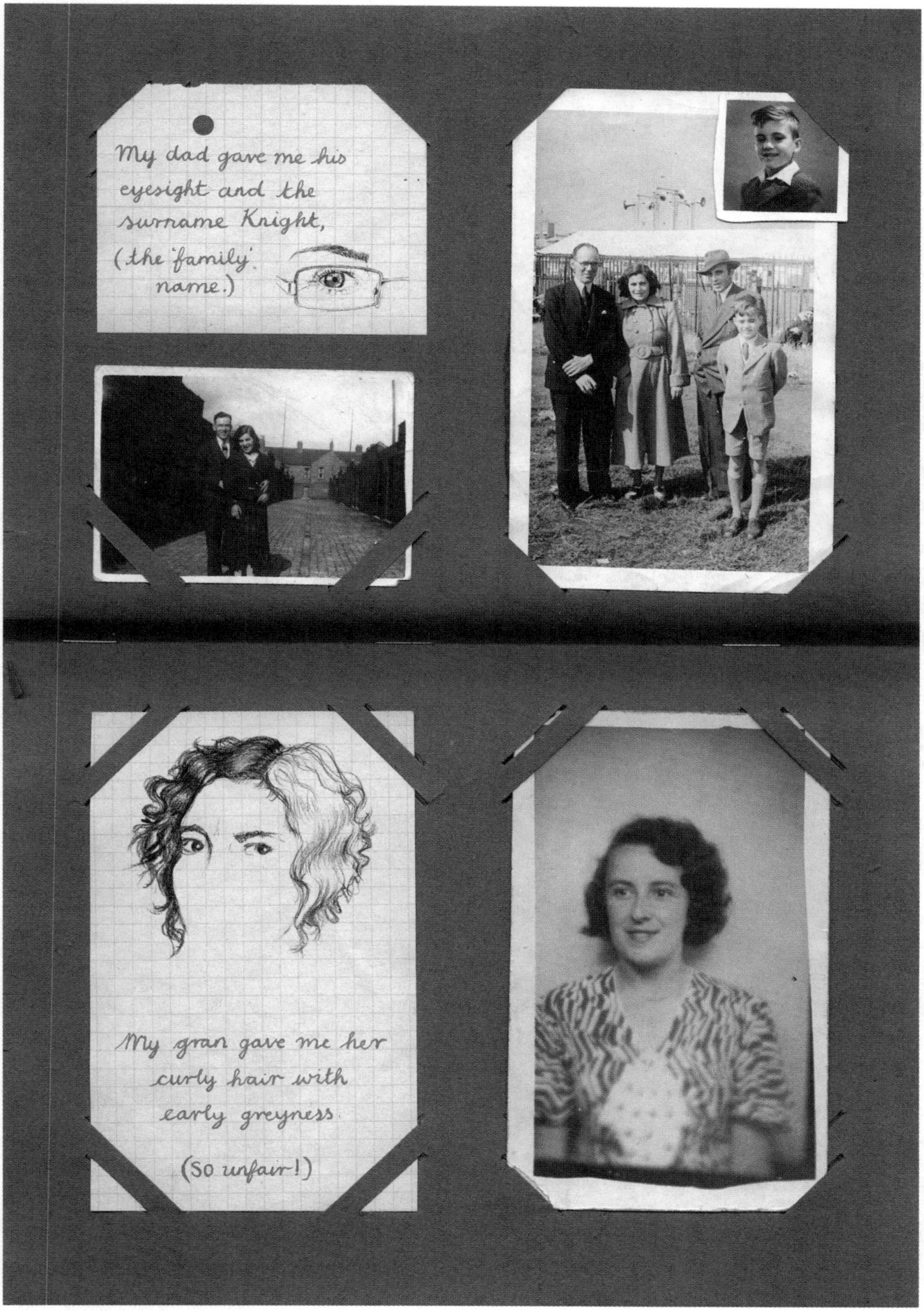
My dad gave me his eyesight and the surname Knight, (the 'family' name.)
My gran gave me her curly hair with early greyness.
(So unfair!)

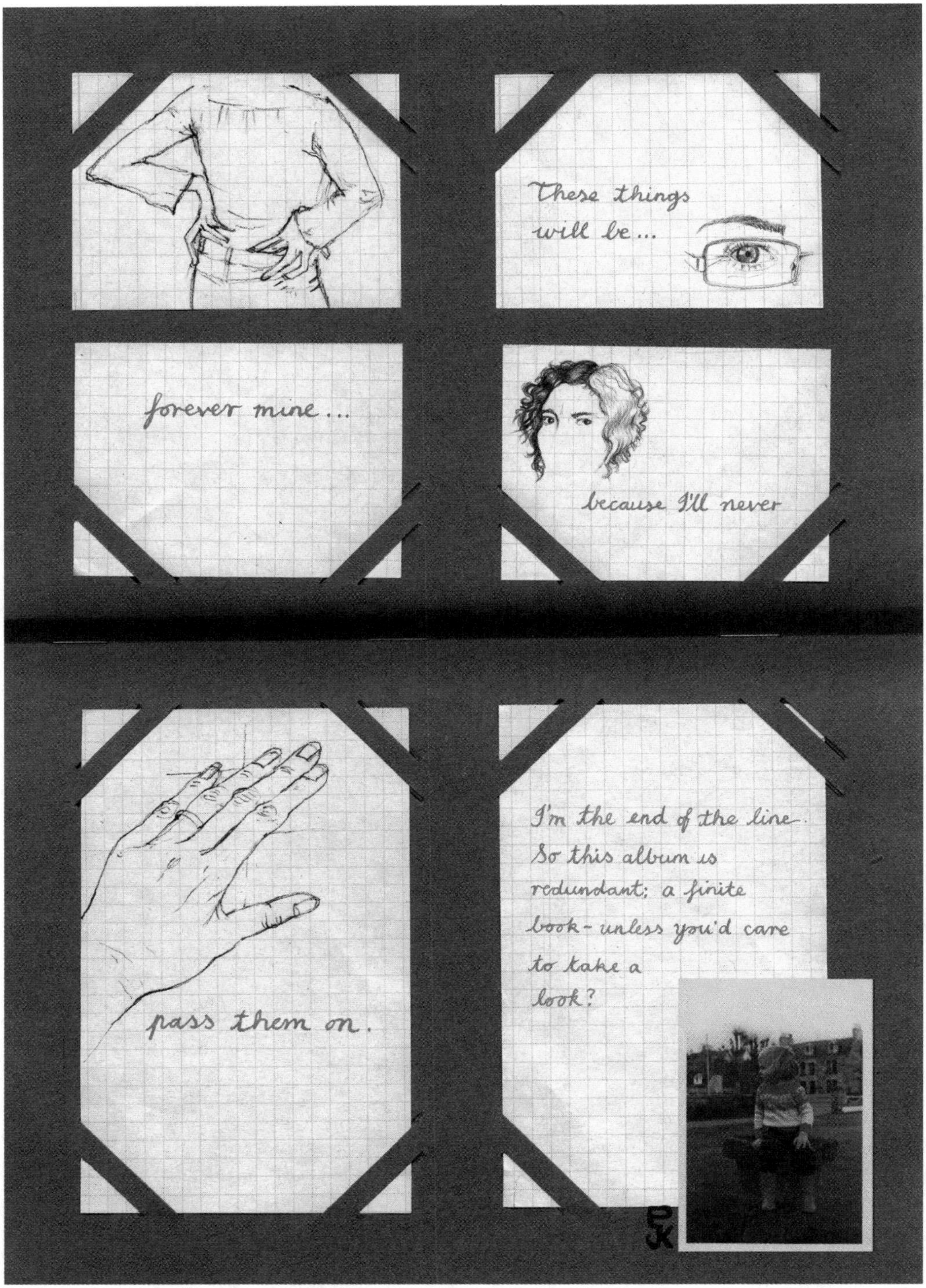
These things
will be...
forever mine...
because I'll never
pass them on.
I'm the end of the line.
So this album is
redundant: a finite
book - unless you'd care
to take a
look?

Present / Perfect

(2016)

Jenell Johnson

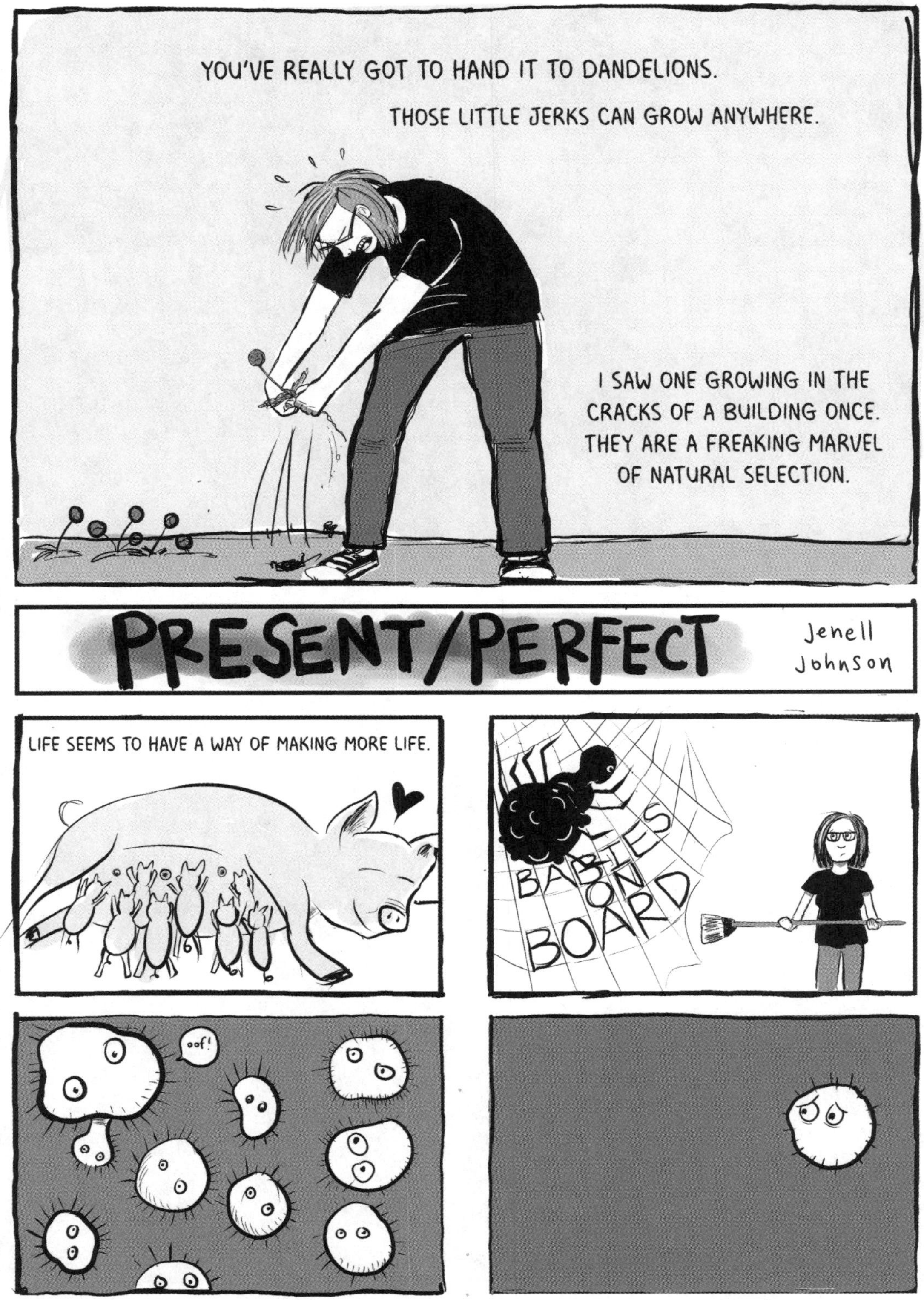
YOU'VE REALLY GOT TO HAND IT TO DANDELIONS.
THOSE LITTLE JERKS CAN GROW ANYWHERE.
I SAW ONE GROWING IN THE CRACKS OF A BUILDING ONCE. THEY ARE A FREAKING MARVEL OF NATURAL SELECTION.
PRESENT/PERFECT
Jenell Johnson
LIFE SEEMS TO HAVE A WAY OF MAKING MORE LIFE.
BABIES ON BOARD
oof!

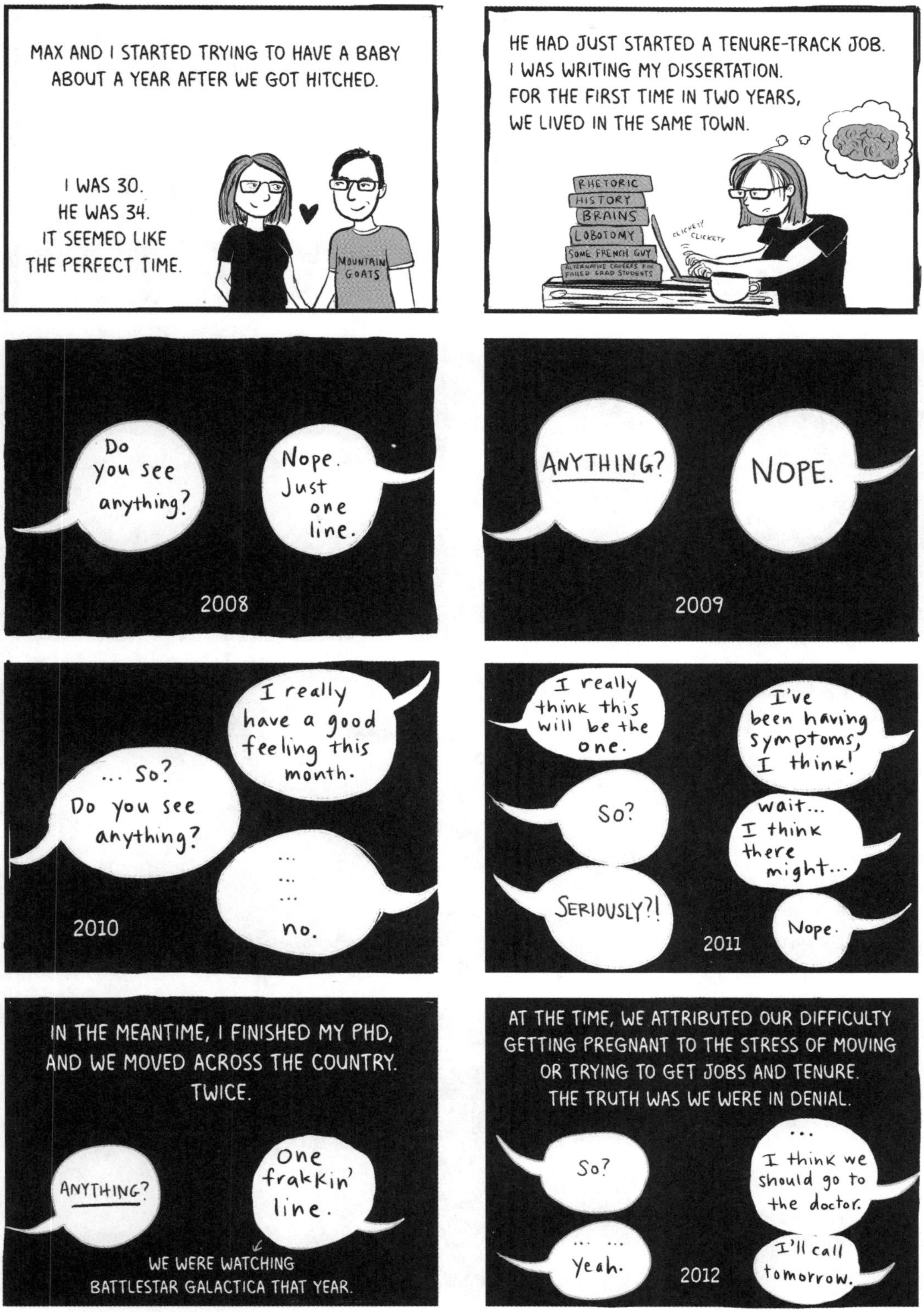
MAX AND I STARTED TRYING TO HAVE A BABY ABOUT A YEAR AFTER WE GOT HITCHED.
I WAS 30. HE WAS 34. IT SEEMED LIKE THE PERFECT TIME.
MOUNTAIN GOATS
HE HAD JUST STARTED A TENURE-TRACK JOB. I WAS WRITING MY DISSERTATION. FOR THE FIRST TIME IN TWO YEARS, WE LIVED IN THE SAME TOWN.
RHETORIC
HISTORY
BRAINS
LOBOTOMY
SOME FRENCH GUY
ALTERNATIVE CAREERS FOR FAILED GRAD STUDENTS
CLICKETY CLICKETY
Do you see anything?
Nope. Just one line.
2008
ANYTHING?
NOPE.
2009
I really have a good feeling this month.
... So? Do you see anything?
... ... no.
2010
I really think this will be the one.
I've been having symptoms, I think!
So?
wait... I think there might...
SERIOUSLY?!
Nope.
2011
IN THE MEANTIME, I FINISHED MY PHD, AND WE MOVED ACROSS THE COUNTRY. TWICE.
ANYTHING?
One frakkin' line.
WE WERE WATCHING BATTLESTAR GALACTICA THAT YEAR.
AT THE TIME, WE ATTRIBUTED OUR DIFFICULTY GETTING PREGNANT TO THE STRESS OF MOVING OR TRYING TO GET JOBS AND TENURE. THE TRUTH WAS WE WERE IN DENIAL.
So?
... I think we should go to the doctor.
... ... Yeah.
I'll call tomorrow.
2012

FOR THE NEXT SIX MONTHS, WE WENT THROUGH DOZENS OF TESTS TO TRY AND FIGURE OUT WHAT WAS GOING ON. SOME HURT. MANY WERE AWKWARD AND EMBARRASSING. VERY FEW WERE COVERED BY INSURANCE.

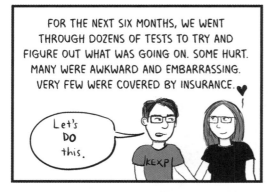

Let's **DO** this.

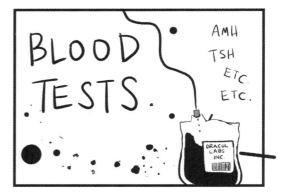

BLOOD TESTS.

AMH TSH ETC. ETC.

DRACUL LABS INC.

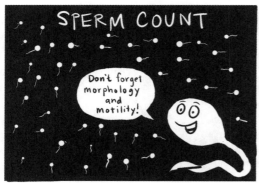

SPERM COUNT

Don't forget morphology and motility!

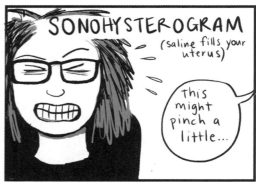

SONOHYSTEROGRAM

(saline fills your uterus)

This might pinch a little...

HYSTEROSCOPY

IN THIS TEST, A CAMERA IS SNAKED THROUGH THE CERVIX TO GET A PEEK AT THE UTERUS. I HAD TWO. ONE WHILE UNDER GENERAL-ISH ANESTHESIA—WITH A BONUS POLYPECTOMY FOR A POLYP THAT TURNED OUT NOT TO EXIST. OH, AND A BIOPSY FOR GOOD MEASURE. I WAS WIDE AWAKE DURING THE SECOND.

DURING THESE TESTS, I LEARNED I HAVE A "SENSITIVE CERVIX," WHICH BASICALLY MEANT THAT IT HATED TO BE TOUCHED, LET ALONE ENTERED.

I ALSO IMAGINED IT MEANT MY CERVIX ENJOYED SMOKING CLOVE CIGARETTES, READING PABLO NERUDA, AND LISTENING TO MORRISSEY'S SOLO WORK.

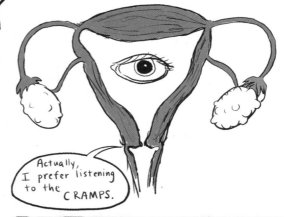

Actually, I prefer listening to the CRAMPS.

AFTER THE TESTS, WE GOT THE TERRIBLE NEWS.

THERE WAS NO NEWS.

OUR INFERTILITY HAD NO KNOWN MEDICAL EXPLANATION.

ERRATA

Pages 103–4

The panels on these pages were erroneously transposed. After reading page 102, please flip to page 104.

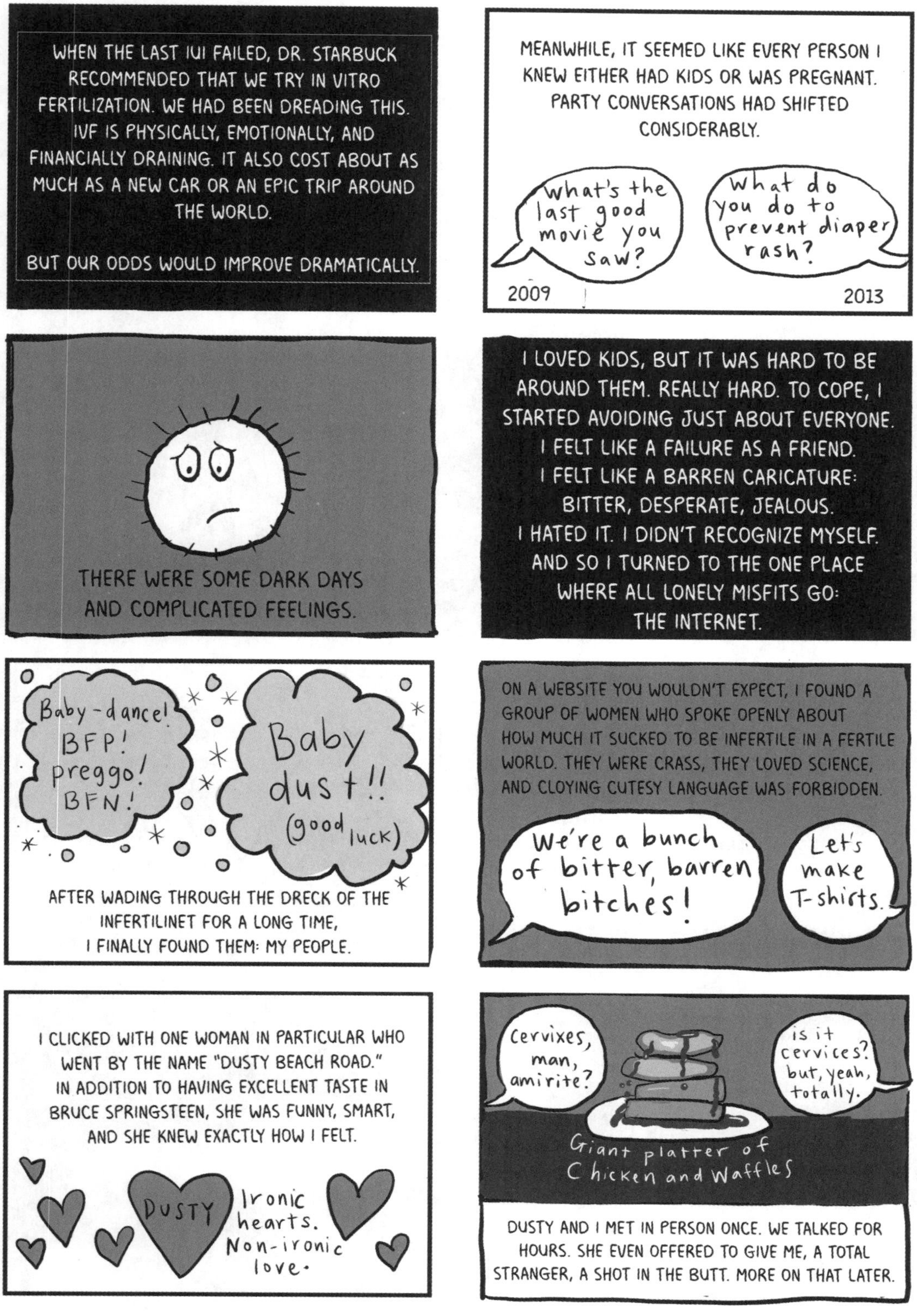
WHEN THE LAST IUI FAILED, DR. STARBUCK RECOMMENDED THAT WE TRY IN VITRO FERTILIZATION. WE HAD BEEN DREADING THIS. IVF IS PHYSICALLY, EMOTIONALLY, AND FINANCIALLY DRAINING. IT ALSO COST ABOUT AS MUCH AS A NEW CAR OR AN EPIC TRIP AROUND THE WORLD.
BUT OUR ODDS WOULD IMPROVE DRAMATICALLY.
MEANWHILE, IT SEEMED LIKE EVERY PERSON I KNEW EITHER HAD KIDS OR WAS PREGNANT. PARTY CONVERSATIONS HAD SHIFTED CONSIDERABLY.
What's the last good movie you saw?
What do you do to prevent diaper rash?
2009
2013
THERE WERE SOME DARK DAYS AND COMPLICATED FEELINGS.
I LOVED KIDS, BUT IT WAS HARD TO BE AROUND THEM. REALLY HARD. TO COPE, I STARTED AVOIDING JUST ABOUT EVERYONE. I FELT LIKE A FAILURE AS A FRIEND. I FELT LIKE A BARREN CARICATURE: BITTER, DESPERATE, JEALOUS. I HATED IT. I DIDN'T RECOGNIZE MYSELF. AND SO I TURNED TO THE ONE PLACE WHERE ALL LONELY MISFITS GO: THE INTERNET.
Baby-dance! BFP! preggo! BFN!
Baby dust!! (good luck)
AFTER WADING THROUGH THE DRECK OF THE INFERTILINET FOR A LONG TIME, I FINALLY FOUND THEM: MY PEOPLE.
ON A WEBSITE YOU WOULDN'T EXPECT, I FOUND A GROUP OF WOMEN WHO SPOKE OPENLY ABOUT HOW MUCH IT SUCKED TO BE INFERTILE IN A FERTILE WORLD. THEY WERE CRASS, THEY LOVED SCIENCE, AND CLOYING CUTESY LANGUAGE WAS FORBIDDEN.
We're a bunch of bitter, barren bitches!
Let's make T-shirts.
I CLICKED WITH ONE WOMAN IN PARTICULAR WHO WENT BY THE NAME "DUSTY BEACH ROAD." IN ADDITION TO HAVING EXCELLENT TASTE IN BRUCE SPRINGSTEEN, SHE WAS FUNNY, SMART, AND SHE KNEW EXACTLY HOW I FELT.
DUSTY
Ironic hearts. Non-ironic love.
Cervixes, man, amirite?
is it cervices? but, yeah, totally.
Giant platter of Chicken and Waffles
DUSTY AND I MET IN PERSON ONCE. WE TALKED FOR HOURS. SHE EVEN OFFERED TO GIVE ME, A TOTAL STRANGER, A SHOT IN THE BUTT. MORE ON THAT LATER.

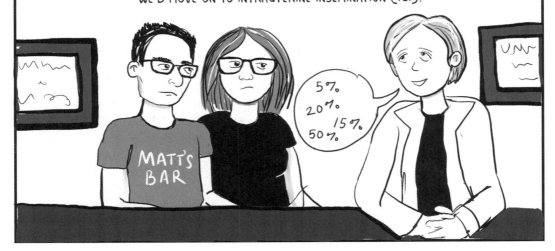

WE WERE REFERRED TO A REPRODUCTIVE ENDOCRINOLOGIST.

OUR RE, "DR. STARBUCK" (WE CALLED HER THIS BECAUSE SHE BORE A STRIKING RESEMBLANCE TO KATEE SACKHOFF) GAVE US SOME ADDITIONAL BAD NEWS. OUR ODDS OF CONCEIVING ON OUR OWN WERE ABOUT 5 PERCENT, IF THAT. SHE RECOMMENDED THAT WE BEGIN TREATMENT. WE'D START WITH HORMONAL ASSISTANCE, AND IF THAT DIDN'T WORK, WE'D MOVE ON TO INTRAUTERINE INSEMINATION (IUI).

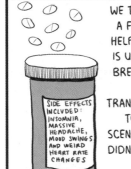

WE TRIED ON OUR OWN FOR A FEW MONTHS WITH THE HELP OF LETRAZOLE, WHICH IS USUALLY USED TO TREAT BREAST CANCER. THIS WAS COMBINED WITH TRANSVAGINAL ULTRASOUNDS TO AVOID "OCTOMOM" SCENARIOS. I OVULATED, BUT DIDN'T GET PREGNANT. NEXT STOP: IUI.

SIDE EFFECTS INCLUDED: INSOMNIA, MASSIVE HEADACHE, MOOD SWINGS AND WEIRD HEART RATE CHANGES

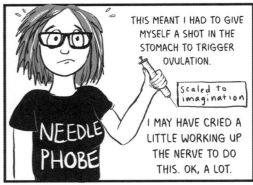

THIS MEANT I HAD TO GIVE MYSELF A SHOT IN THE STOMACH TO TRIGGER OVULATION.

Scaled to imagination

I MAY HAVE CRIED A LITTLE WORKING UP THE NERVE TO DO THIS. OK, A LOT.

NEEDLE PHOBE

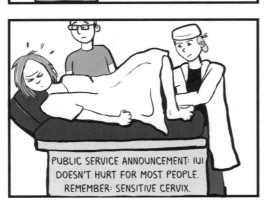

PUBLIC SERVICE ANNOUNCEMENT: IUI DOESN'T HURT FOR MOST PEOPLE. REMEMBER: SENSITIVE CERVIX.

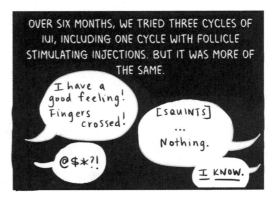

OVER SIX MONTHS, WE TRIED THREE CYCLES OF IUI, INCLUDING ONE CYCLE WITH FOLLICLE STIMULATING INJECTIONS. BUT IT WAS MORE OF THE SAME.

I have a good feeling! Fingers crossed!

@$*?!

[SQUINTS] ... Nothing.

I KNOW.

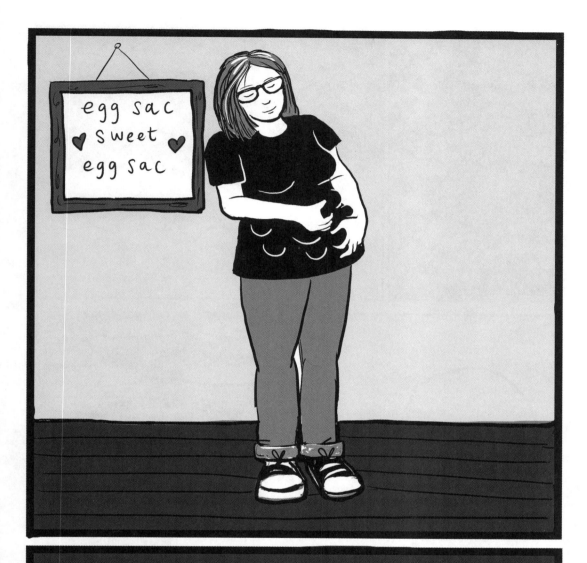

AFTER A LOT OF TALKING, MAX AND I DECIDED TO GO AHEAD WITH IVF. AFTER CASHING IN OUR LIFE SAVINGS, WE RECEIVED A GIANT BOX OF DRUGS IN THE MAIL, WHICH CAME WITH LOTS AND LOTS OF NEEDLES AND A BIOHAZARD BOX TO PUT THEM IN. AND HERSHEY'S KISSES. I SUPPOSE THAT WAS SUPPOSED TO BE NICE, BUT IT FELT PATRONIZING.

FIRST, BIRTH CONTROL PILLS (!) TO SUPPRESS OVULATION. THEN DAILY INJECTIONS OF LUPRON FOR TWO WEEKS, THEN INJECTIONS OF MENOPUR (WHICH HAS ITS ORIGINS IN THE URINE OF POST-MENOPAUSAL NUNS) COMBINED WITH ANOTHER HEAVY DUTY FOLLICLE STIMULATOR. THEN DAILY PROGESTERONE SHOTS IN THE BUTT. MORE ON THAT SOON.

THE WHOLE POINT OF THE HORMONES WAS TO MAKE ME INTO A WALKING, TALKING, EGG SAC. MY BELLY SWELLED SO FAST THAT I GOT STRETCH MARKS. I STILL HAVE THEM.

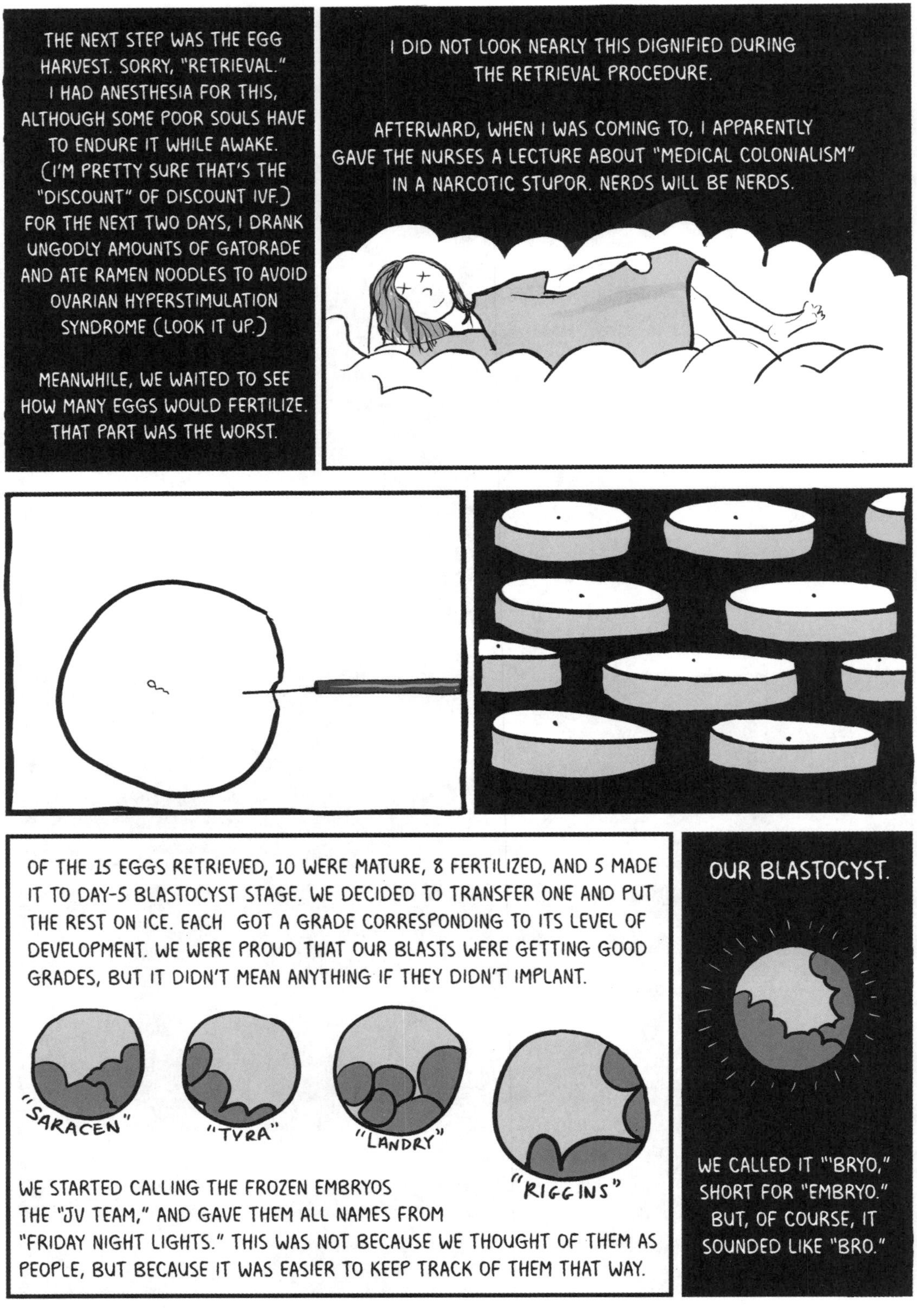

THE NEXT STEP WAS THE EGG HARVEST. SORRY, "RETRIEVAL." I HAD ANESTHESIA FOR THIS, ALTHOUGH SOME POOR SOULS HAVE TO ENDURE IT WHILE AWAKE. (I'M PRETTY SURE THAT'S THE "DISCOUNT" OF DISCOUNT IVF.) FOR THE NEXT TWO DAYS, I DRANK UNGODLY AMOUNTS OF GATORADE AND ATE RAMEN NOODLES TO AVOID OVARIAN HYPERSTIMULATION SYNDROME (LOOK IT UP.)

MEANWHILE, WE WAITED TO SEE HOW MANY EGGS WOULD FERTILIZE. THAT PART WAS THE WORST.

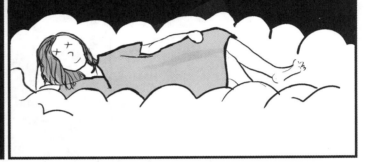

I DID NOT LOOK NEARLY THIS DIGNIFIED DURING THE RETRIEVAL PROCEDURE.

AFTERWARD, WHEN I WAS COMING TO, I APPARENTLY GAVE THE NURSES A LECTURE ABOUT "MEDICAL COLONIALISM" IN A NARCOTIC STUPOR. NERDS WILL BE NERDS.

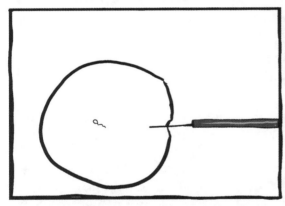

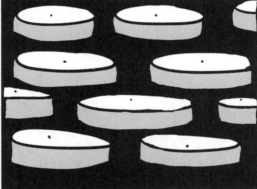

OF THE 15 EGGS RETRIEVED, 10 WERE MATURE, 8 FERTILIZED, AND 5 MADE IT TO DAY-5 BLASTOCYST STAGE. WE DECIDED TO TRANSFER ONE AND PUT THE REST ON ICE. EACH GOT A GRADE CORRESPONDING TO ITS LEVEL OF DEVELOPMENT. WE WERE PROUD THAT OUR BLASTS WERE GETTING GOOD GRADES, BUT IT DIDN'T MEAN ANYTHING IF THEY DIDN'T IMPLANT.

"SARACEN"

"TYRA"

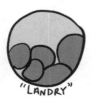
"LANDRY"

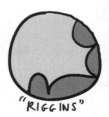
"RIGGINS"

WE STARTED CALLING THE FROZEN EMBRYOS THE "JV TEAM," AND GAVE THEM ALL NAMES FROM "FRIDAY NIGHT LIGHTS." THIS WAS NOT BECAUSE WE THOUGHT OF THEM AS PEOPLE, BUT BECAUSE IT WAS EASIER TO KEEP TRACK OF THEM THAT WAY.

OUR BLASTOCYST.

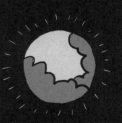

WE CALLED IT "'BRYO," SHORT FOR "EMBRYO." BUT, OF COURSE, IT SOUNDED LIKE "BRO."

THE ONE THING IVF NEWBIES DREAD MORE THAN ANYTHING ARE PROGESTERONE SHOTS. UNLIKE THE DOZENS-TO-HUNDREDS OF OTHER HORMONE INJECTIONS, WHICH ARE ADMINISTERED UNDER THE SKIN, PROGESTERONE MUST BE SLOWLY INJECTED INTO A MUSCLE. ALTHOUGH I HAVE KNOWN A FEW PEOPLE WHO CAN INJECT THEMSELVES IN THE THIGH (SPECIFICALLY, SOME OF MY BADASS TRANS FRIENDS WHO TAKE HORMONES), I SIMPLY COULDN'T DO IT.
THE NEEDLE IS HUGE. AND THICK. AND I'M A CHICKEN.
THE WEEK BEFORE OUR EMBRYO TRANSFER, MAX WATCHED DOZENS OF YOUTUBE VIDEOS. THEN HE PRACTICED BY JABBING A LARGE PORK BUTT ROAST.
THEN WE RAN AROUND THE HOUSE SINGING DIFFERENT BUTT-THEMED SONGS TO PSYCH OURSELVES UP. AND THEN HE STABBED ME WITHOUT FLINCHING.
READER, I HARDLY FELT A THING.

WE MADE THE BUTT INTO PULLED PORK SANDWICHES.

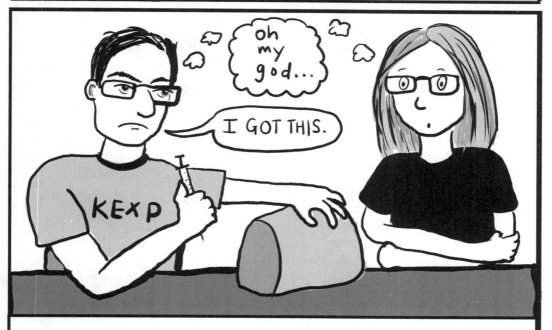

IF WE GOT PREGNANT, WE WOULD HAVE TO DO BUTT SHOTS EACH DAY FOR THE WHOLE FIRST TRIMESTER. WE HOPED IT WOULD BECOME A TOUCHING NIGHTLY RITUAL.

THIS IS WHERE I WILL NOTE THAT IVF COMPLETELY "CURED" MY NEEDLE PHOBIA.
I GOT SO GOOD AT GIVING MYSELF INJECTIONS, IN FACT, THAT I COULD PUT PANCAKE BATTER IN A PAN, RUN TO THE BATHROOM, DO THE SHOT, AND BE BACK IN TIME TO FLIP THE PANCAKE.

I'M NOT KIDDING. I'M REALLY THAT GOOD AT INJECTIONS.

I'M ALSO REALLY GOOD AT MAKING PANCAKES.

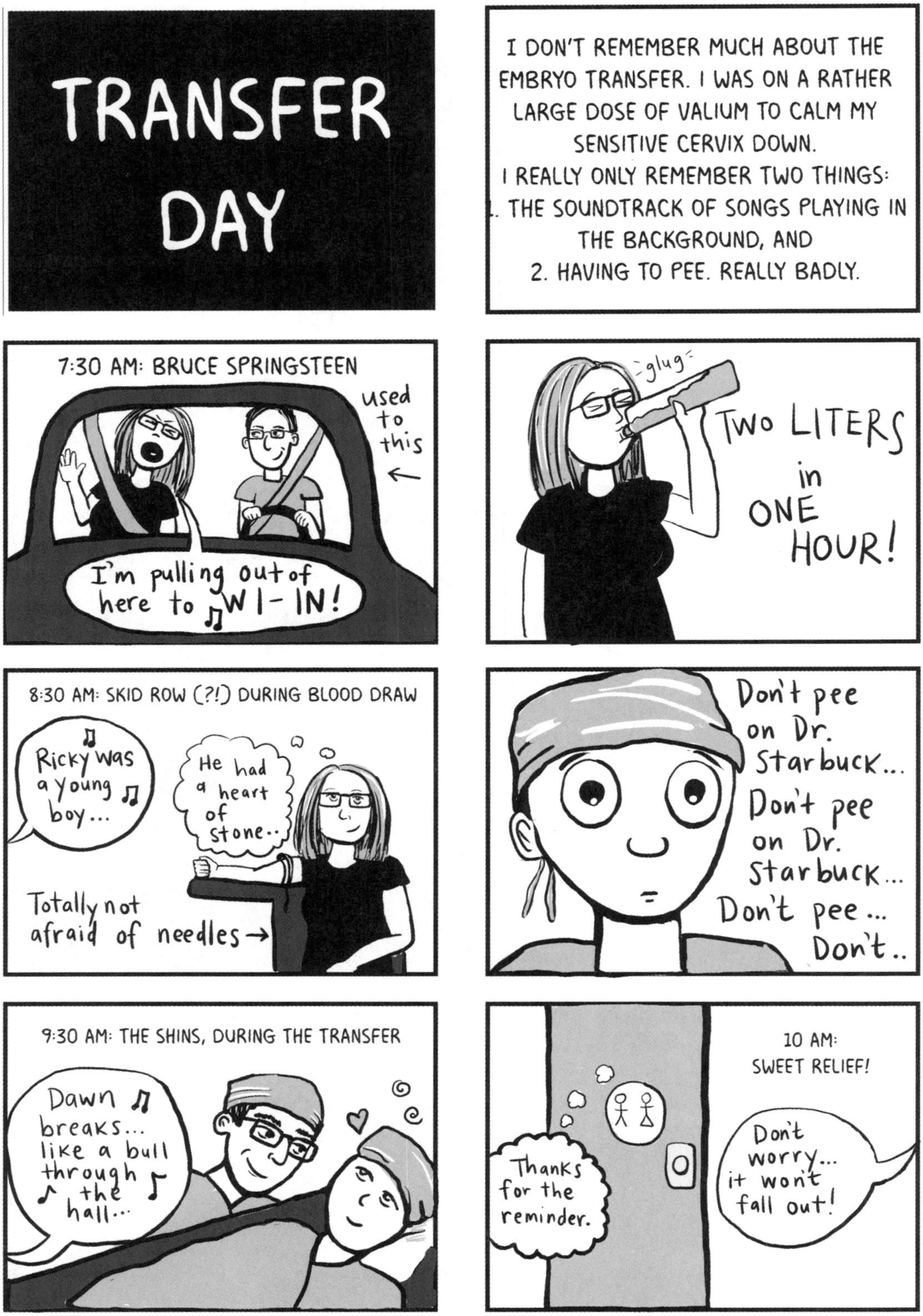
TRANSFER DAY
I DON'T REMEMBER MUCH ABOUT THE EMBRYO TRANSFER. I WAS ON A RATHER LARGE DOSE OF VALIUM TO CALM MY SENSITIVE CERVIX DOWN.
I REALLY ONLY REMEMBER TWO THINGS:
1. THE SOUNDTRACK OF SONGS PLAYING IN THE BACKGROUND, AND
2. HAVING TO PEE. REALLY BADLY.
7:30 AM: BRUCE SPRINGSTEEN
used to this
I'm pulling out of here to WI-IN!
glug
TWO LITERS in ONE HOUR!
8:30 AM: SKID ROW (?!) DURING BLOOD DRAW
Ricky was a young boy...
He had a heart of stone...
Totally not afraid of needles
Don't pee on Dr. Starbuck... Don't pee on Dr. Starbuck... Don't pee... Don't..
9:30 AM: THE SHINS, DURING THE TRANSFER
Dawn breaks... like a bull through the hall...
10 AM: SWEET RELIEF!
Thanks for the reminder.
Don't worry... it won't fall out!

WE WAITED.
AND WAITED.
AND WAITED.
AND WAITED.
AND THEN.
pregastick
Really?
Yes.
whoosh
whoosh
Dandelion Fertility Clinic
World's most expensive complimentary onesie.
PREGNANCY 101
RAISING COOL KIDS

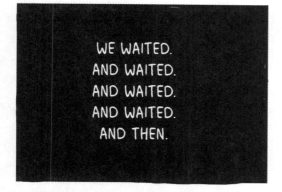

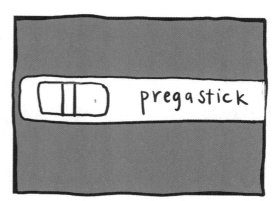

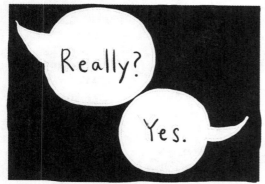

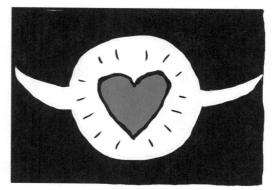

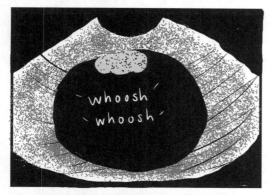

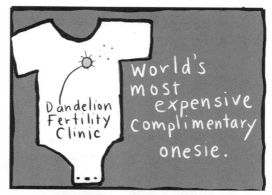

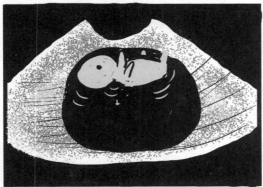

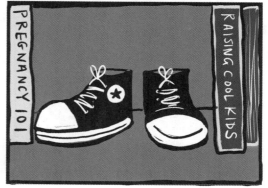

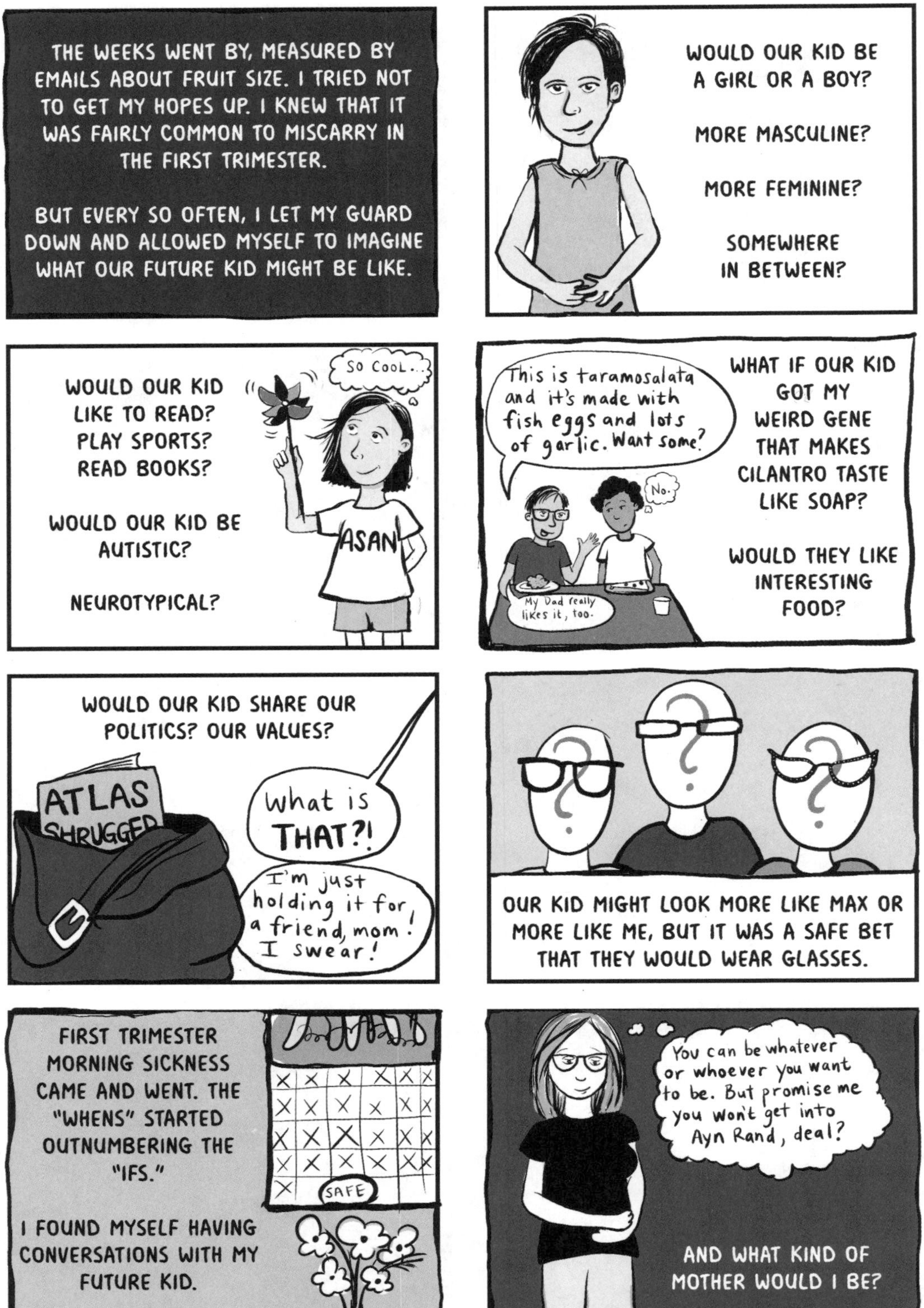
THE WEEKS WENT BY, MEASURED BY EMAILS ABOUT FRUIT SIZE. I TRIED NOT TO GET MY HOPES UP. I KNEW THAT IT WAS FAIRLY COMMON TO MISCARRY IN THE FIRST TRIMESTER.
BUT EVERY SO OFTEN, I LET MY GUARD DOWN AND ALLOWED MYSELF TO IMAGINE WHAT OUR FUTURE KID MIGHT BE LIKE.
WOULD OUR KID BE A GIRL OR A BOY?
MORE MASCULINE?
MORE FEMININE?
SOMEWHERE IN BETWEEN?
WOULD OUR KID LIKE TO READ? PLAY SPORTS? READ BOOKS?
WOULD OUR KID BE AUTISTIC?
NEUROTYPICAL?
SO COOL...
ASAN
This is taramosalata and it's made with fish eggs and lots of garlic. Want some?
No.
My Dad really likes it, too.
WHAT IF OUR KID GOT MY WEIRD GENE THAT MAKES CILANTRO TASTE LIKE SOAP?
WOULD THEY LIKE INTERESTING FOOD?
WOULD OUR KID SHARE OUR POLITICS? OUR VALUES?
ATLAS SHRUGGED
What is THAT?!
I'm just holding it for a friend, mom! I swear!
OUR KID MIGHT LOOK MORE LIKE MAX OR MORE LIKE ME, BUT IT WAS A SAFE BET THAT THEY WOULD WEAR GLASSES.
FIRST TRIMESTER MORNING SICKNESS CAME AND WENT. THE "WHENS" STARTED OUTNUMBERING THE "IFS."
I FOUND MYSELF HAVING CONVERSATIONS WITH MY FUTURE KID.
SAFE
You can be whatever or whoever you want to be. But promise me you won't get into Ayn Rand, deal?
AND WHAT KIND OF MOTHER WOULD I BE?

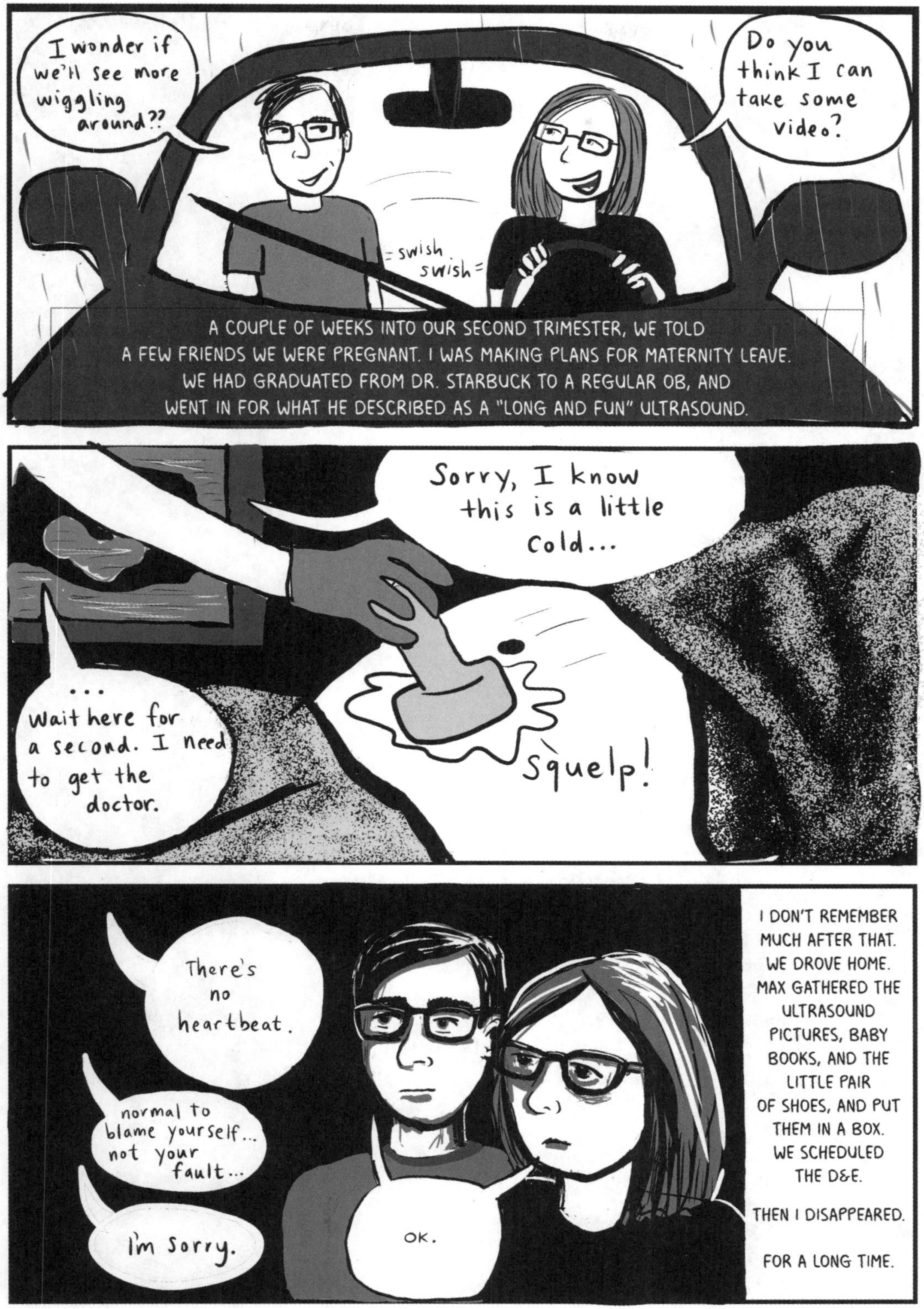
I wonder if we'll see more wiggling around??
Do you think I can take some video?
swish swish
A COUPLE OF WEEKS INTO OUR SECOND TRIMESTER, WE TOLD A FEW FRIENDS WE WERE PREGNANT. I WAS MAKING PLANS FOR MATERNITY LEAVE. WE HAD GRADUATED FROM DR. STARBUCK TO A REGULAR OB, AND WENT IN FOR WHAT HE DESCRIBED AS A "LONG AND FUN" ULTRASOUND.
Sorry, I know this is a little cold...
Squelp!
... Wait here for a second. I need to get the doctor.
There's no heartbeat.
normal to blame yourself... not your fault...
I'm sorry.
OK.
I DON'T REMEMBER MUCH AFTER THAT. WE DROVE HOME. MAX GATHERED THE ULTRASOUND PICTURES, BABY BOOKS, AND THE LITTLE PAIR OF SHOES, AND PUT THEM IN A BOX. WE SCHEDULED THE D&E.
THEN I DISAPPEARED.
FOR A LONG TIME.

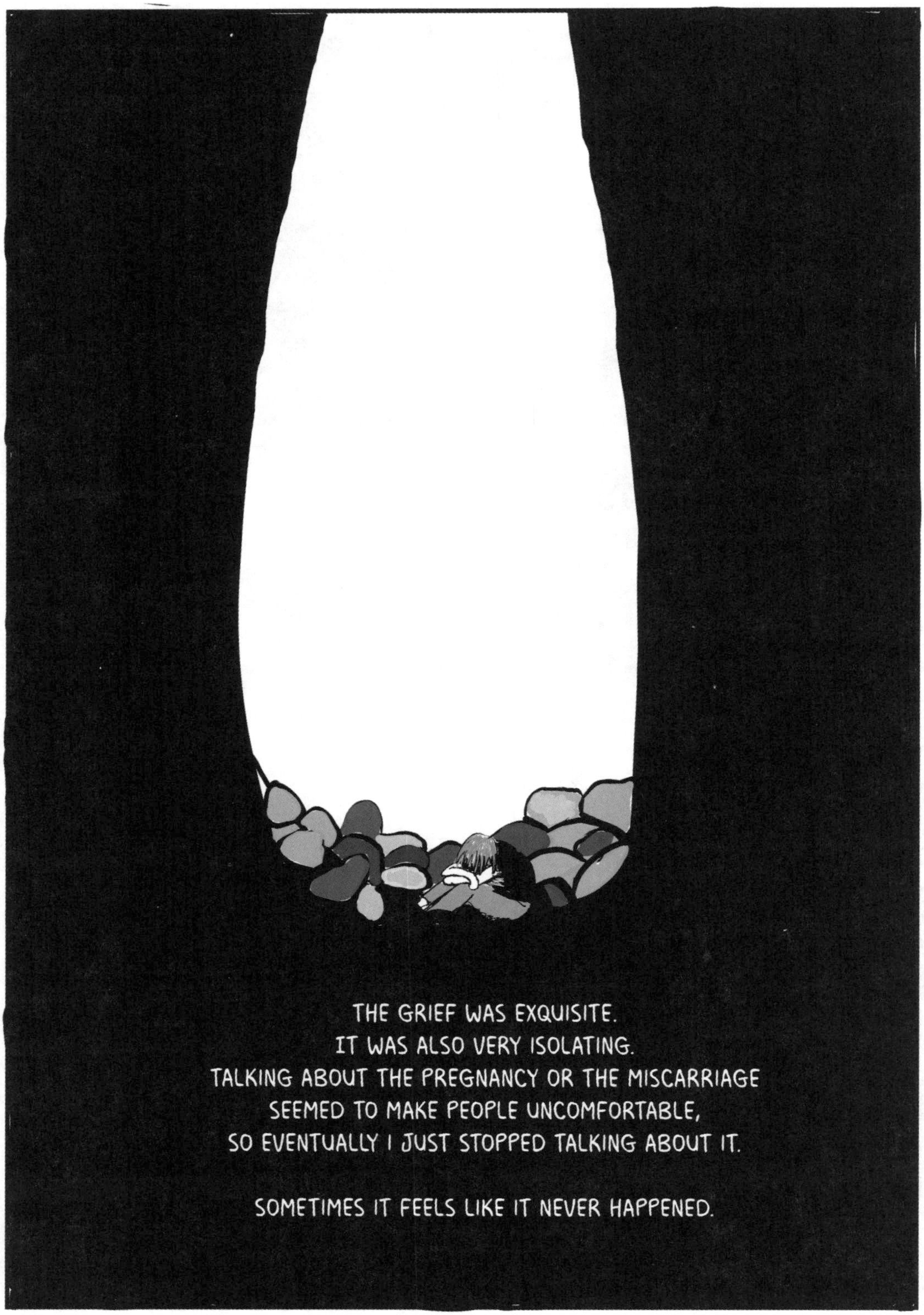
THE GRIEF WAS EXQUISITE.
IT WAS ALSO VERY ISOLATING.
TALKING ABOUT THE PREGNANCY OR THE MISCARRIAGE
SEEMED TO MAKE PEOPLE UNCOMFORTABLE,
SO EVENTUALLY I JUST STOPPED TALKING ABOUT IT.
SOMETIMES IT FEELS LIKE IT NEVER HAPPENED.

WE TOOK SOME TIME OFF BEFORE MOVING ON TO THE NEXT TRANSFER. WE THOUGHT WE MIGHT BE ABLE TO SNAG ONE OF THOSE POST-MISCARRIAGE MIRACLE BABIES PEOPLE KEPT TELLING US ABOUT. NOPE. SO WE MOVED FORWARD WITH THE JV TEAM. EACH FROZEN EMBRYO TRANSFER MEANT MORE HORMONE INJECTIONS, AND BONUS DAILY ESTROGEN PATCHES (ABOUT 4X THE DOSE POST-MENOPAUSAL PEOPLE USE).
AND, OF COURSE, NIGHTLY BUTT SHOTS.

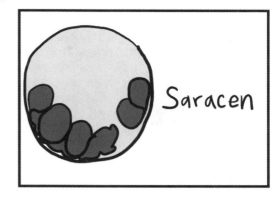

Saracen

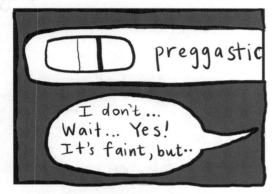

preggastic

I don't... Wait... Yes! It's faint, but...

THIS TRANSFER RESULTED IN A CHEMICAL PREGNANCY — A VERY EARLY MISCARRIAGE. WE WERE DISAPPOINTED, BUT NOTHING LIKE THE GRIEF OF THE PREVIOUS MISCARRIAGE.
DR. STARBUCK RECOMMENDED THAT WE TRANSFER TWO, WHICH CAME WITH THE RISK OF MULTIPLES. WE DECIDED TO TAKE THE RISK IF IT MEANT BETTER ODDS.

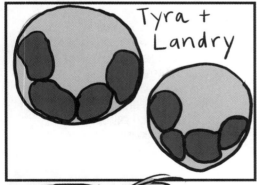

Tyra + Landry

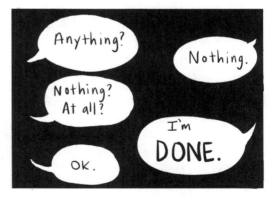

Anything?

Nothing.

Nothing? At all?

OK.

I'm DONE.

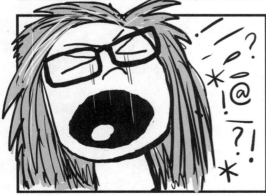

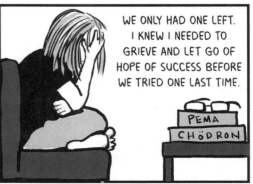

WE ONLY HAD ONE LEFT. I KNEW I NEEDED TO GRIEVE AND LET GO OF HOPE OF SUCCESS BEFORE WE TRIED ONE LAST TIME.

PEMA
CHÖDRON

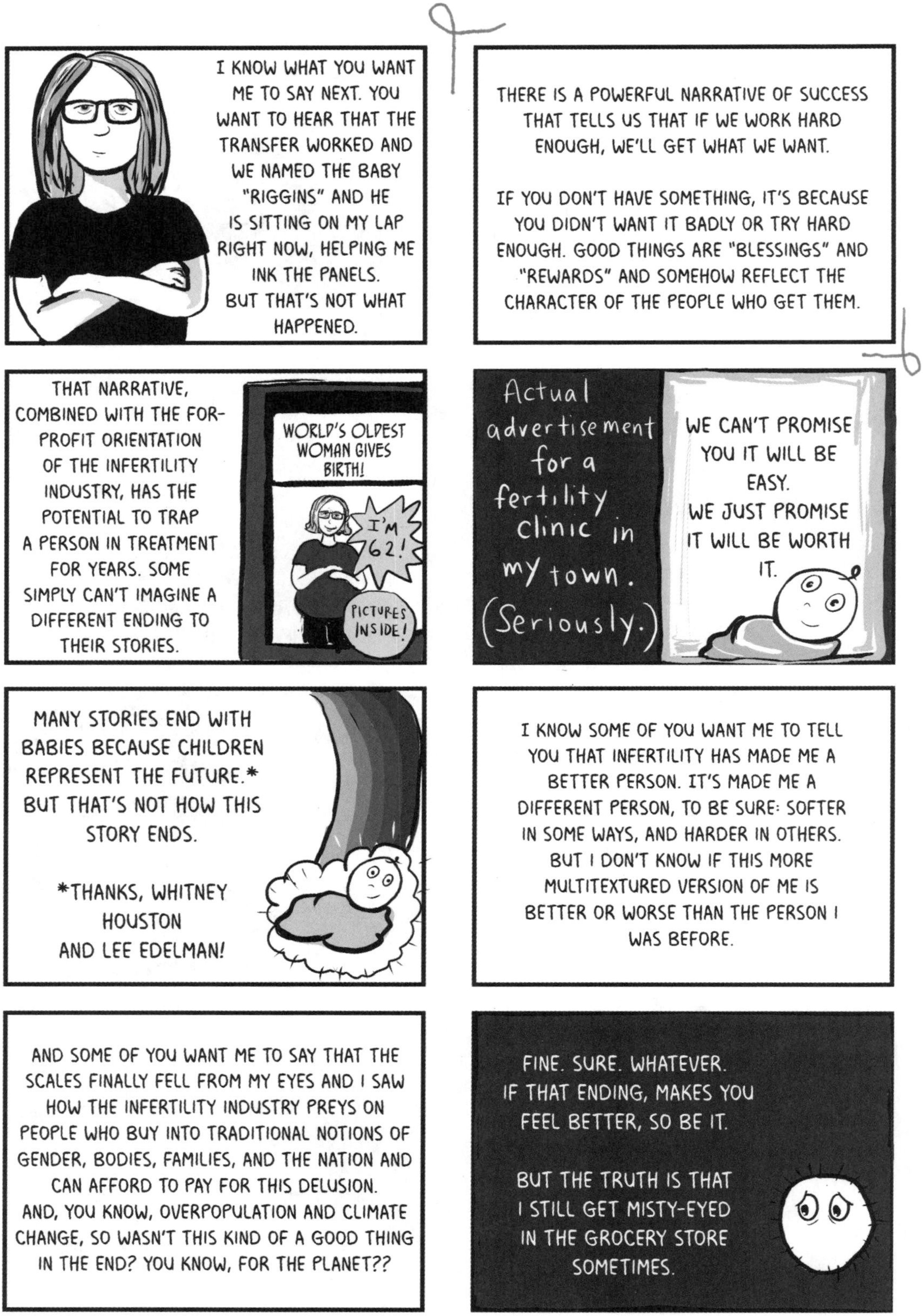
I KNOW WHAT YOU WANT ME TO SAY NEXT. YOU WANT TO HEAR THAT THE TRANSFER WORKED AND WE NAMED THE BABY "RIGGINS" AND HE IS SITTING ON MY LAP RIGHT NOW, HELPING ME INK THE PANELS. BUT THAT'S NOT WHAT HAPPENED.
THERE IS A POWERFUL NARRATIVE OF SUCCESS THAT TELLS US THAT IF WE WORK HARD ENOUGH, WE'LL GET WHAT WE WANT.
IF YOU DON'T HAVE SOMETHING, IT'S BECAUSE YOU DIDN'T WANT IT BADLY OR TRY HARD ENOUGH. GOOD THINGS ARE "BLESSINGS" AND "REWARDS" AND SOMEHOW REFLECT THE CHARACTER OF THE PEOPLE WHO GET THEM.
THAT NARRATIVE, COMBINED WITH THE FOR-PROFIT ORIENTATION OF THE INFERTILITY INDUSTRY, HAS THE POTENTIAL TO TRAP A PERSON IN TREATMENT FOR YEARS. SOME SIMPLY CAN'T IMAGINE A DIFFERENT ENDING TO THEIR STORIES.
WORLD'S OLDEST WOMAN GIVES BIRTH!
I'M 62!
PICTURES INSIDE!
Actual advertisement for a fertility clinic in my town. (Seriously.)
WE CAN'T PROMISE YOU IT WILL BE EASY. WE JUST PROMISE IT WILL BE WORTH IT.
MANY STORIES END WITH BABIES BECAUSE CHILDREN REPRESENT THE FUTURE.* BUT THAT'S NOT HOW THIS STORY ENDS.
*THANKS, WHITNEY HOUSTON AND LEE EDELMAN!
I KNOW SOME OF YOU WANT ME TO TELL YOU THAT INFERTILITY HAS MADE ME A BETTER PERSON. IT'S MADE ME A DIFFERENT PERSON, TO BE SURE: SOFTER IN SOME WAYS, AND HARDER IN OTHERS. BUT I DON'T KNOW IF THIS MORE MULTITEXTURED VERSION OF ME IS BETTER OR WORSE THAN THE PERSON I WAS BEFORE.
AND SOME OF YOU WANT ME TO SAY THAT THE SCALES FINALLY FELL FROM MY EYES AND I SAW HOW THE INFERTILITY INDUSTRY PREYS ON PEOPLE WHO BUY INTO TRADITIONAL NOTIONS OF GENDER, BODIES, FAMILIES, AND THE NATION AND CAN AFFORD TO PAY FOR THIS DELUSION. AND, YOU KNOW, OVERPOPULATION AND CLIMATE CHANGE, SO WASN'T THIS KIND OF A GOOD THING IN THE END? YOU KNOW, FOR THE PLANET??
FINE. SURE. WHATEVER. IF THAT ENDING, MAKES YOU FEEL BETTER, SO BE IT.
BUT THE TRUTH IS THAT I STILL GET MISTY-EYED IN THE GROCERY STORE SOMETIMES.

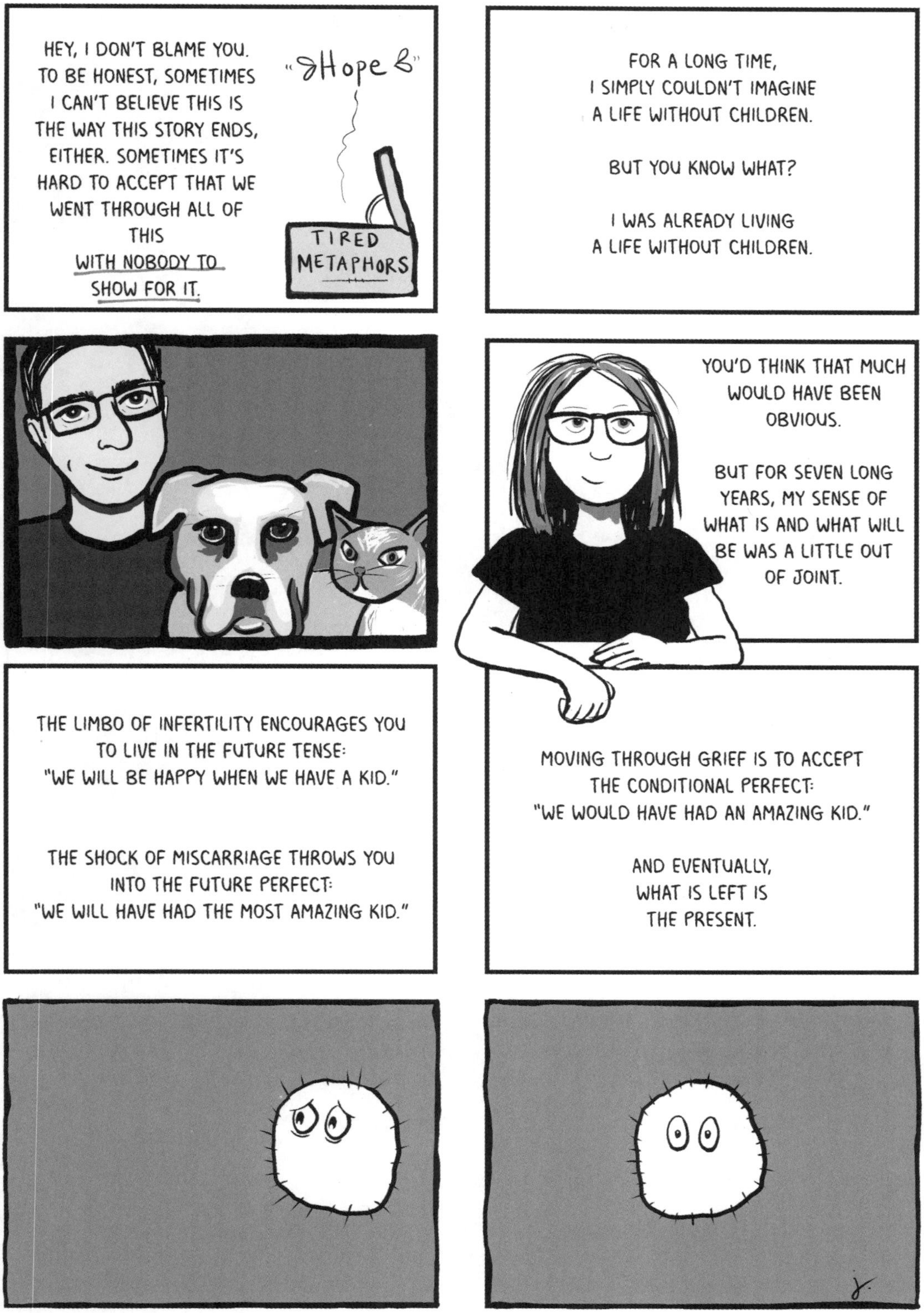

HEY, I DON'T BLAME YOU. TO BE HONEST, SOMETIMES I CAN'T BELIEVE THIS IS THE WAY THIS STORY ENDS, EITHER. SOMETIMES IT'S HARD TO ACCEPT THAT WE WENT THROUGH ALL OF THIS <u>WITH NOBODY TO SHOW FOR IT.</u>

FOR A LONG TIME, I SIMPLY COULDN'T IMAGINE A LIFE WITHOUT CHILDREN.

BUT YOU KNOW WHAT?

I WAS ALREADY LIVING A LIFE WITHOUT CHILDREN.

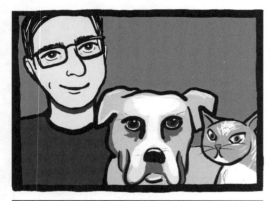

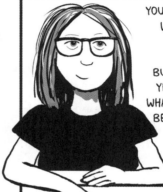

YOU'D THINK THAT MUCH WOULD HAVE BEEN OBVIOUS.

BUT FOR SEVEN LONG YEARS, MY SENSE OF WHAT IS AND WHAT WILL BE WAS A LITTLE OUT OF JOINT.

THE LIMBO OF INFERTILITY ENCOURAGES YOU TO LIVE IN THE FUTURE TENSE: "WE WILL BE HAPPY WHEN WE HAVE A KID."

THE SHOCK OF MISCARRIAGE THROWS YOU INTO THE FUTURE PERFECT: "WE WILL HAVE HAD THE MOST AMAZING KID."

MOVING THROUGH GRIEF IS TO ACCEPT THE CONDITIONAL PERFECT: "WE WOULD HAVE HAD AN AMAZING KID."

AND EVENTUALLY, WHAT IS LEFT IS THE PRESENT.

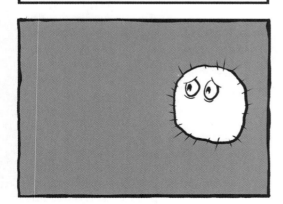

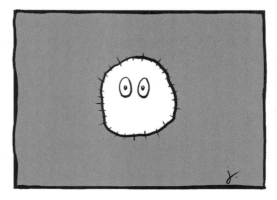

A Significant Loss: The Story of My Miscarriage

(2014)

Endrené Shepherd

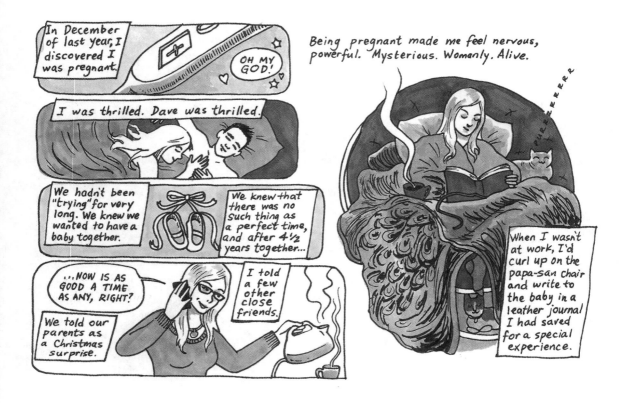

In December of last year, I discovered I was pregnant.

OH MY GOD!

I was thrilled. Dave was thrilled.

We hadn't been "trying" for very long. We knew we wanted to have a baby together.

We knew that there was no such thing as a perfect time, and after 4½ years together...

...NOW IS AS GOOD A TIME AS ANY, RIGHT?

I told a few other close friends.

We told our parents as a Christmas surprise.

Being pregnant made me feel nervous, powerful. Mysterious. Womanly. Alive.

PURRRRRR

When I wasn't at work, I'd curl up on the papa-san chair and write to the baby in a leather journal I had saved for a special experience.

I had an ap on my phone that gave me weekly updates on the baby's status.
I happily told Dave everything I learned.
IT'S AS BIG AS A GRAPE!
COOL!
My mom marked off stuff in the Sears catalogue that she thought we might want for the baby. I felt determined that we could get most of what we needed from Craigslist. No point in buying things new if we would only use some of them for a few months.
CHANGE BABY HERE!
At work, I filled Post-Its with baby names.
hmm
mm
I had one day when I felt 'fluey', but otherwise, I was healthy. I felt buoyed by my secret... a baby was coming!
Dave laid his head on my tummy and said,
HI BABY!
It was all so beautiful.

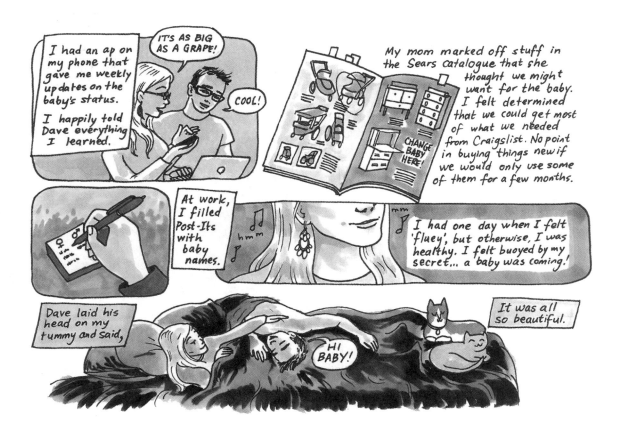

1
2
3
I was looking forward to the end of the first trimester.
YOU'VE GOTTA HAVE A SHOT! IT'S YOUR BIRTHDAY!
AH. UHM, I'M ON ANTIBIOTICS?
OH! TOO BAD!
I was getting tired of lying about why I couldn't drink alcohol, or eat sushi or smoked salmon, or rare steak. I couldn't easily explain why I was suddenly allergic to my own cats, or why I was so day-dreamy.
A week shy of the end of the first trimester, I told all of my coworkers..
(she had already guessed!)
I was really pleased by how supportive and enthusiastic everyone was!
The very next day...
I DON'T WANT TO WAKE UP...

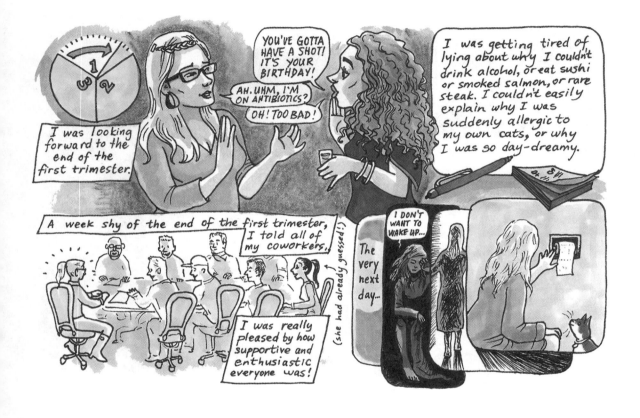

DAVE! DAAAVE!
Huzzn?
I THINK I NEED TO GO TO THE HOSPITAL...
THERE'S BLOOD...
IT COULD BE NOTHING....
BUT I DON'T KNOW...
We went to the ER.
WE'VE GOT YOU BOOKED FOR AN ULTRASOUND AT AROUND 10AM.
I was nervous and cold. I was thankful that at least the Emergency Room wasn't busy and I got my own room, with a door. It was comforting to have Dave stay by my side, and the nurses were kind.
I tried hard to stay positive.
I BROUGHT YOU A WARM BLANKET.
THANK YOU.
Wrapped in blankets, I was wheeled down to the ultrasound room.
The ultrasound tech's face was impassive. She hardly spoke.
THE DOCTOR WILL HAVE A LOOK, AND THEN SHARE THE RESULTS WITH YOU.

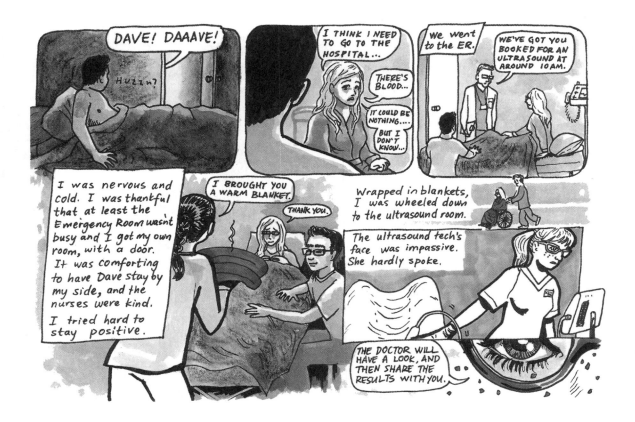

I was wheeled back to the room.

She didn't show me the baby. Not a very good sign...

...still, I was hopeful.

But not optimistic.

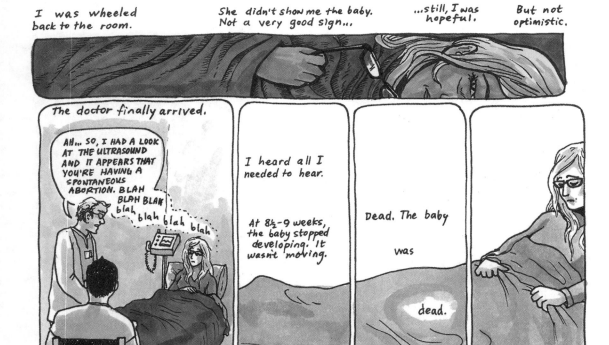

The doctor finally arrived.

AH... SO, I HAD A LOOK AT THE ULTRASOUND AND IT APPEARS THAT YOU'RE HAVING A SPONTANEOUS ABORTION. BLAH BLAH BLAH blah blah blah blah

I heard all I needed to hear.

At 8½-9 weeks, the baby stopped developing. It wasn't moving.

Dead. The baby

was

dead.

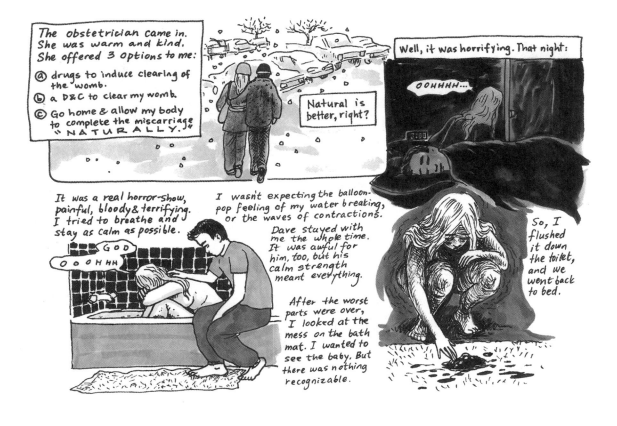

The obstetrician came in. She was warm and kind. She offered 3 options to me:

ⓐ drugs to induce clearing of the womb.

ⓑ a D&C to clear my womb.

ⓒ Go home & allow my body to complete the miscarriage "NATURALLY."

Natural is better, right?

Well, it was horrifying. That night:

OOHHHH...

It was a real horror-show, painful, bloody & terrifying. I tried to breathe and stay as calm as possible.

GOD

OOOHHH

I wasn't expecting the balloon-pop feeling of my water breaking, or the waves of contractions.

Dave stayed with me the whole time. It was awful for him, too, but his calm strength meant everything.

After the worst parts were over, I looked at the mess on the bath mat. I wanted to see the baby. But there was nothing recognizable.

So, I flushed it down the toilet, and we went back to bed.

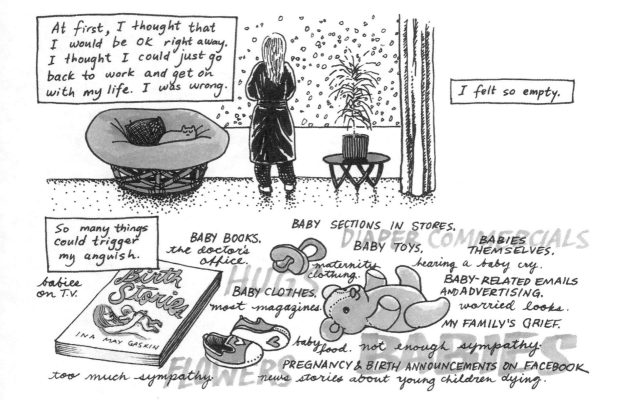

At first, I thought that I would be OK right away. I thought I could just go back to work and get on with my life. I was wrong.

I felt so empty.

So many things could trigger my anguish.

BABY SECTIONS IN STORES.
BABY BOOKS. the doctor's office.
DIAPER COMMERCIALS
BABY TOYS. BABIES THEMSELVES.
maternity clothing. hearing a baby cry.
HUGS
babies on T.V.
BABY CLOTHES.
BABY-RELATED EMAILS AND ADVERTISING.
most magazines.
worried looks.
MY FAMILY'S GRIEF.
baby food. not enough sympathy.
BABIES
too much sympathy. PREGNANCY & BIRTH ANNOUNCEMENTS ON FACEBOOK
FLOWERS news stories about young children dying.

Birth Stories INA MAY GASKIN

I posted a vague status update on FB, asking for kind thoughts as I went through a hard time.
I told the inner circle (and a few kind & curious souls) what was happening.
SIGH.
As I opened up to others, they opened up to me.
It turned out that I had joined one of the planet's most miserable (mostly secret) societies.
Talking to women, almost every one of them with a child had had at least one miscarriage.
Miscarriage isn't normally one of those things introduced as a conversational topic.
I LOST 3 BABIES BEFORE MY SON WAS BORN...
I'VE HAD FIVE. IT NEVER GOT EASIER.
I STILL HAVE THE ULTRASOUND...
I DIDN'T EVEN KNOW I WAS PREGNANT...
I WAS FIVE MONTHS ALONG, SO I THOUGHT I WAS SAFE...
I NAMED THEM BOTH.
Talking about it eased my sense of isolation.

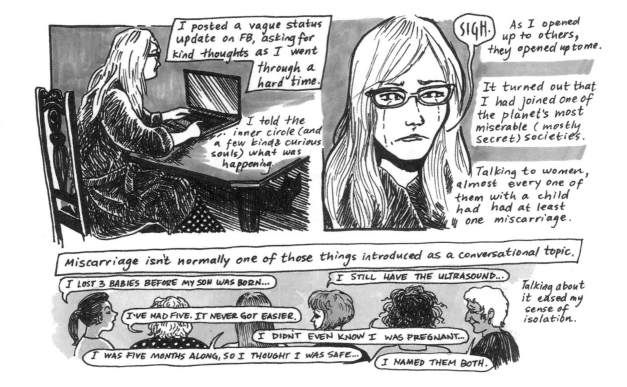

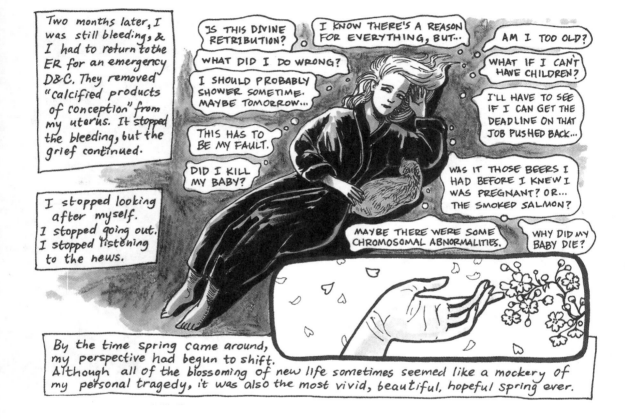

Two months later, I was still bleeding, & I had to return to the ER for an emergency D&C. They removed "calcified products of conception" from my uterus. It stopped the bleeding, but the grief continued.

I stopped looking after myself. I stopped going out. I stopped listening to the news.

IS THIS DIVINE RETRIBUTION?

WHAT DID I DO WRONG?

I SHOULD PROBABLY SHOWER SOMETIME. MAYBE TOMORROW...

THIS HAS TO BE MY FAULT.

DID I KILL MY BABY?

I KNOW THERE'S A REASON FOR EVERYTHING, BUT...

AM I TOO OLD?

WHAT IF I CAN'T HAVE CHILDREN?

I'LL HAVE TO SEE IF I CAN GET THE DEADLINE ON THAT JOB PUSHED BACK...

WAS IT THOSE BEERS I HAD BEFORE I KNEW I WAS PREGNANT? OR... THE SMOKED SALMON?

MAYBE THERE WERE SOME CHROMOSOMAL ABNORMALITIES.

WHY DID MY BABY DIE?

By the time spring came around, my perspective had begun to shift. Although all of the blossoming of new life sometimes seemed like a mockery of my personal tragedy, it was also the most vivid, beautiful, hopeful spring ever.

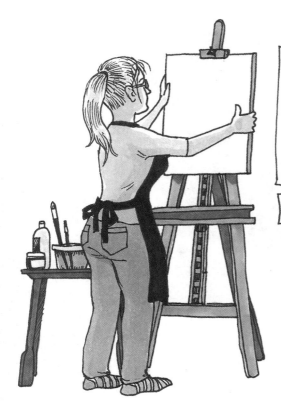

It's almost been a year now, and I mostly feel OK. I can talk about this experience without bursting into tears, most days. I'm not pregnant again, even though that's the advice that well-meaning people generally give. I'll always be sad to have lost that baby. That specific baby. I'm not in a hurry to replace him.
I'd still like to have kids, but it's OK if it's not in the cards. Who knows, right?
ALL YOU NEED IS LOVE
I'll be OK.

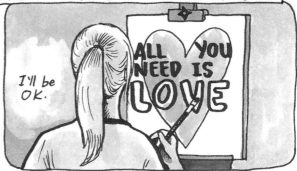

"Losing Thomas and Ella: A Father's Story"

(2015)

Marcus B. Weaver-Hightower

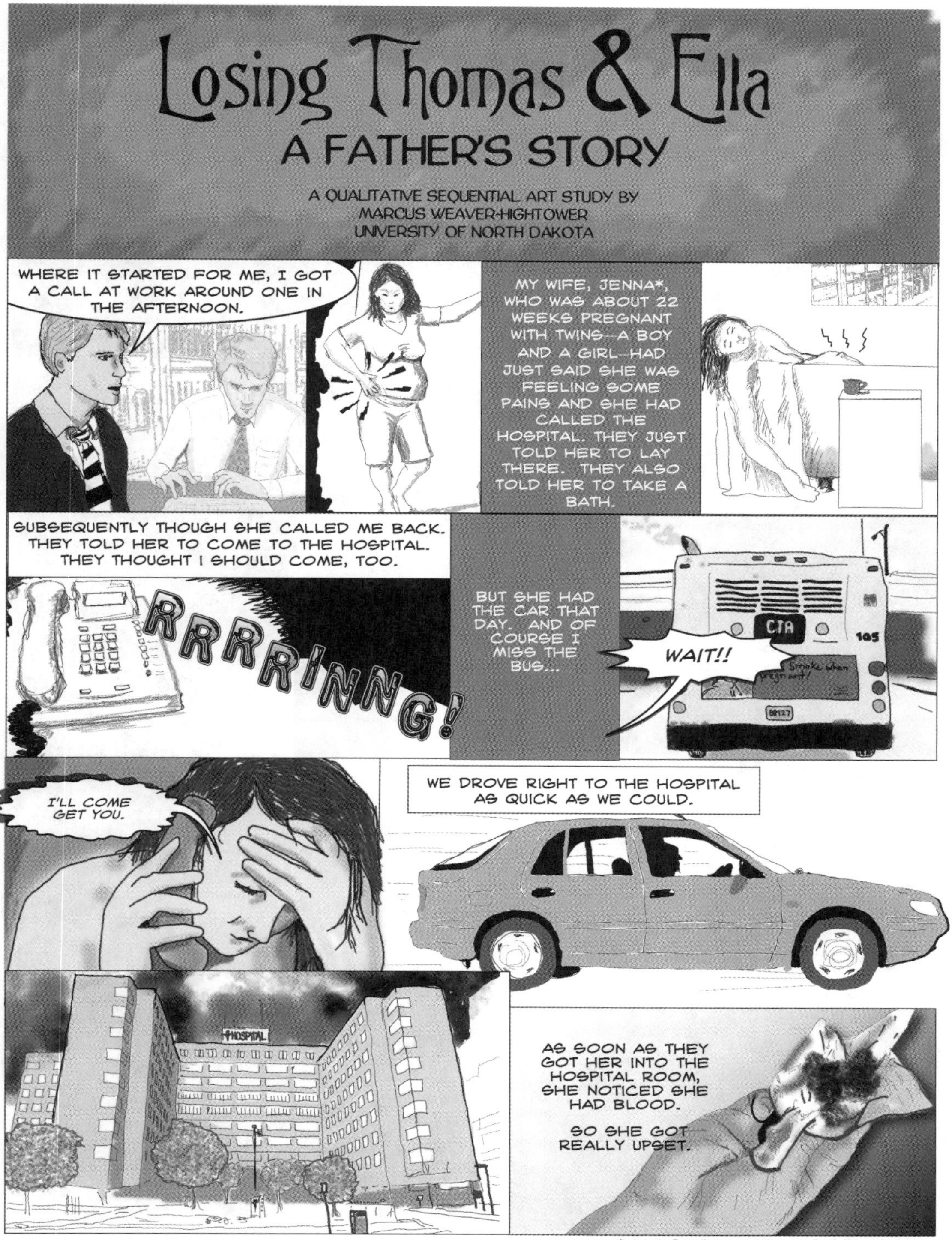
Losing Thomas & Ella
A FATHER'S STORY
A QUALITATIVE SEQUENTIAL ART STUDY BY MARCUS WEAVER-HIGHTOWER UNIVERSITY OF NORTH DAKOTA
WHERE IT STARTED FOR ME, I GOT A CALL AT WORK AROUND ONE IN THE AFTERNOON.
MY WIFE, JENNA*, WHO WAS ABOUT 22 WEEKS PREGNANT WITH TWINS—A BOY AND A GIRL—HAD JUST SAID SHE WAS FEELING SOME PAINS AND SHE HAD CALLED THE HOSPITAL. THEY JUST TOLD HER TO LAY THERE. THEY ALSO TOLD HER TO TAKE A BATH.
SUBSEQUENTLY THOUGH SHE CALLED ME BACK. THEY TOLD HER TO COME TO THE HOSPITAL. THEY THOUGHT I SHOULD COME, TOO.
RRRRINNG!
BUT SHE HAD THE CAR THAT DAY. AND OF COURSE I MISS THE BUS...
CTA
105
WAIT!!
I'LL COME GET YOU.
WE DROVE RIGHT TO THE HOSPITAL AS QUICK AS WE COULD.
HOSPITAL
AS SOON AS THEY GOT HER INTO THE HOSPITAL ROOM, SHE NOTICED SHE HAD BLOOD.
SO SHE GOT REALLY UPSET.

* PSEUDONYMS ARE USED THROUGHOUT.

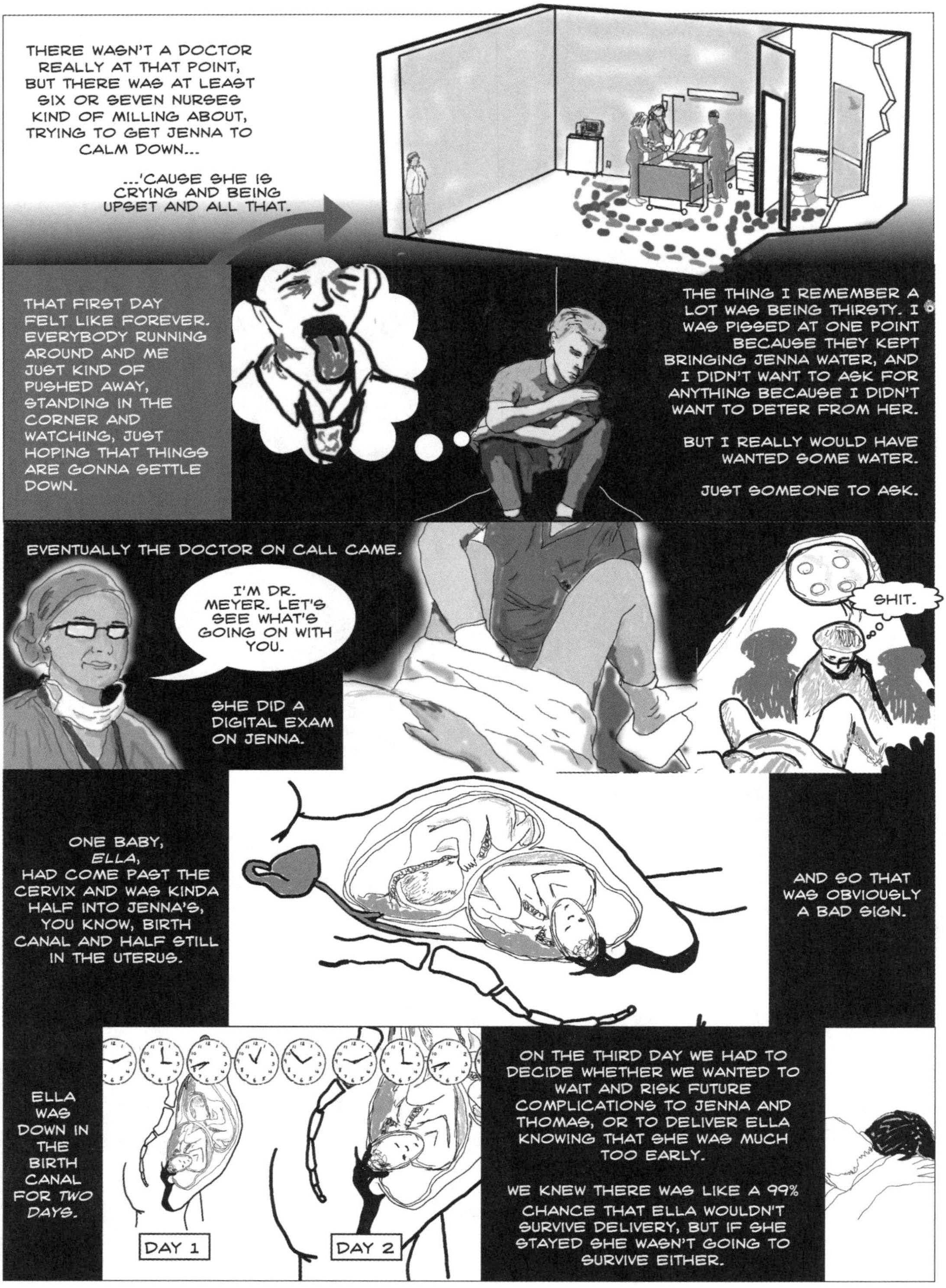
THERE WASN'T A DOCTOR REALLY AT THAT POINT, BUT THERE WAS AT LEAST SIX OR SEVEN NURSES KIND OF MILLING ABOUT, TRYING TO GET JENNA TO CALM DOWN...
...'CAUSE SHE IS CRYING AND BEING UPSET AND ALL THAT.
THAT FIRST DAY FELT LIKE FOREVER. EVERYBODY RUNNING AROUND AND ME JUST KIND OF PUSHED AWAY, STANDING IN THE CORNER AND WATCHING, JUST HOPING THAT THINGS ARE GONNA SETTLE DOWN.
THE THING I REMEMBER A LOT WAS BEING THIRSTY. I WAS PISSED AT ONE POINT BECAUSE THEY KEPT BRINGING JENNA WATER, AND I DIDN'T WANT TO ASK FOR ANYTHING BECAUSE I DIDN'T WANT TO DETER FROM HER.
BUT I REALLY WOULD HAVE WANTED SOME WATER.
JUST SOMEONE TO ASK.
EVENTUALLY THE DOCTOR ON CALL CAME.
I'M DR. MEYER. LET'S SEE WHAT'S GOING ON WITH YOU.
SHE DID A DIGITAL EXAM ON JENNA.
SHIT.
ONE BABY, *ELLA*, HAD COME PAST THE CERVIX AND WAS KINDA HALF INTO JENNA'S, YOU KNOW, BIRTH CANAL AND HALF STILL IN THE UTERUS.
AND SO THAT WAS OBVIOUSLY A BAD SIGN.
ELLA WAS DOWN IN THE BIRTH CANAL FOR *TWO DAYS*.
DAY 1
DAY 2
ON THE THIRD DAY WE HAD TO DECIDE WHETHER WE WANTED TO WAIT AND RISK FUTURE COMPLICATIONS TO JENNA AND THOMAS, OR TO DELIVER ELLA KNOWING THAT SHE WAS MUCH TOO EARLY.
WE KNEW THERE WAS LIKE A 99% CHANCE THAT ELLA WOULDN'T SURVIVE DELIVERY, BUT IF SHE STAYED SHE WASN'T GOING TO SURVIVE EITHER.

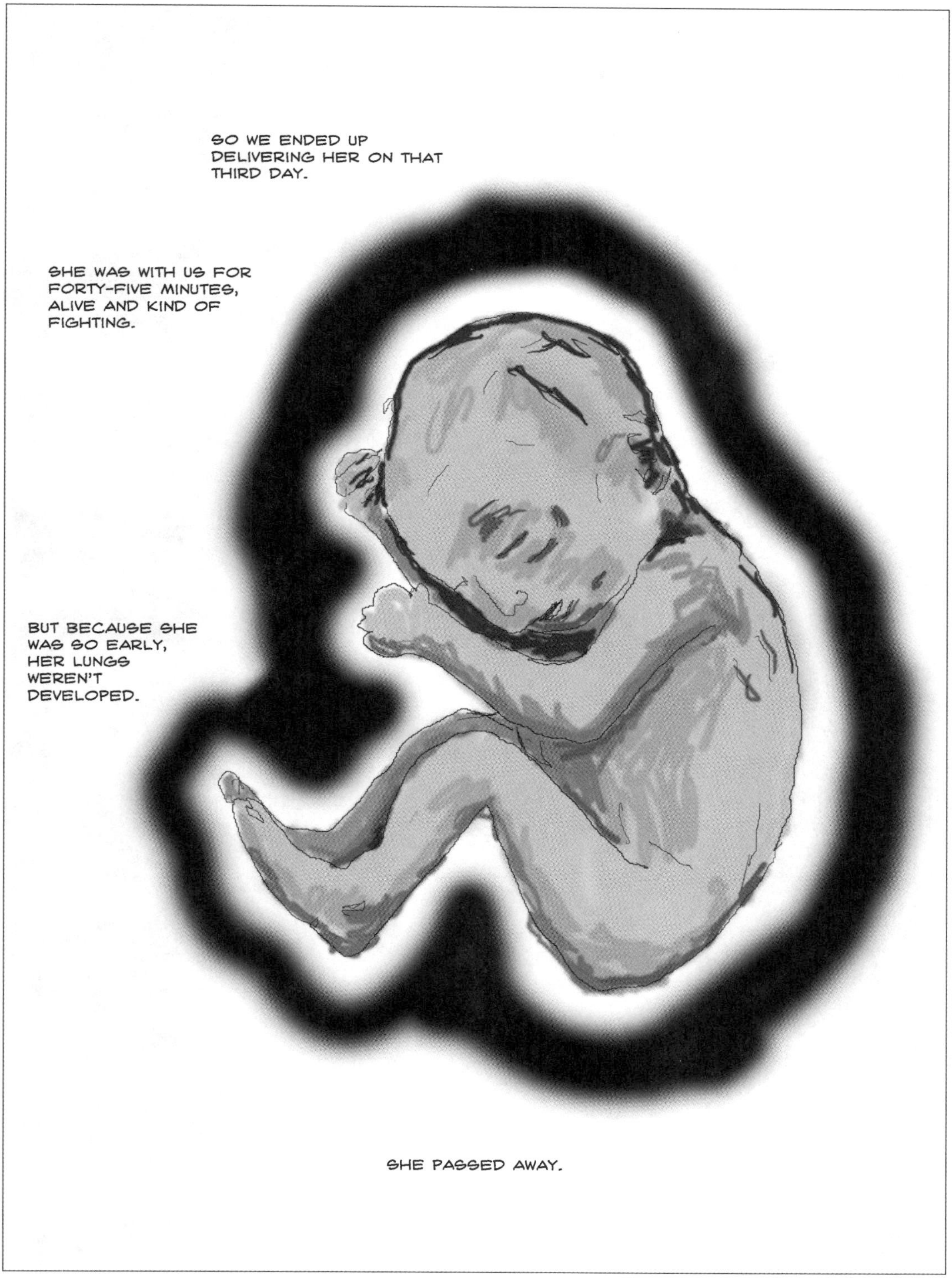
SO WE ENDED UP DELIVERING HER ON THAT THIRD DAY.
SHE WAS WITH US FOR FORTY-FIVE MINUTES, ALIVE AND KIND OF FIGHTING.
BUT BECAUSE SHE WAS SO EARLY, HER LUNGS WEREN'T DEVELOPED.
SHE PASSED AWAY.

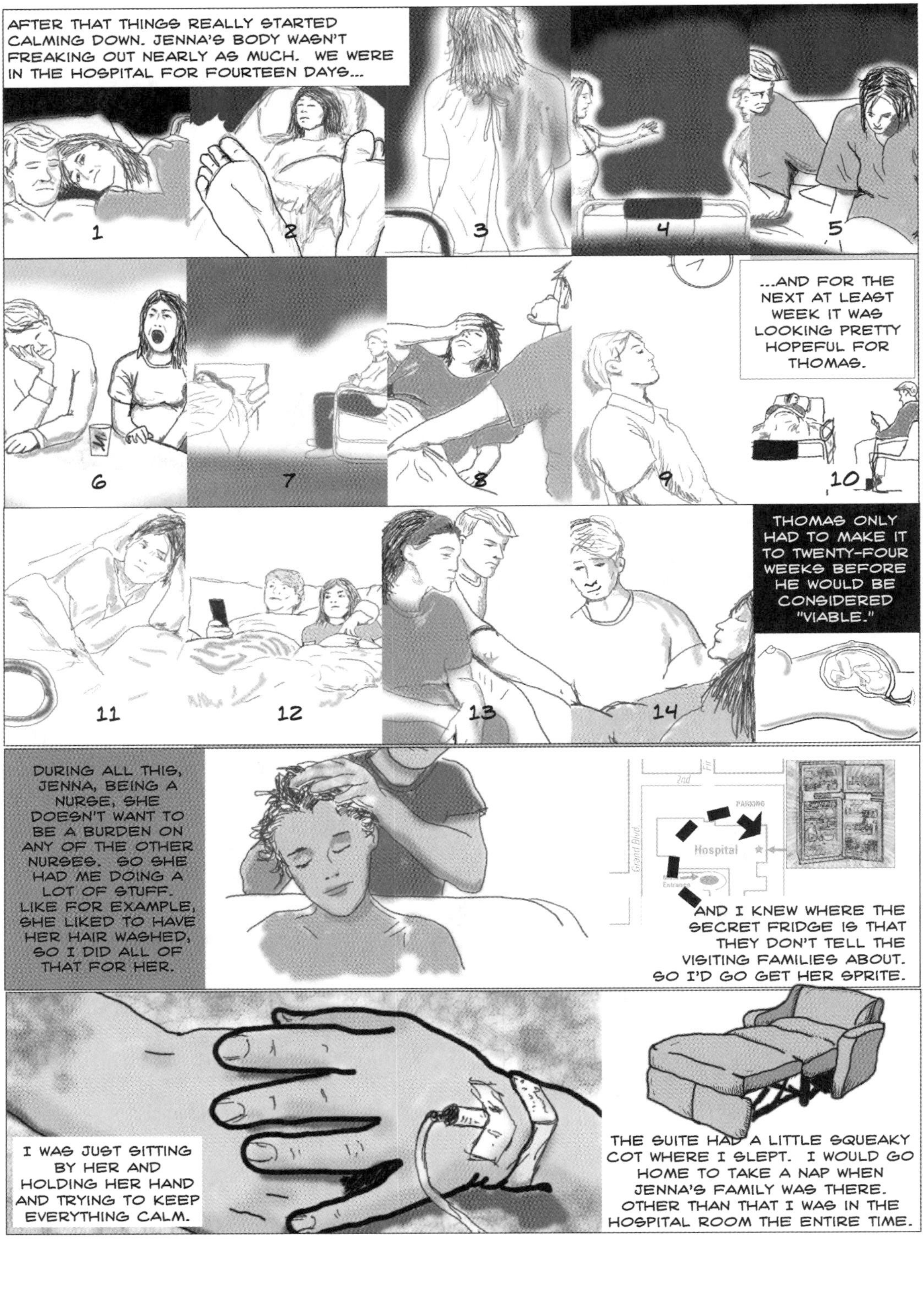
AFTER THAT THINGS REALLY STARTED CALMING DOWN. JENNA'S BODY WASN'T FREAKING OUT NEARLY AS MUCH. WE WERE IN THE HOSPITAL FOR FOURTEEN DAYS...
...AND FOR THE NEXT AT LEAST WEEK IT WAS LOOKING PRETTY HOPEFUL FOR THOMAS.
THOMAS ONLY HAD TO MAKE IT TO TWENTY-FOUR WEEKS BEFORE HE WOULD BE CONSIDERED "VIABLE."
DURING ALL THIS, JENNA, BEING A NURSE, SHE DOESN'T WANT TO BE A BURDEN ON ANY OF THE OTHER NURSES. SO SHE HAD ME DOING A LOT OF STUFF. LIKE FOR EXAMPLE, SHE LIKED TO HAVE HER HAIR WASHED, SO I DID ALL OF THAT FOR HER.
PARKING
Hospital
Grand Blvd
AND I KNEW WHERE THE SECRET FRIDGE IS THAT THEY DON'T TELL THE VISITING FAMILIES ABOUT. SO I'D GO GET HER SPRITE.
I WAS JUST SITTING BY HER AND HOLDING HER HAND AND TRYING TO KEEP EVERYTHING CALM.
THE SUITE HAD A LITTLE SQUEAKY COT WHERE I SLEPT. I WOULD GO HOME TO TAKE A NAP WHEN JENNA'S FAMILY WAS THERE. OTHER THAN THAT I WAS IN THE HOSPITAL ROOM THE ENTIRE TIME.

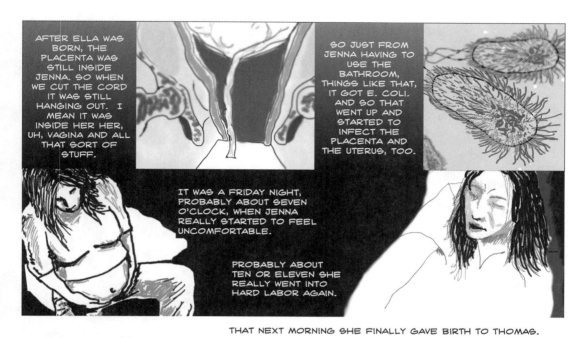

AFTER ELLA WAS BORN, THE PLACENTA WAS STILL INSIDE JENNA. SO WHEN WE CUT THE CORD IT WAS STILL HANGING OUT. I MEAN IT WAS INSIDE HER HER, UH, VAGINA AND ALL THAT SORT OF STUFF.

SO JUST FROM JENNA HAVING TO USE THE BATHROOM, THINGS LIKE THAT, IT GOT E. COLI. AND SO THAT WENT UP AND STARTED TO INFECT THE PLACENTA AND THE UTERUS, TOO.

IT WAS A FRIDAY NIGHT, PROBABLY ABOUT SEVEN O'CLOCK, WHEN JENNA REALLY STARTED TO FEEL UNCOMFORTABLE.

PROBABLY ABOUT TEN OR ELEVEN SHE REALLY WENT INTO HARD LABOR AGAIN.

THAT NEXT MORNING SHE FINALLY GAVE BIRTH TO THOMAS.

HE CAME OUT INSIDE THE SACK.*

WHEN THE DOCTOR OPENED THE SACK, THOMAS WAS ALREADY STILLBORN.

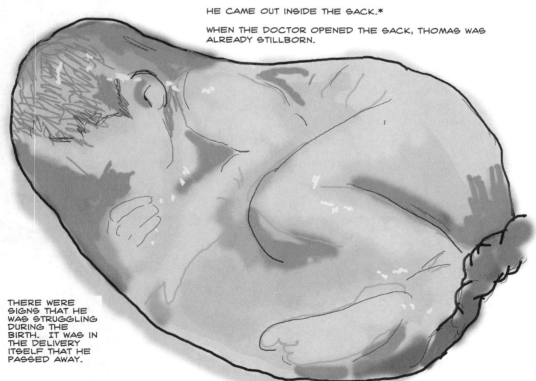

THERE WERE SIGNS THAT HE WAS STRUGGLING DURING THE BIRTH. IT WAS IN THE DELIVERY ITSELF THAT HE PASSED AWAY.

*Also called a "veiled" or "en-caul" birth.

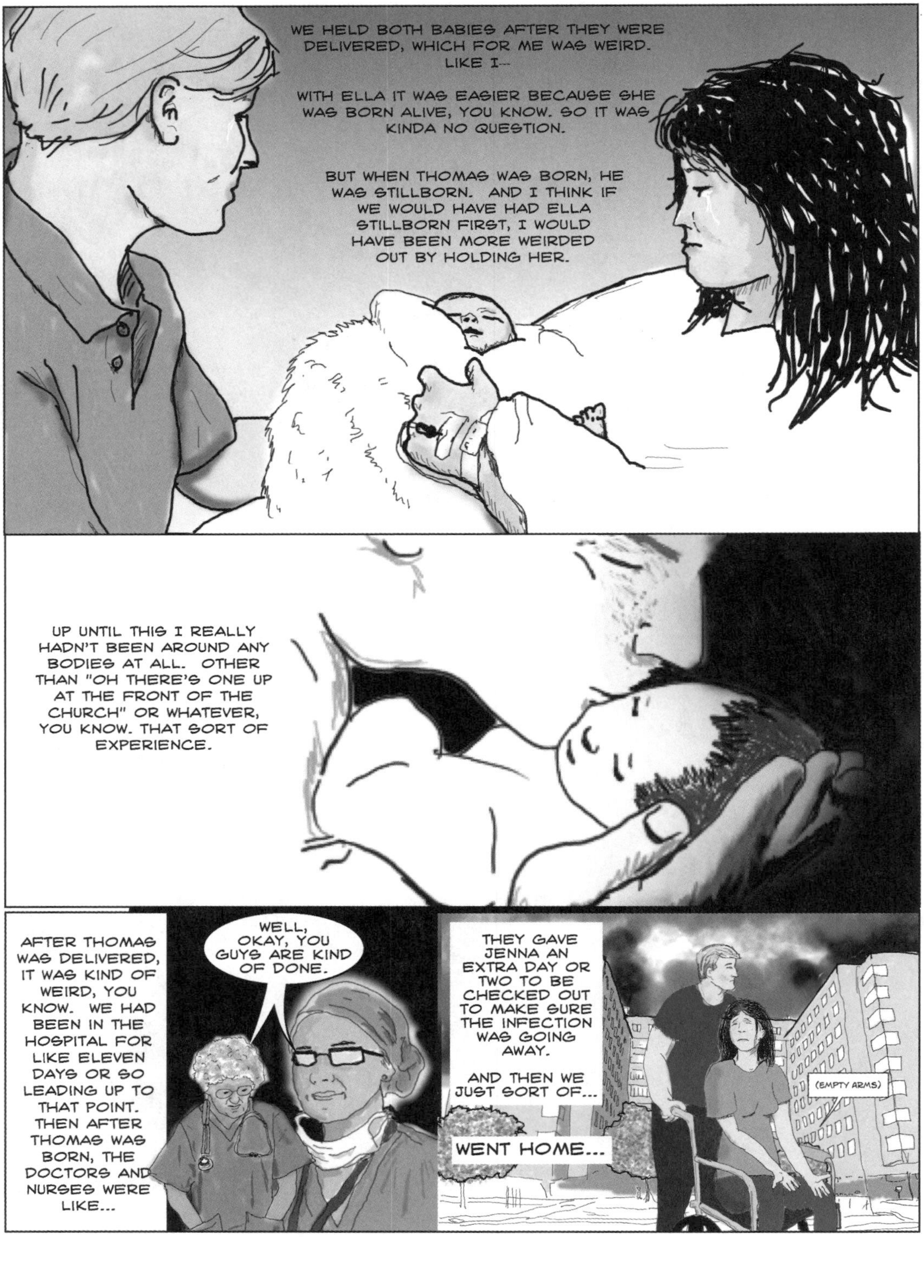
WE HELD BOTH BABIES AFTER THEY WERE DELIVERED, WHICH FOR ME WAS WEIRD. LIKE I--
WITH ELLA IT WAS EASIER BECAUSE SHE WAS BORN ALIVE, YOU KNOW. SO IT WAS KINDA NO QUESTION.
BUT WHEN THOMAS WAS BORN, HE WAS STILLBORN. AND I THINK IF WE WOULD HAVE HAD ELLA STILLBORN FIRST, I WOULD HAVE BEEN MORE WEIRDED OUT BY HOLDING HER.
UP UNTIL THIS I REALLY HADN'T BEEN AROUND ANY BODIES AT ALL. OTHER THAN "OH THERE'S ONE UP AT THE FRONT OF THE CHURCH" OR WHATEVER, YOU KNOW. THAT SORT OF EXPERIENCE.
AFTER THOMAS WAS DELIVERED, IT WAS KIND OF WEIRD, YOU KNOW. WE HAD BEEN IN THE HOSPITAL FOR LIKE ELEVEN DAYS OR SO LEADING UP TO THAT POINT. THEN AFTER THOMAS WAS BORN, THE DOCTORS AND NURSES WERE LIKE...
WELL, OKAY, YOU GUYS ARE KIND OF DONE.
THEY GAVE JENNA AN EXTRA DAY OR TWO TO BE CHECKED OUT TO MAKE SURE THE INFECTION WAS GOING AWAY.
AND THEN WE JUST SORT OF...
WENT HOME...
(EMPTY ARMS)

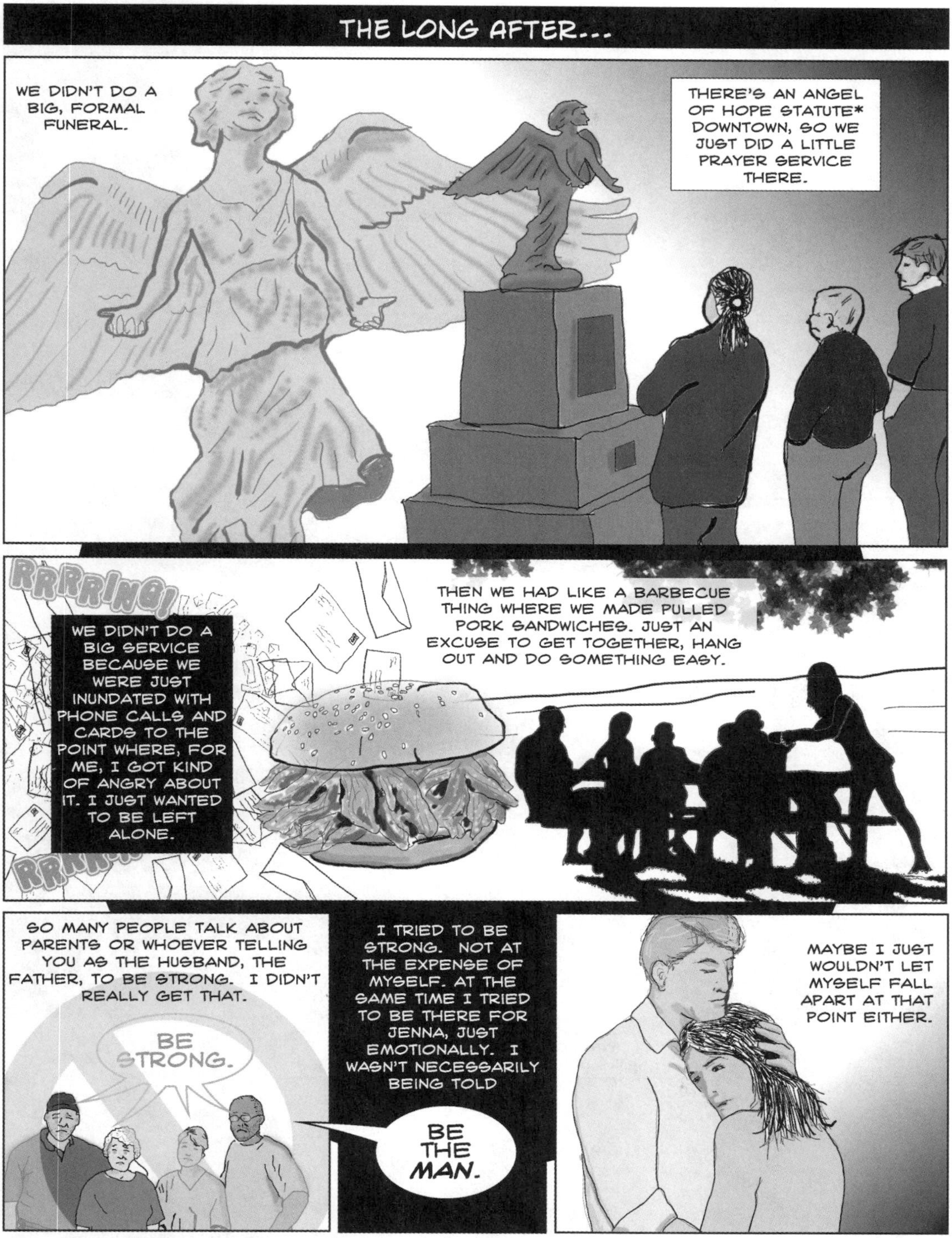
THE LONG AFTER...
WE DIDN'T DO A BIG, FORMAL FUNERAL.
THERE'S AN ANGEL OF HOPE STATUTE* DOWNTOWN, SO WE JUST DID A LITTLE PRAYER SERVICE THERE.
RRRRING!
WE DIDN'T DO A BIG SERVICE BECAUSE WE WERE JUST INUNDATED WITH PHONE CALLS AND CARDS TO THE POINT WHERE, FOR ME, I GOT KIND OF ANGRY ABOUT IT. I JUST WANTED TO BE LEFT ALONE.
THEN WE HAD LIKE A BARBECUE THING WHERE WE MADE PULLED PORK SANDWICHES. JUST AN EXCUSE TO GET TOGETHER, HANG OUT AND DO SOMETHING EASY.
SO MANY PEOPLE TALK ABOUT PARENTS OR WHOEVER TELLING YOU AS THE HUSBAND, THE FATHER, TO BE STRONG. I DIDN'T REALLY GET THAT.
BE STRONG.
I TRIED TO BE STRONG. NOT AT THE EXPENSE OF MYSELF. AT THE SAME TIME I TRIED TO BE THERE FOR JENNA, JUST EMOTIONALLY. I WASN'T NECESSARILY BEING TOLD
BE THE MAN.
MAYBE I JUST WOULDN'T LET MYSELF FALL APART AT THAT POINT EITHER.

* SO-CALLED "CHRISTMAS BOX ANGEL STATUES" HAVE BEEN ERECTED WORLDWIDE TO COMMEMORATE DEAD CHILDREN, BASED ON A NOVEL BY RICHARD PAUL EVANS (1993).

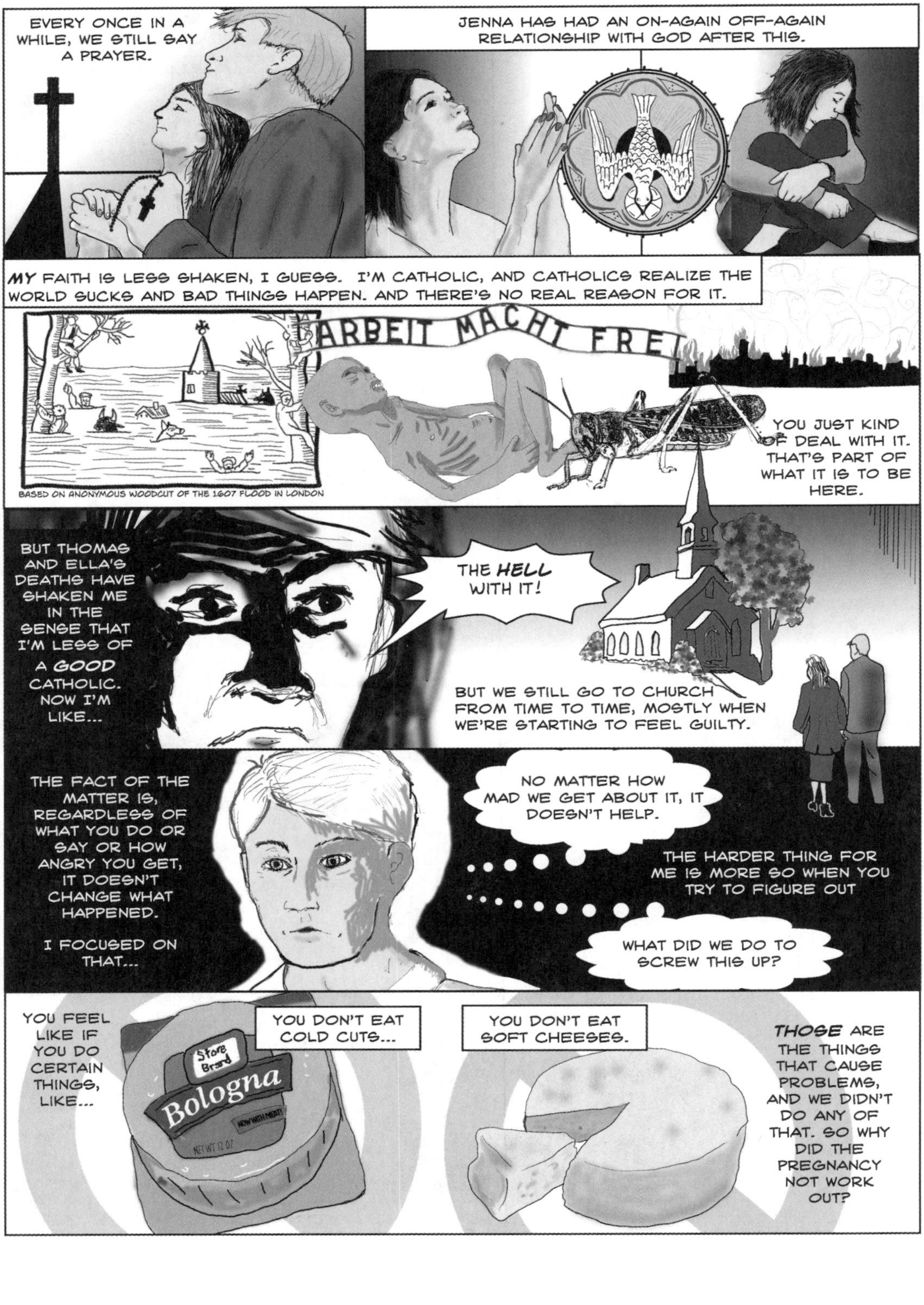
EVERY ONCE IN A WHILE, WE STILL SAY A PRAYER.
JENNA HAS HAD AN ON-AGAIN OFF-AGAIN RELATIONSHIP WITH GOD AFTER THIS.
MY FAITH IS LESS SHAKEN, I GUESS. I'M CATHOLIC, AND CATHOLICS REALIZE THE WORLD SUCKS AND BAD THINGS HAPPEN. AND THERE'S NO REAL REASON FOR IT.
ARBEIT MACHT FREI
BASED ON ANONYMOUS WOODCUT OF THE 1607 FLOOD IN LONDON
YOU JUST KIND OF DEAL WITH IT. THAT'S PART OF WHAT IT IS TO BE HERE.
BUT THOMAS AND ELLA'S DEATHS HAVE SHAKEN ME IN THE SENSE THAT I'M LESS OF A GOOD CATHOLIC. NOW I'M LIKE...
THE HELL WITH IT!
BUT WE STILL GO TO CHURCH FROM TIME TO TIME, MOSTLY WHEN WE'RE STARTING TO FEEL GUILTY.
THE FACT OF THE MATTER IS, REGARDLESS OF WHAT YOU DO OR SAY OR HOW ANGRY YOU GET, IT DOESN'T CHANGE WHAT HAPPENED.
I FOCUSED ON THAT...
NO MATTER HOW MAD WE GET ABOUT IT, IT DOESN'T HELP.
THE HARDER THING FOR ME IS MORE SO WHEN YOU TRY TO FIGURE OUT
WHAT DID WE DO TO SCREW THIS UP?
YOU FEEL LIKE IF YOU DO CERTAIN THINGS, LIKE...
YOU DON'T EAT COLD CUTS...
Store Brand
Bologna
NOW WITH MEAT!
NET WT 12 OZ
YOU DON'T EAT SOFT CHEESES.
THOSE ARE THE THINGS THAT CAUSE PROBLEMS, AND WE DIDN'T DO ANY OF THAT. SO WHY DID THE PREGNANCY NOT WORK OUT?

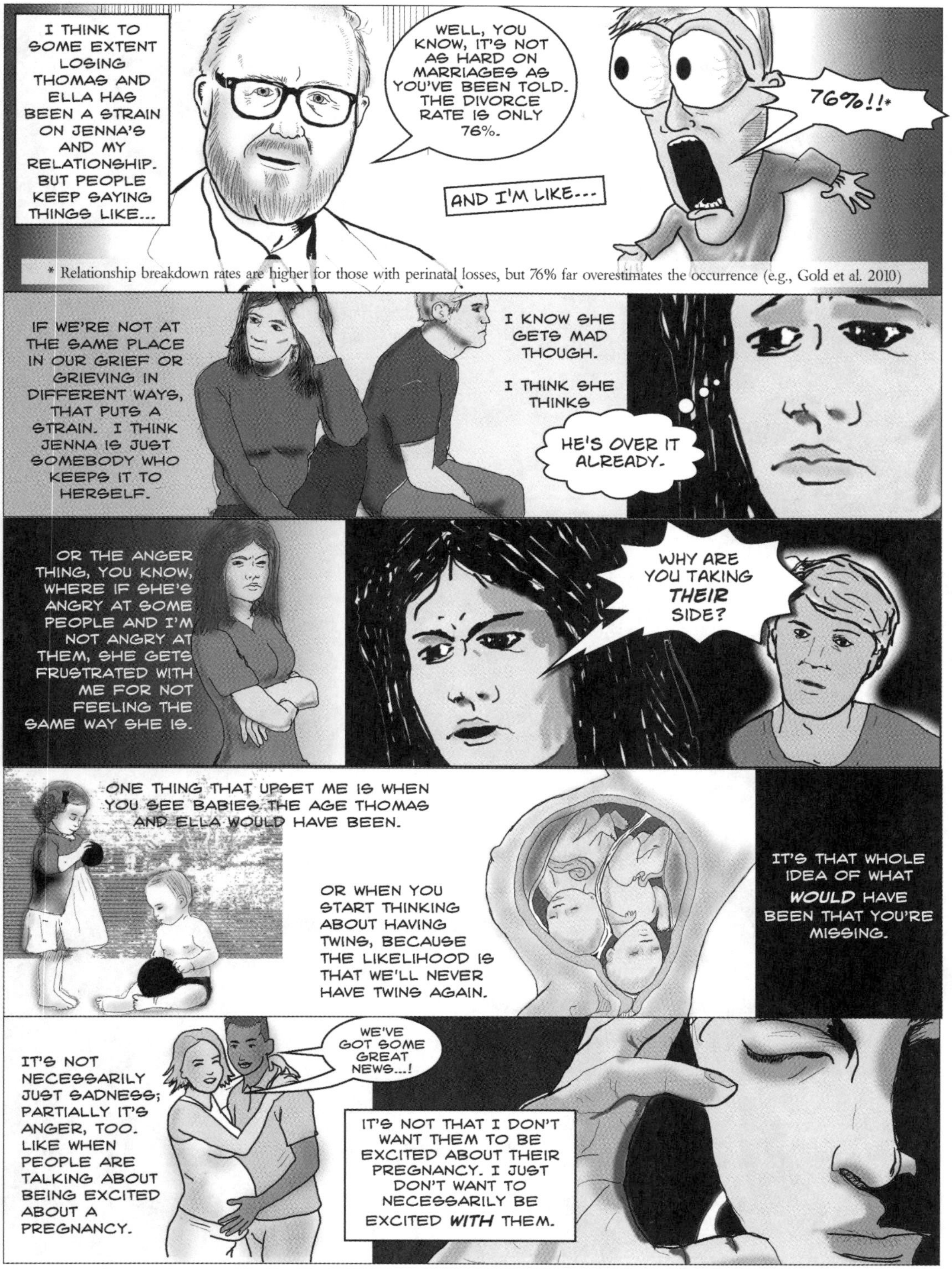
I THINK TO SOME EXTENT LOSING THOMAS AND ELLA HAS BEEN A STRAIN ON JENNA'S AND MY RELATIONSHIP. BUT PEOPLE KEEP SAYING THINGS LIKE...
WELL, YOU KNOW, IT'S NOT AS HARD ON MARRIAGES AS YOU'VE BEEN TOLD. THE DIVORCE RATE IS ONLY 76%.
AND I'M LIKE...
76%!!*
* Relationship breakdown rates are higher for those with perinatal losses, but 76% far overestimates the occurrence (e.g., Gold et al. 2010)
IF WE'RE NOT AT THE SAME PLACE IN OUR GRIEF OR GRIEVING IN DIFFERENT WAYS, THAT PUTS A STRAIN. I THINK JENNA IS JUST SOMEBODY WHO KEEPS IT TO HERSELF.
I KNOW SHE GETS MAD THOUGH.
I THINK SHE THINKS
HE'S OVER IT ALREADY.
OR THE ANGER THING, YOU KNOW, WHERE IF SHE'S ANGRY AT SOME PEOPLE AND I'M NOT ANGRY AT THEM, SHE GETS FRUSTRATED WITH ME FOR NOT FEELING THE SAME WAY SHE IS.
WHY ARE YOU TAKING THEIR SIDE?
ONE THING THAT UPSET ME IS WHEN YOU SEE BABIES THE AGE THOMAS AND ELLA WOULD HAVE BEEN.
OR WHEN YOU START THINKING ABOUT HAVING TWINS, BECAUSE THE LIKELIHOOD IS THAT WE'LL NEVER HAVE TWINS AGAIN.
IT'S THAT WHOLE IDEA OF WHAT WOULD HAVE BEEN THAT YOU'RE MISSING.
IT'S NOT NECESSARILY JUST SADNESS; PARTIALLY IT'S ANGER, TOO. LIKE WHEN PEOPLE ARE TALKING ABOUT BEING EXCITED ABOUT A PREGNANCY.
WE'VE GOT SOME GREAT NEWS...!
IT'S NOT THAT I DON'T WANT THEM TO BE EXCITED ABOUT THEIR PREGNANCY. I JUST DON'T WANT TO NECESSARILY BE EXCITED WITH THEM.

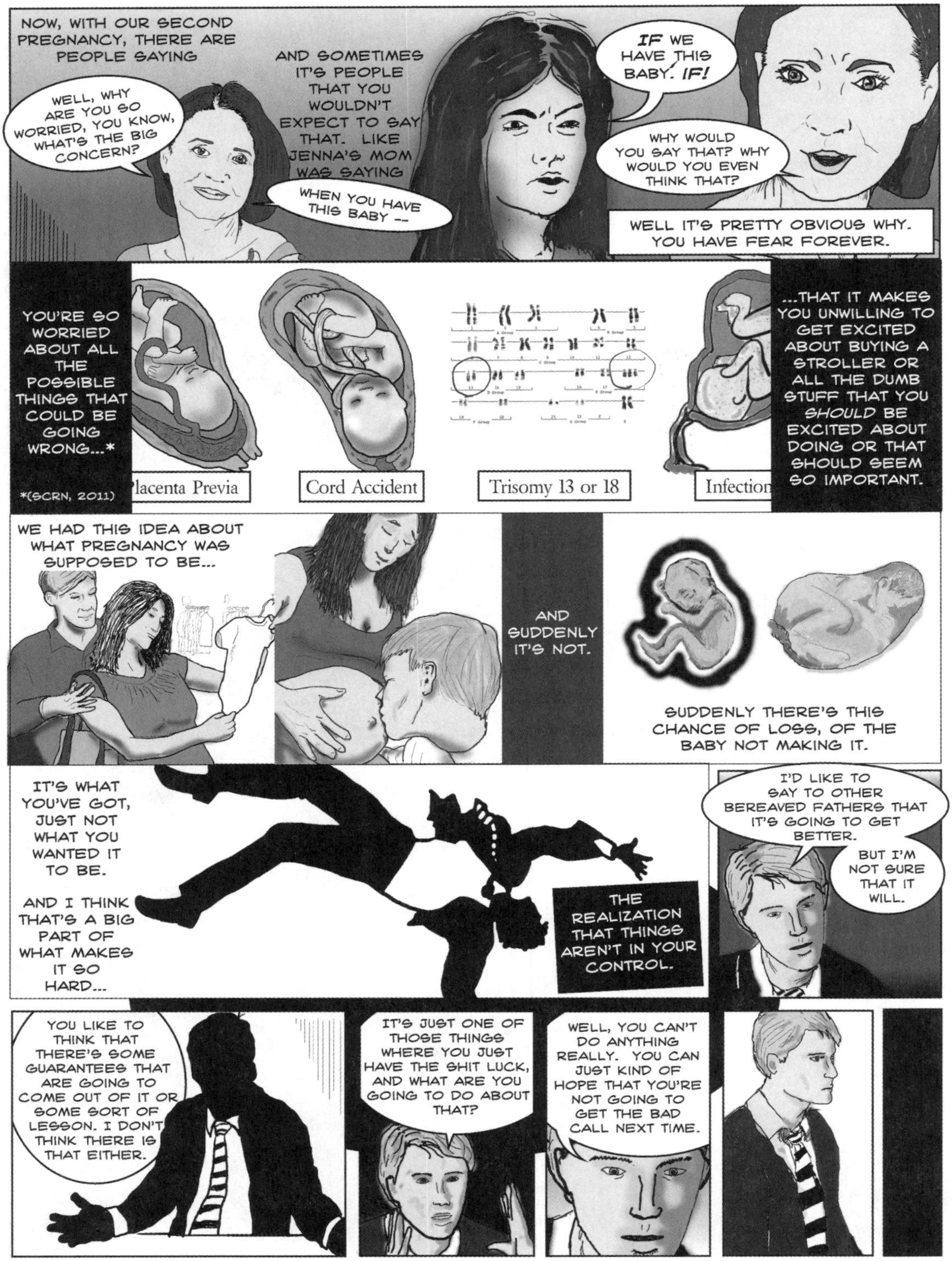
NOW, WITH OUR SECOND PREGNANCY, THERE ARE PEOPLE SAYING
WELL, WHY ARE YOU SO WORRIED, YOU KNOW, WHAT'S THE BIG CONCERN?
AND SOMETIMES IT'S PEOPLE THAT YOU WOULDN'T EXPECT TO SAY THAT. LIKE JENNA'S MOM WAS SAYING
WHEN YOU HAVE THIS BABY --
IF WE HAVE THIS BABY. IF!
WHY WOULD YOU SAY THAT? WHY WOULD YOU EVEN THINK THAT?
WELL IT'S PRETTY OBVIOUS WHY. YOU HAVE FEAR FOREVER.
YOU'RE SO WORRIED ABOUT ALL THE POSSIBLE THINGS THAT COULD BE GOING WRONG...*
*(SCRN, 2011)
Placenta Previa
Cord Accident
Trisomy 13 or 18
Infection
...THAT IT MAKES YOU UNWILLING TO GET EXCITED ABOUT BUYING A STROLLER OR ALL THE DUMB STUFF THAT YOU SHOULD BE EXCITED ABOUT DOING OR THAT SHOULD SEEM SO IMPORTANT.
WE HAD THIS IDEA ABOUT WHAT PREGNANCY WAS SUPPOSED TO BE...
AND SUDDENLY IT'S NOT.
SUDDENLY THERE'S THIS CHANCE OF LOSS, OF THE BABY NOT MAKING IT.
IT'S WHAT YOU'VE GOT, JUST NOT WHAT YOU WANTED IT TO BE.
AND I THINK THAT'S A BIG PART OF WHAT MAKES IT SO HARD...
THE REALIZATION THAT THINGS AREN'T IN YOUR CONTROL.
I'D LIKE TO SAY TO OTHER BEREAVED FATHERS THAT IT'S GOING TO GET BETTER.
BUT I'M NOT SURE THAT IT WILL.
YOU LIKE TO THINK THAT THERE'S SOME GUARANTEES THAT ARE GOING TO COME OUT OF IT OR SOME SORT OF LESSON. I DON'T THINK THERE IS THAT EITHER.
IT'S JUST ONE OF THOSE THINGS WHERE YOU JUST HAVE THE SHIT LUCK, AND WHAT ARE YOU GOING TO DO ABOUT THAT?
WELL, YOU CAN'T DO ANYTHING REALLY. YOU CAN JUST KIND OF HOPE THAT YOU'RE NOT GOING TO GET THE BAD CALL NEXT TIME.

Pregnant Butch: Nine Long Months Spent in Drag

(2014)

A. K. Summers

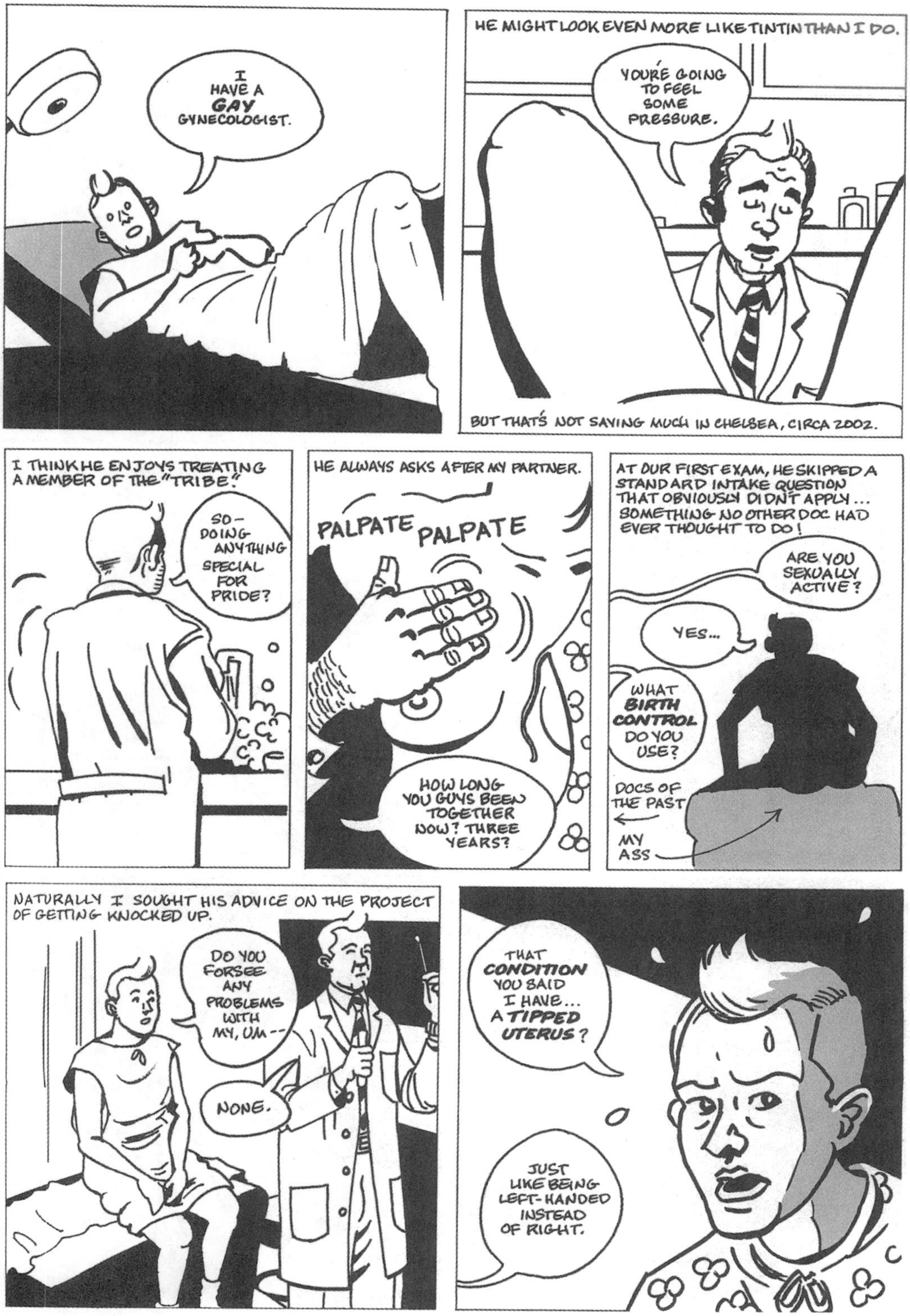
I HAVE A GAY GYNECOLOGIST.
HE MIGHT LOOK EVEN MORE LIKE TINTIN THAN I DO.
YOU'RE GOING TO FEEL SOME PRESSURE.
BUT THAT'S NOT SAYING MUCH IN CHELSEA, CIRCA 2002.
I THINK HE ENJOYS TREATING A MEMBER OF THE "TRIBE."
SO- DOING ANYTHING SPECIAL FOR PRIDE?
HE ALWAYS ASKS AFTER MY PARTNER.
PALPATE PALPATE
HOW LONG YOU GUYS BEEN TOGETHER NOW? THREE YEARS?
AT OUR FIRST EXAM, HE SKIPPED A STANDARD INTAKE QUESTION THAT OBVIOUSLY DIDN'T APPLY... SOMETHING NO OTHER DOC HAD EVER THOUGHT TO DO!
ARE YOU SEXUALLY ACTIVE?
YES...
WHAT BIRTH CONTROL DO YOU USE?
DOCS OF THE PAST
MY ASS
NATURALLY I SOUGHT HIS ADVICE ON THE PROJECT OF GETTING KNOCKED UP.
DO YOU FORSEE ANY PROBLEMS WITH MY, UM--
NONE.
THAT CONDITION YOU SAID I HAVE... A TIPPED UTERUS?
JUST LIKE BEING LEFT-HANDED INSTEAD OF RIGHT.

HE WAS STRANGELY RETICENT, READY TO MOVE ON TO THE NEXT PATIENT.
ANYTHING ELSE?
I PRESSED ON. THIS *IS* ROCKET SCIENCE AND YOU ARE A *GAY ROCKET SCIENTIST*!
Yup
Also this here
Don't forget
HOW SHOULD WE GO ABOUT IT?
A LONG PAUSE, AND THEN
MY RECOMMENDATION WOULD BE TO *HARVEST* EGGS FROM YOUR PARTNER, *FERTILIZE* THEM WITH ANONYMOUS DONOR SPERM AND *IMPLANT* THEM IN YOUR UTERUS. THAT WAY THERE COULD BE NO *LEGAL CHALLENGE* TO EITHER OF YOUR PARENTAL RIGHTS.
KOFF
I WAS THUNDERSTRUCK. I FELT AS THOUGH I'D STUMBLED ON THE *BOYS FROM BRAZIL*.*
OH MY GOD WHERE ARE MY PANTS?!
I... I... WAS *ADOPTED*. I REALLY WANT A *BIOLOGICAL CONNECTION* TO MY CHILD...
* SCI-FI MOVIE ABOUT HITLER CLONES
KNOW YER LADY PARTS
TO TELL YOU THE TRUTH, IT SOUNDS A LITTLE TOO *INVASIVE* FOR ME--
-- BUT THANKS FOR THE ADVICE.
IF THAT'S *ALL*...
...COME AND SEE ME WHEN YOU'RE *PREGNANT*.

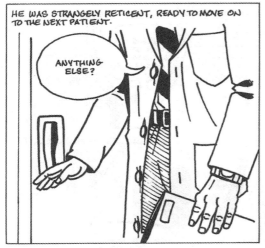

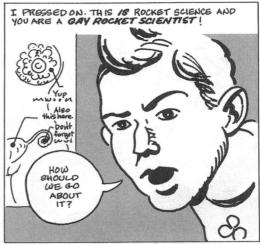

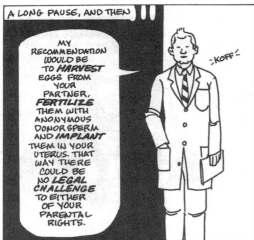

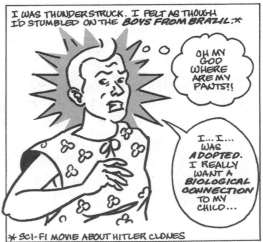

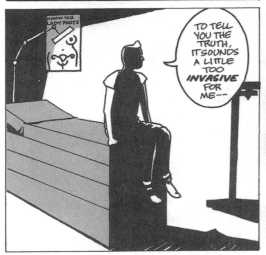

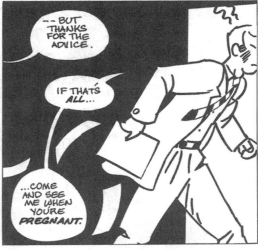

THE WISE CRONES

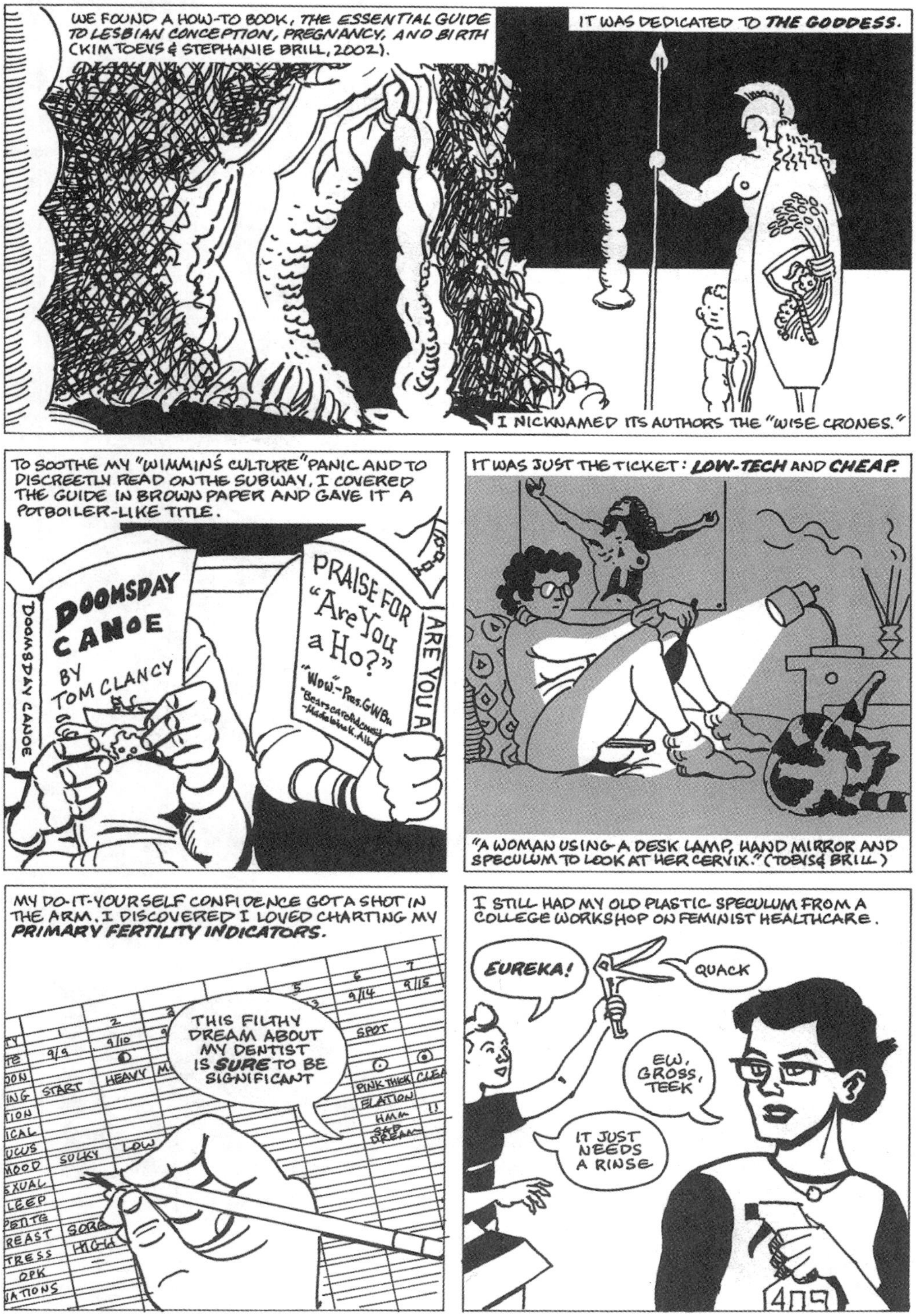
WE FOUND A HOW-TO BOOK, THE ESSENTIAL GUIDE TO LESBIAN CONCEPTION, PREGNANCY, AND BIRTH (KIM TOEVS & STEPHANIE BRILL, 2002).
IT WAS DEDICATED TO THE GODDESS.
I NICKNAMED ITS AUTHORS THE "WISE CRONES."
TO SOOTHE MY "WIMMIN'S CULTURE" PANIC AND TO DISCREETLY READ ON THE SUBWAY, I COVERED THE GUIDE IN BROWN PAPER AND GAVE IT A POTBOILER-LIKE TITLE.
DOOMSDAY CANOE BY TOM CLANCY
DOOMSDAY CANOE
PRAISE FOR "Are You a Ho?"
"WOW." - Pres. G.W.Bu
ARE YOU A
IT WAS JUST THE TICKET: LOW-TECH AND CHEAP.
"A WOMAN USING A DESK LAMP, HAND MIRROR AND SPECULUM TO LOOK AT HER CERVIX." (TOEVS & BRILL)
MY DO-IT-YOURSELF CONFIDENCE GOT A SHOT IN THE ARM. I DISCOVERED I LOVED CHARTING MY PRIMARY FERTILITY INDICATORS.
THIS FILTHY DREAM ABOUT MY DENTIST IS SURE TO BE SIGNIFICANT
9/9 9/10 9/14 9/15
START HEAVY
SPOT
PINK THICK
ELATION
HMM
SAD DREAM
SULKY LOW
MOOD
SEXUAL
SLEEP
BREAST
STRESS
OPK
I STILL HAD MY OLD PLASTIC SPECULUM FROM A COLLEGE WORKSHOP ON FEMINIST HEALTHCARE.
EUREKA!
QUACK
EW, GROSS, TEEK
IT JUST NEEDS A RINSE
409

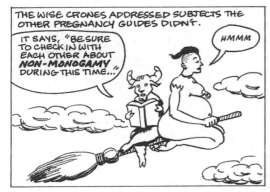

THE WISE CRONES ADDRESSED SUBJECTS THE OTHER PREGNANCY GUIDES DIDN'T.

IT SAYS, "BE SURE TO CHECK IN WITH EACH OTHER ABOUT *NON-MONOGAMY* DURING THIS TIME..."

HMMM

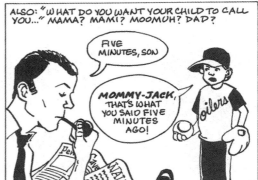

ALSO: "WHAT DO YOU WANT YOUR CHILD TO CALL YOU..." MAMA? MAMI? MOOMUH? DAD?

FIVE MINUTES, SON

MOMMY-JACK, THAT'S WHAT YOU SAID FIVE MINUTES AGO!

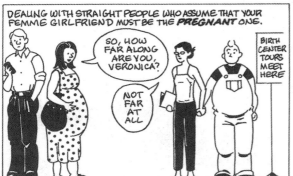

DEALING WITH STRAIGHT PEOPLE WHO ASSUME THAT YOUR FEMME GIRLFRIEND MUST BE THE *PREGNANT* ONE.

SO, HOW FAR ALONG ARE YOU, VERONICA?

NOT FAR AT ALL

BIRTH CENTER TOURS MEET HERE

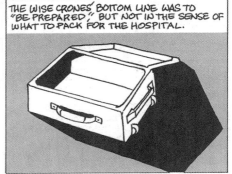

THE WISE CRONES' BOTTOM LINE WAS TO "BE PREPARED," BUT NOT IN THE SENSE OF WHAT TO PACK FOR THE HOSPITAL.

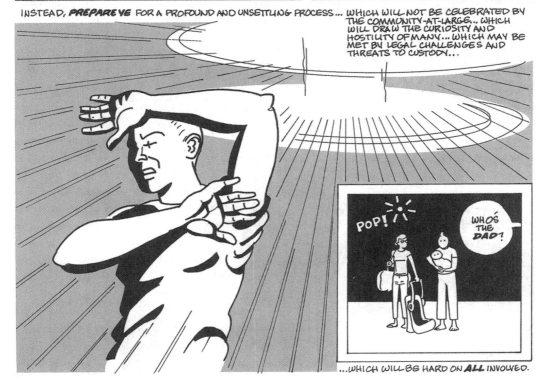

INSTEAD, *PREPARE YE* FOR A PROFOUND AND UNSETTLING PROCESS... WHICH WILL NOT BE CELEBRATED BY THE COMMUNITY-AT-LARGE... WHICH WILL DRAW THE CURIOSITY AND HOSTILITY OF MANY... WHICH MAY BE MET BY LEGAL CHALLENGES AND THREATS TO CUSTODY...

POP!

WHO'S THE *DAD*?

...WHICH WILL BE HARD ON *ALL* INVOLVED.

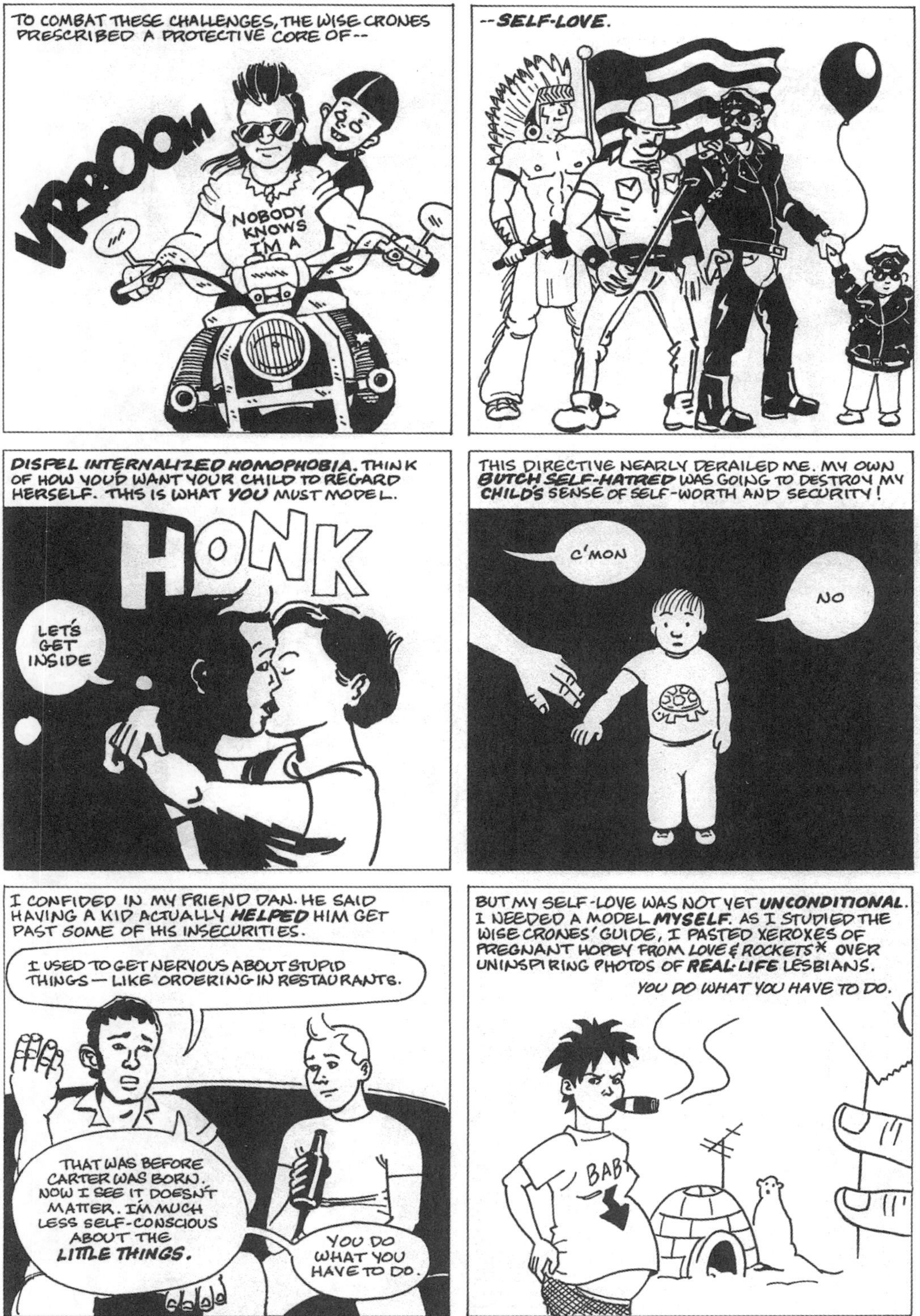
TO COMBAT THESE CHALLENGES, THE WISE CRONES PRESCRIBED A PROTECTIVE CORE OF--
VRROOM
NOBODY KNOWS I'M A
--SELF-LOVE.
DISPEL INTERNALIZED HOMOPHOBIA. THINK OF HOW YOU'D WANT YOUR CHILD TO REGARD HERSELF. THIS IS WHAT YOU MUST MODEL.
HONK
LET'S GET INSIDE
THIS DIRECTIVE NEARLY DERAILED ME. MY OWN BUTCH SELF-HATRED WAS GOING TO DESTROY MY CHILD'S SENSE OF SELF-WORTH AND SECURITY!
C'MON
NO
I CONFIDED IN MY FRIEND DAN. HE SAID HAVING A KID ACTUALLY HELPED HIM GET PAST SOME OF HIS INSECURITIES.
I USED TO GET NERVOUS ABOUT STUPID THINGS — LIKE ORDERING IN RESTAURANTS.
THAT WAS BEFORE CARTER WAS BORN. NOW I SEE IT DOESN'T MATTER. I'M MUCH LESS SELF-CONSCIOUS ABOUT THE LITTLE THINGS.
YOU DO WHAT YOU HAVE TO DO.
BUT MY SELF-LOVE WAS NOT YET UNCONDITIONAL. I NEEDED A MODEL MYSELF. AS I STUDIED THE WISE CRONES' GUIDE, I PASTED XEROXES OF PREGNANT HOPEY FROM LOVE & ROCKETS* OVER UNINSPIRING PHOTOS OF REAL-LIFE LESBIANS.
YOU DO WHAT YOU HAVE TO DO.
BABY

*© JAIME HERNANDEZ, LOVE & ROCKETS, 1988.

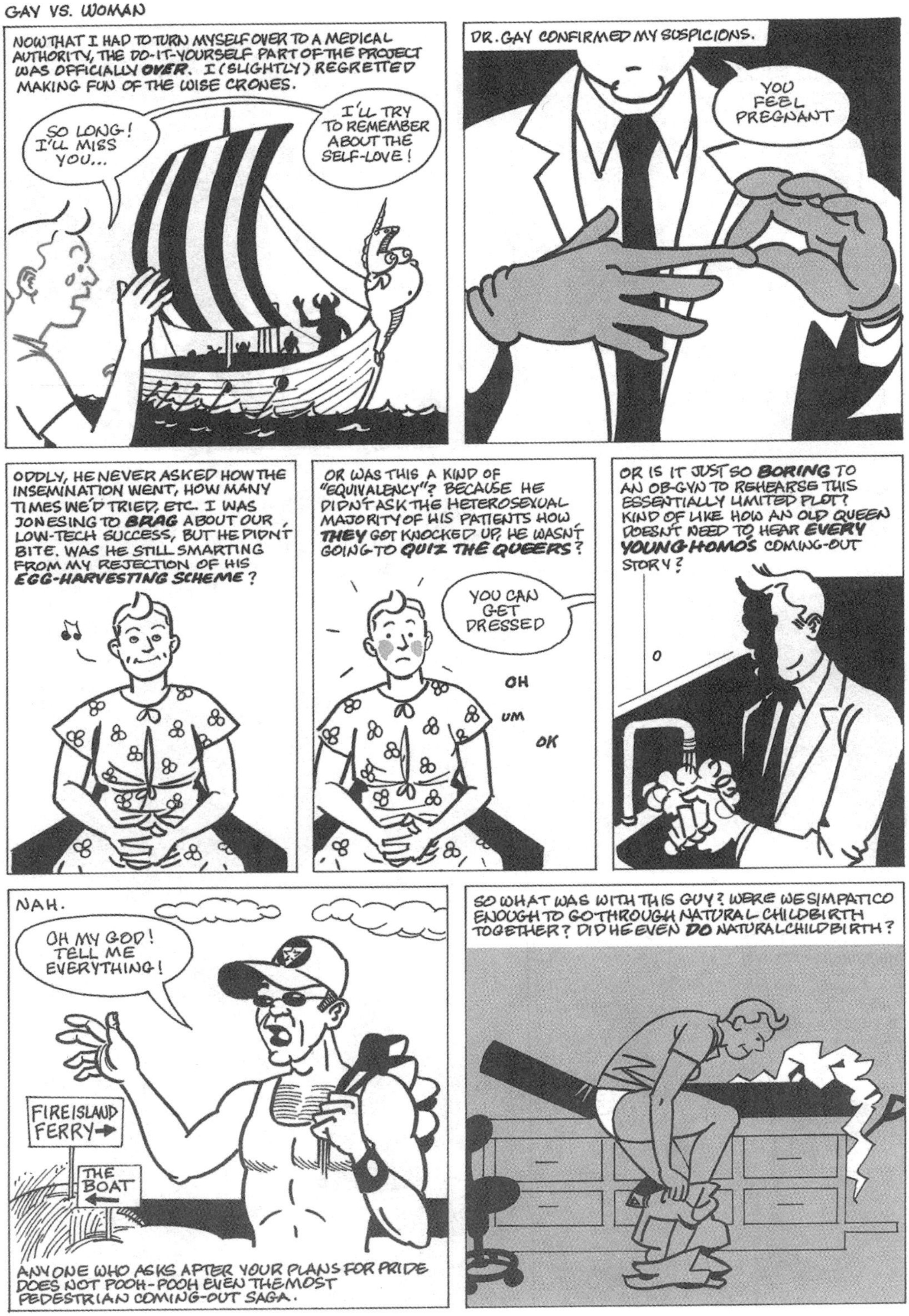
GAY VS. WOMAN
NOW THAT I HAD TO TURN MYSELF OVER TO A MEDICAL AUTHORITY, THE DO-IT-YOURSELF PART OF THE PROJECT WAS OFFICIALLY OVER. I (SLIGHTLY) REGRETTED MAKING FUN OF THE WISE CRONES.
SO LONG! I'LL MISS YOU...
I'LL TRY TO REMEMBER ABOUT THE SELF-LOVE!
DR. GAY CONFIRMED MY SUSPICIONS.
YOU FEEL PREGNANT
ODDLY, HE NEVER ASKED HOW THE INSEMINATION WENT, HOW MANY TIMES WE'D TRIED, ETC. I WAS JONESING TO BRAG ABOUT OUR LOW-TECH SUCCESS, BUT HE DIDN'T BITE. WAS HE STILL SMARTING FROM MY REJECTION OF HIS EGG-HARVESTING SCHEME?
OR WAS THIS A KIND OF "EQUIVALENCY"? BECAUSE HE DIDN'T ASK THE HETEROSEXUAL MAJORITY OF HIS PATIENTS HOW THEY GOT KNOCKED UP, HE WASN'T GOING TO QUIZ THE QUEERS?
YOU CAN GET DRESSED
OH
UM
OK
OR IS IT JUST SO BORING TO AN OB-GYN TO REHEARSE THIS ESSENTIALLY LIMITED PLOT? KIND OF LIKE HOW AN OLD QUEEN DOESN'T NEED TO HEAR EVERY YOUNG HOMO'S COMING-OUT STORY?
NAH.
OH MY GOD! TELL ME EVERYTHING!
FIRE ISLAND FERRY →
THE BOAT ←
ANYONE WHO ASKS AFTER YOUR PLANS FOR PRIDE DOES NOT POOH-POOH EVEN THE MOST PEDESTRIAN COMING-OUT SAGA.
SO WHAT WAS WITH THIS GUY? WERE WE SIMPATICO ENOUGH TO GO THROUGH NATURAL CHILDBIRTH TOGETHER? DID HE EVEN DO NATURAL CHILDBIRTH?

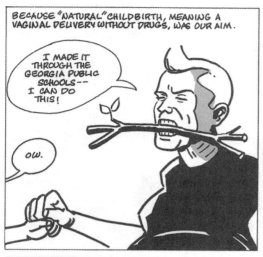

BECAUSE "NATURAL" CHILDBIRTH, MEANING A VAGINAL DELIVERY WITHOUT DRUGS, WAS OUR AIM.

I MADE IT THROUGH THE GEORGIA PUBLIC SCHOOLS-- I CAN DO THIS!

OW.

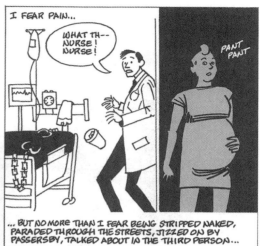

I FEAR PAIN...

WHAT TH-- NURSE! NURSE!

PANT PANT

... BUT NO MORE THAN I FEAR BEING STRIPPED NAKED, PARADED THROUGH THE STREETS, JIZZED ON BY PASSERSBY, TALKED ABOUT IN THE THIRD PERSON...

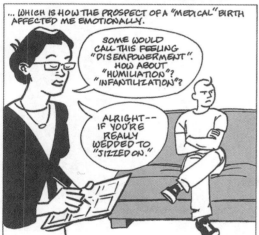

... WHICH IS HOW THE PROSPECT OF A "MEDICAL" BIRTH AFFECTED ME EMOTIONALLY.

SOME WOULD CALL THIS FEELING "DISEMPOWERMENT". HOW ABOUT "HUMILIATION"? "INFANTILIZATION"?

ALRIGHT-- IF YOU'RE REALLY WEDDED TO "JIZZED ON."

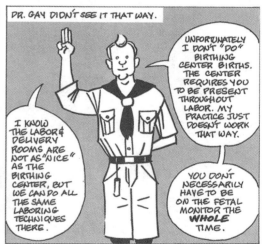

DR. GAY DIDN'T SEE IT THAT WAY.

I KNOW THE LABOR & DELIVERY ROOMS ARE NOT AS "NICE" AS THE BIRTHING CENTER, BUT WE CAN DO ALL THE SAME LABORING TECHNIQUES THERE.

UNFORTUNATELY I DON'T "DO" BIRTHING CENTER BIRTHS. THE CENTER REQUIRES YOU TO BE PRESENT THROUGHOUT LABOR. MY PRACTICE JUST DOESN'T WORK THAT WAY.

YOU DON'T NECESSARILY HAVE TO BE ON THE FETAL MONITOR THE WHOLE TIME.

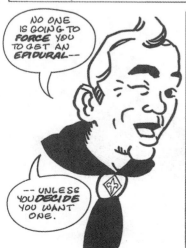

NO ONE IS GOING TO FORCE YOU TO GET AN EPIDURAL--

-- UNLESS YOU DECIDE YOU WANT ONE.

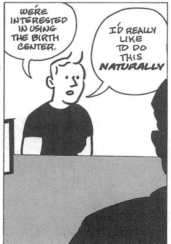

WE'RE INTERESTED IN USING THE BIRTH CENTER.

I'D REALLY LIKE TO DO THIS NATURALLY

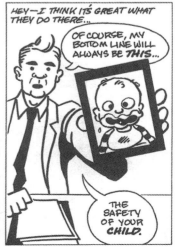

HEY-- I THINK IT'S GREAT WHAT THEY DO THERE...

OF COURSE, MY BOTTOM LINE WILL ALWAYS BE THIS...

THE SAFETY OF YOUR CHILD.

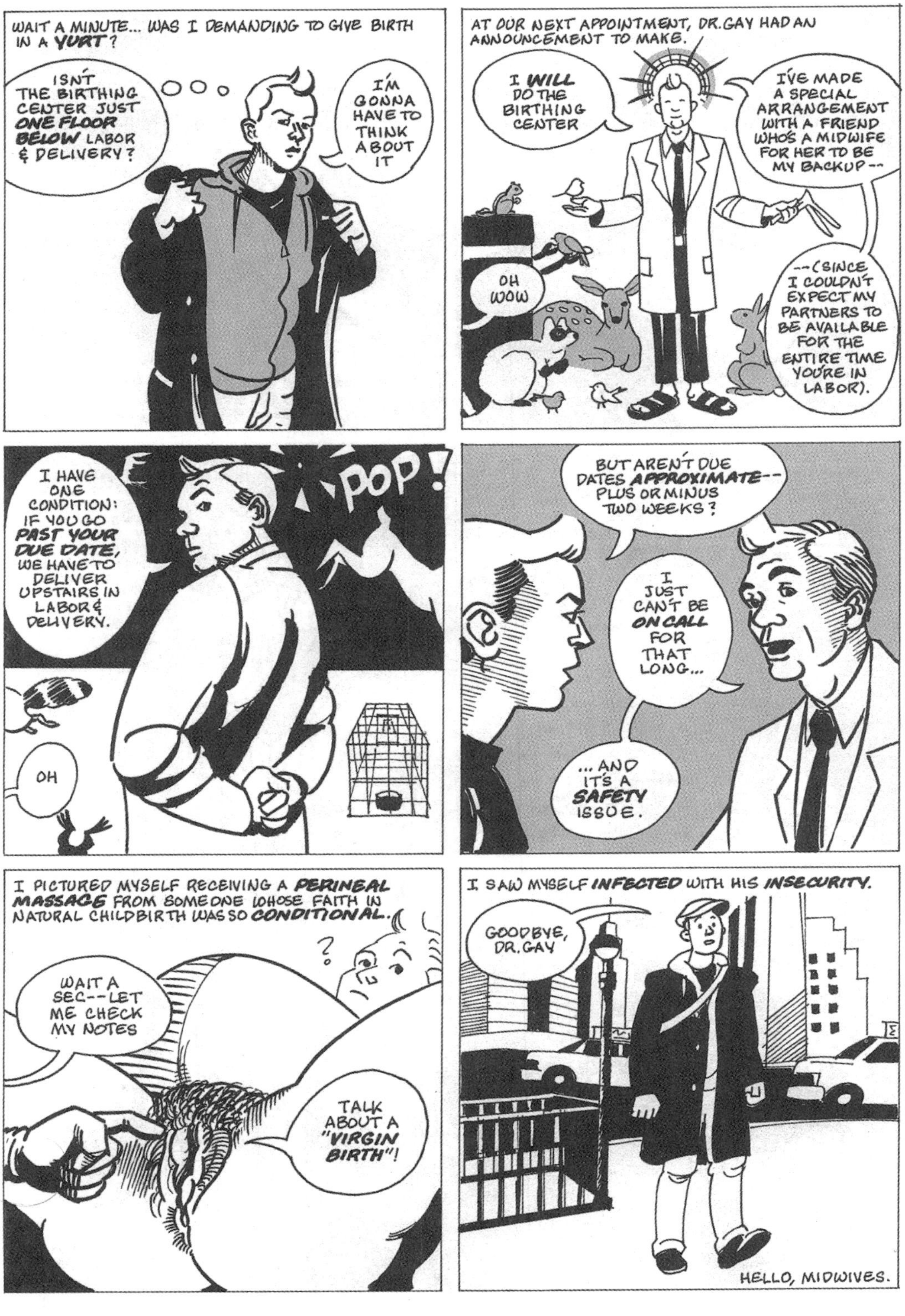
WAIT A MINUTE... WAS I DEMANDING TO GIVE BIRTH IN A YURT?
ISN'T THE BIRTHING CENTER JUST ONE FLOOR BELOW LABOR & DELIVERY?
I'M GONNA HAVE TO THINK ABOUT IT
AT OUR NEXT APPOINTMENT, DR. GAY HAD AN ANNOUNCEMENT TO MAKE.
I WILL DO THE BIRTHING CENTER
I'VE MADE A SPECIAL ARRANGEMENT WITH A FRIEND WHO'S A MIDWIFE FOR HER TO BE MY BACKUP--
--(SINCE I COULDN'T EXPECT MY PARTNERS TO BE AVAILABLE FOR THE ENTIRE TIME YOU'RE IN LABOR).
OH WOW
I HAVE ONE CONDITION: IF YOU GO PAST YOUR DUE DATE, WE HAVE TO DELIVER UPSTAIRS IN LABOR & DELIVERY.
POP!
OH
BUT AREN'T DUE DATES APPROXIMATE-- PLUS OR MINUS TWO WEEKS?
I JUST CAN'T BE ON CALL FOR THAT LONG...
...AND IT'S A SAFETY ISSUE.
I PICTURED MYSELF RECEIVING A PERINEAL MASSAGE FROM SOMEONE WHOSE FAITH IN NATURAL CHILDBIRTH WAS SO CONDITIONAL.
?
WAIT A SEC--LET ME CHECK MY NOTES
TALK ABOUT A "VIRGIN BIRTH"!
I SAW MYSELF INFECTED WITH HIS INSECURITY.
GOODBYE, DR. GAY
HELLO, MIDWIVES.

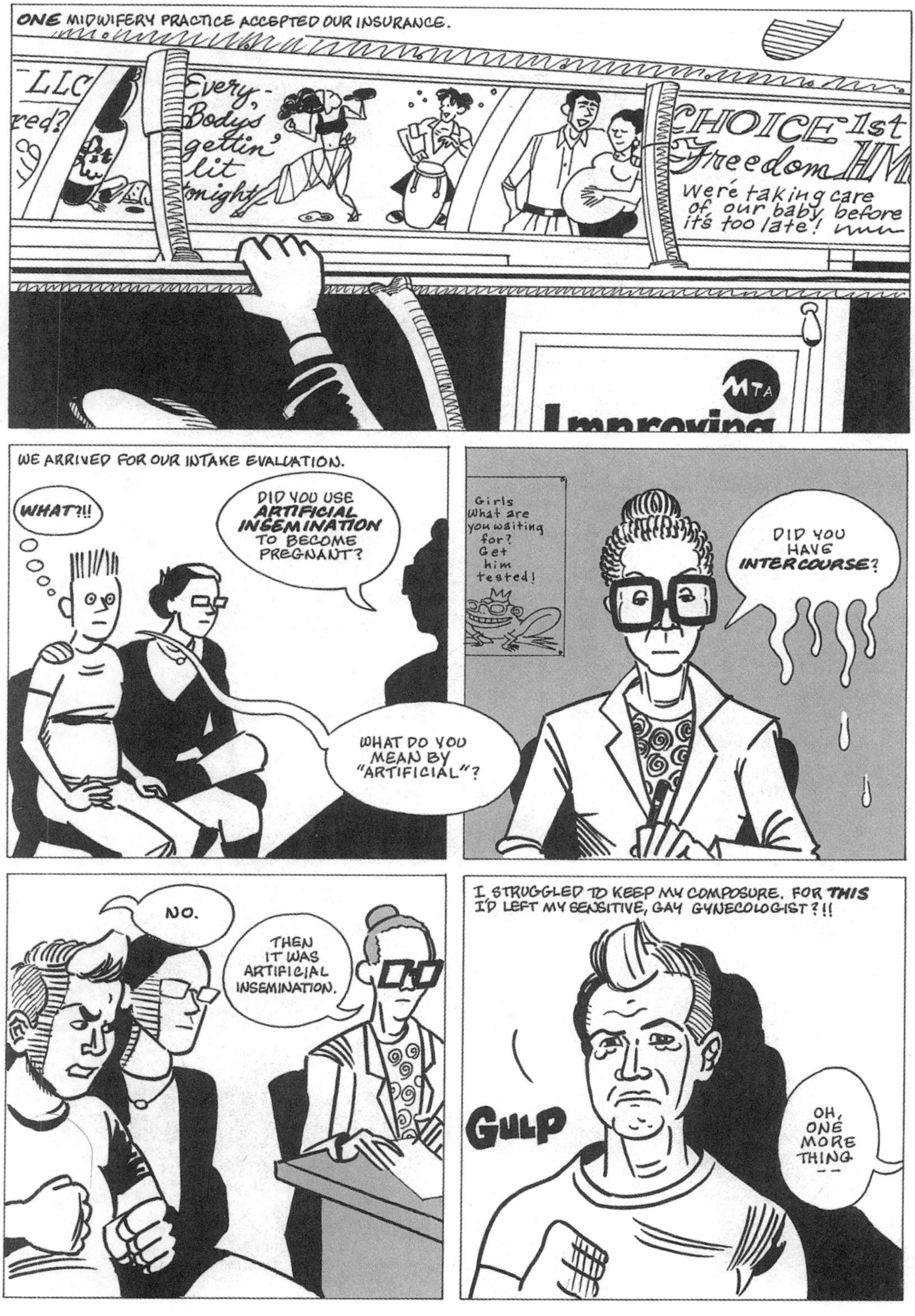
ONE MIDWIFERY PRACTICE ACCEPTED OUR INSURANCE.
Every-Body's gettin' lit tonight
CHOICE 1st Freedom HM
We're taking care of our baby before it's too late!
MTA
Improving
WE ARRIVED FOR OUR INTAKE EVALUATION.
DID YOU USE ARTIFICIAL INSEMINATION TO BECOME PREGNANT?
WHAT?!!
WHAT DO YOU MEAN BY "ARTIFICIAL"?
Girls What are you waiting for? Get him tested!
DID YOU HAVE INTERCOURSE?
NO.
THEN IT WAS ARTIFICIAL INSEMINATION.
I STRUGGLED TO KEEP MY COMPOSURE. FOR THIS I'D LEFT MY SENSITIVE, GAY GYNECOLOGIST?!!
GULP
OH, ONE MORE THING --

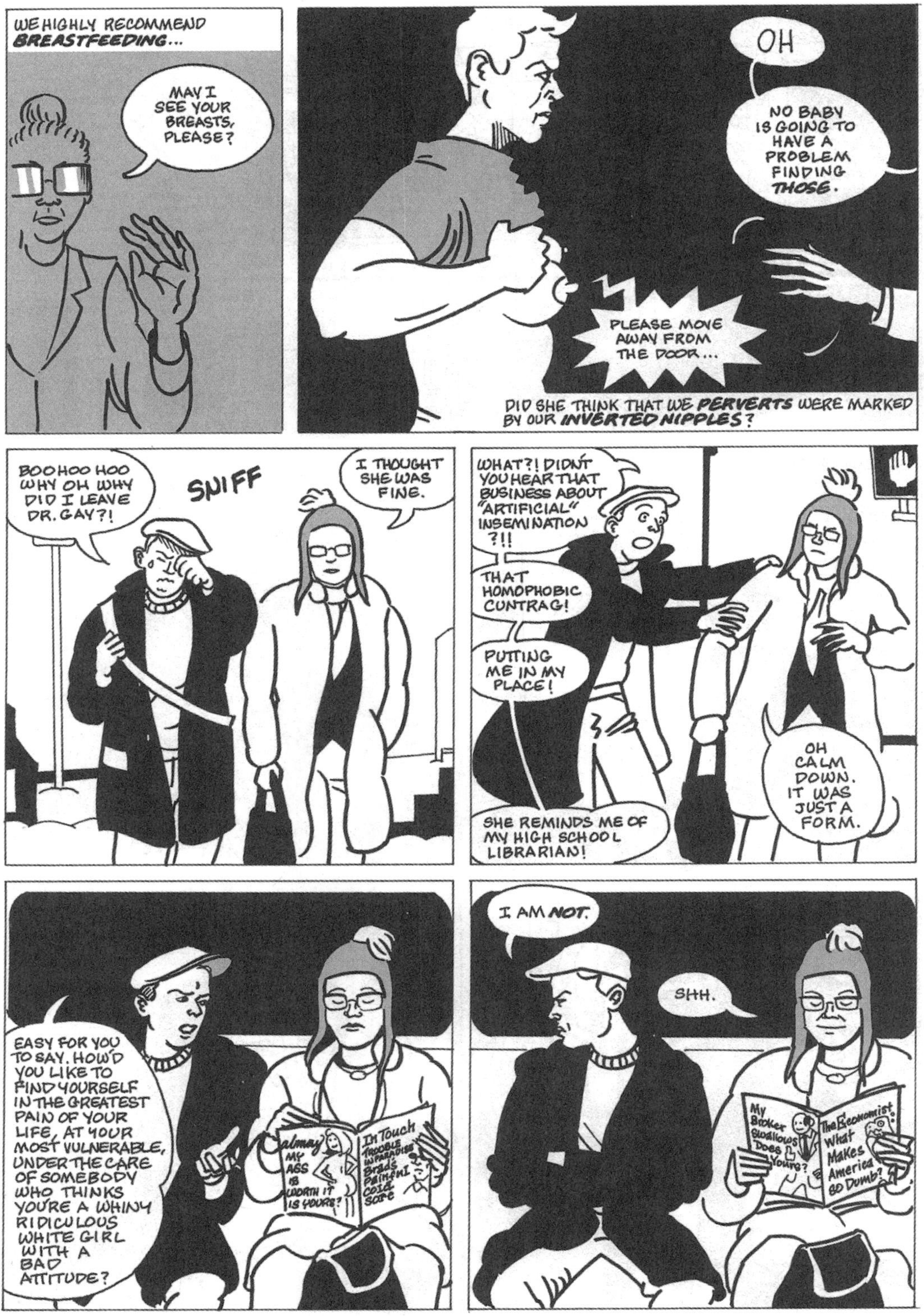
WE HIGHLY RECOMMEND BREASTFEEDING...
MAY I SEE YOUR BREASTS, PLEASE?
OH
NO BABY IS GOING TO HAVE A PROBLEM FINDING THOSE.
PLEASE MOVE AWAY FROM THE DOOR...
DID SHE THINK THAT WE PERVERTS WERE MARKED BY OUR INVERTED NIPPLES?
BOO HOO HOO WHY OH WHY DID I LEAVE DR. GAY?!
SNIFF
I THOUGHT SHE WAS FINE.
WHAT?! DIDN'T YOU HEAR THAT BUSINESS ABOUT "ARTIFICIAL" INSEMINATION ?!!
THAT HOMOPHOBIC CUNTRAG!
PUTTING ME IN MY PLACE!
SHE REMINDS ME OF MY HIGH SCHOOL LIBRARIAN!
OH CALM DOWN. IT WAS JUST A FORM.
EASY FOR YOU TO SAY. HOW'D YOU LIKE TO FIND YOURSELF IN THE GREATEST PAIN OF YOUR LIFE, AT YOUR MOST VULNERABLE, UNDER THE CARE OF SOMEBODY WHO THINKS YOU'RE A WHINY RIDICULOUS WHITE GIRL WITH A BAD ATTITUDE?
almay MY ASS IS WORTH IT IS YOURS?
In Touch TROUBLE IN PARADISE Brad's Painful Colo-scope
I AM NOT.
SHH.
My Broker Swallows Does Yours?
The Economist What Makes America So Dumb?

ORIENTATION

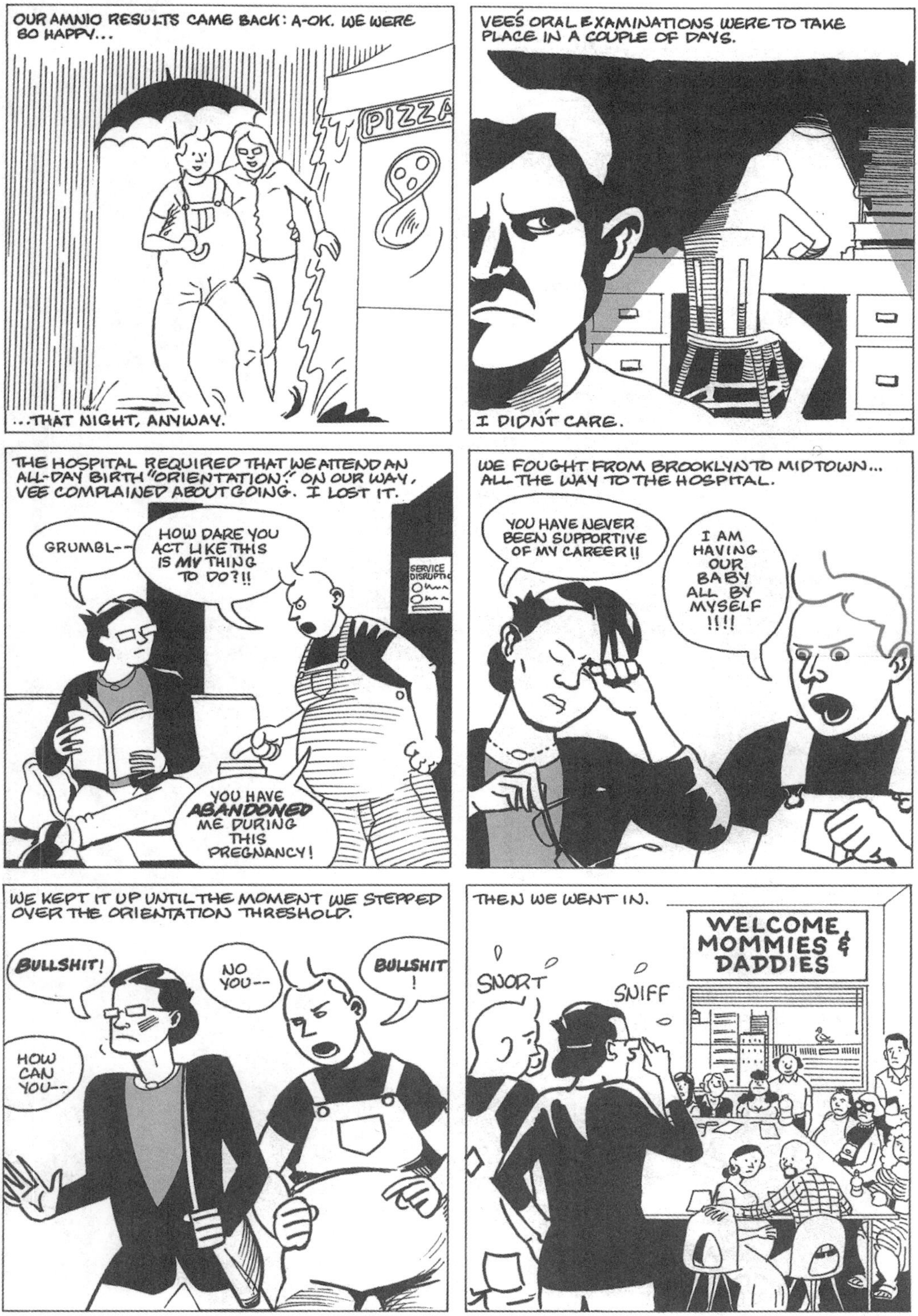
OUR AMNIO RESULTS CAME BACK: A-OK. WE WERE SO HAPPY...
PIZZA
...THAT NIGHT, ANYWAY.
VEE'S ORAL EXAMINATIONS WERE TO TAKE PLACE IN A COUPLE OF DAYS.
I DIDN'T CARE.
THE HOSPITAL REQUIRED THAT WE ATTEND AN ALL-DAY BIRTH "ORIENTATION." ON OUR WAY, VEE COMPLAINED ABOUT GOING. I LOST IT.
GRUMBL--
HOW DARE YOU ACT LIKE THIS IS MY THING TO DO?!!
SERVICE DISRUPTIO
YOU HAVE ABANDONED ME DURING THIS PREGNANCY!
WE FOUGHT FROM BROOKLYN TO MIDTOWN... ALL THE WAY TO THE HOSPITAL.
YOU HAVE NEVER BEEN SUPPORTIVE OF MY CAREER!!
I AM HAVING OUR BABY ALL BY MYSELF !!!!
WE KEPT IT UP UNTIL THE MOMENT WE STEPPED OVER THE ORIENTATION THRESHOLD.
BULLSHIT!
NO YOU--
BULLSHIT !
HOW CAN YOU--
THEN WE WENT IN.
WELCOME, MOMMIES & DADDIES
SNORT
SNIFF

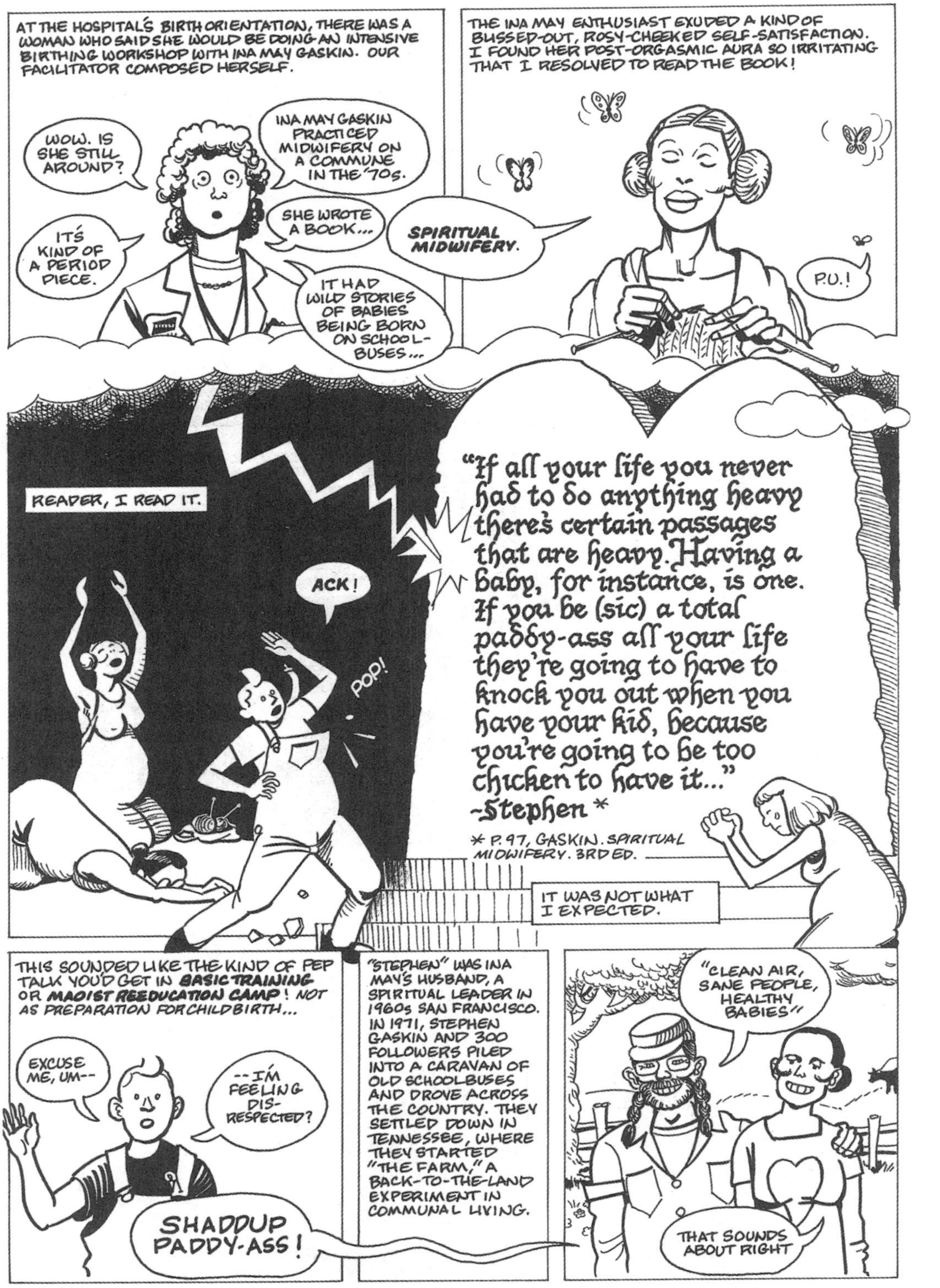
AT THE HOSPITAL'S BIRTH ORIENTATION, THERE WAS A WOMAN WHO SAID SHE WOULD BE DOING AN INTENSIVE BIRTHING WORKSHOP WITH INA MAY GASKIN. OUR FACILITATOR COMPOSED HERSELF.
WOW. IS SHE STILL AROUND?
INA MAY GASKIN PRACTICED MIDWIFERY ON A COMMUNE IN THE '70s.
IT'S KIND OF A PERIOD PIECE.
SHE WROTE A BOOK...
SPIRITUAL MIDWIFERY.
IT HAD WILD STORIES OF BABIES BEING BORN ON SCHOOL-BUSES...
THE INA MAY ENTHUSIAST EXUDED A KIND OF BLISSED-OUT, ROSY-CHEEKED SELF-SATISFACTION. I FOUND HER POST-ORGASMIC AURA SO IRRITATING THAT I RESOLVED TO READ THE BOOK!
P.U.!
READER, I READ IT.
ACK!
POP!
"If all your life you never had to do anything heavy there's certain passages that are heavy. Having a baby, for instance, is one. If you be (sic) a total paddy-ass all your life they're going to have to knock you out when you have your kid, because you're going to be too chicken to have it..." -Stephen *
* P. 97, GASKIN. SPIRITUAL MIDWIFERY. 3RD ED.
IT WAS NOT WHAT I EXPECTED.
THIS SOUNDED LIKE THE KIND OF PEP TALK YOU'D GET IN BASIC TRAINING OR MAOIST REEDUCATION CAMP! NOT AS PREPARATION FOR CHILDBIRTH...
EXCUSE ME, UM--
--I'M FEELING DIS-RESPECTED?
SHADDUP PADDY-ASS!
"STEPHEN" WAS INA MAY'S HUSBAND, A SPIRITUAL LEADER IN 1960s SAN FRANCISCO. IN 1971, STEPHEN GASKIN AND 300 FOLLOWERS PILED INTO A CARAVAN OF OLD SCHOOLBUSES AND DROVE ACROSS THE COUNTRY. THEY SETTLED DOWN IN TENNESSEE, WHERE THEY STARTED "THE FARM," A BACK-TO-THE-LAND EXPERIMENT IN COMMUNAL LIVING.
"CLEAN AIR, SANE PEOPLE, HEALTHY BABIES"
THAT SOUNDS ABOUT RIGHT

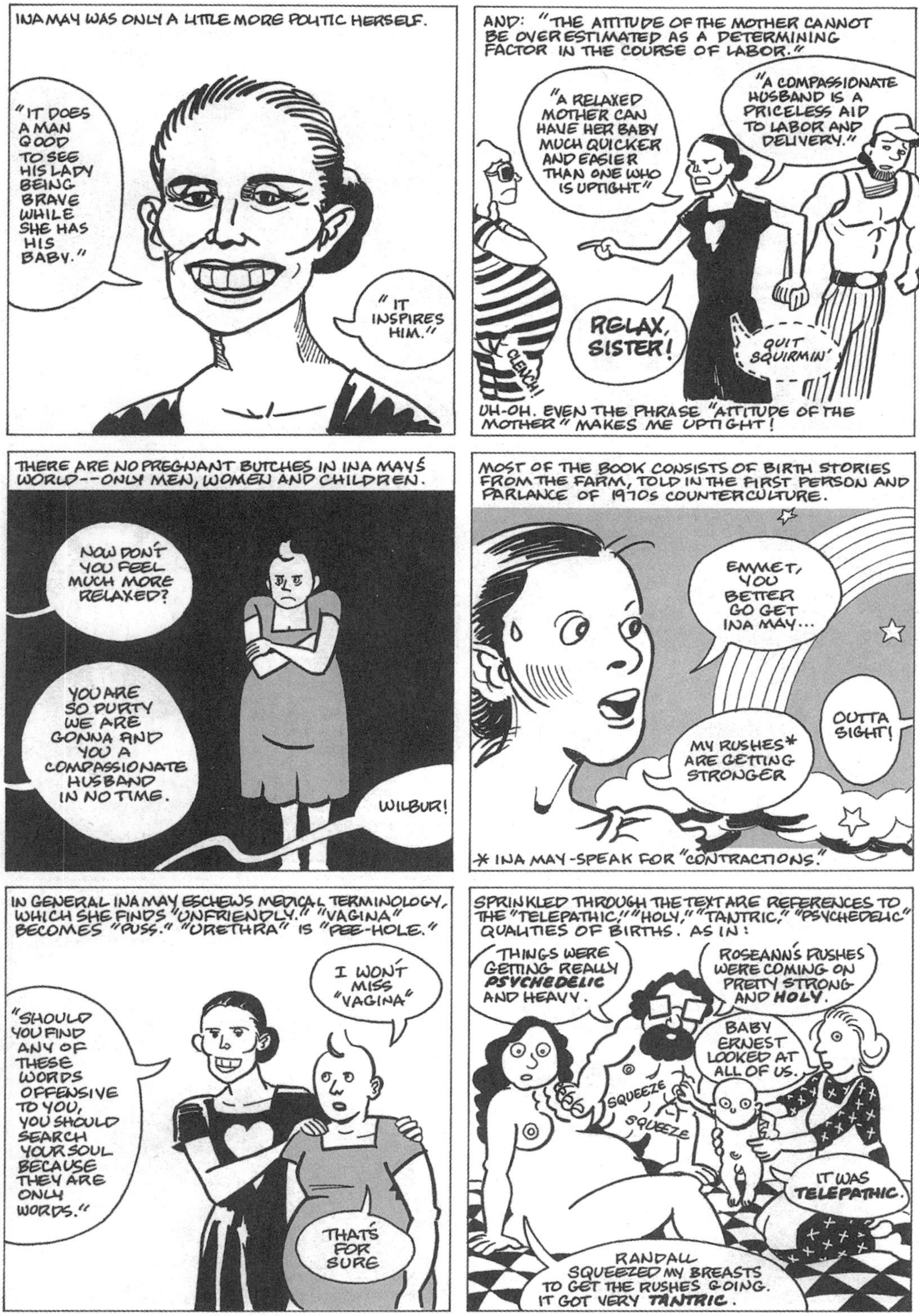
INA MAY WAS ONLY A LITTLE MORE POLITIC HERSELF.
"IT DOES A MAN GOOD TO SEE HIS LADY BEING BRAVE WHILE SHE HAS HIS BABY."
"IT INSPIRES HIM."
AND: "THE ATTITUDE OF THE MOTHER CANNOT BE OVERESTIMATED AS A DETERMINING FACTOR IN THE COURSE OF LABOR."
"A RELAXED MOTHER CAN HAVE HER BABY MUCH QUICKER AND EASIER THAN ONE WHO IS UPTIGHT."
"A COMPASSIONATE HUSBAND IS A PRICELESS AID TO LABOR AND DELIVERY."
RELAX, SISTER!
QUIT SQUIRMIN'
CLENCH!
UH-OH. EVEN THE PHRASE "ATTITUDE OF THE MOTHER" MAKES ME UPTIGHT!
THERE ARE NO PREGNANT BUTCHES IN INA MAY'S WORLD--ONLY MEN, WOMEN AND CHILDREN.
NOW DON'T YOU FEEL MUCH MORE RELAXED?
YOU ARE SO PURTY WE ARE GONNA FIND YOU A COMPASSIONATE HUSBAND IN NO TIME.
WILBUR!
MOST OF THE BOOK CONSISTS OF BIRTH STORIES FROM THE FARM, TOLD IN THE FIRST PERSON AND PARLANCE OF 1970S COUNTERCULTURE.
EMMET, YOU BETTER GO GET INA MAY...
OUTTA SIGHT!
MY RUSHES* ARE GETTING STRONGER
* INA MAY-SPEAK FOR "CONTRACTIONS."
IN GENERAL INA MAY ESCHEWS MEDICAL TERMINOLOGY, WHICH SHE FINDS "UNFRIENDLY." "VAGINA" BECOMES "PUSS." "URETHRA" IS "PEE-HOLE."
I WON'T MISS "VAGINA"
"SHOULD YOU FIND ANY OF THESE WORDS OFFENSIVE TO YOU, YOU SHOULD SEARCH YOUR SOUL BECAUSE THEY ARE ONLY WORDS."
THAT'S FOR SURE
SPRINKLED THROUGH THE TEXT ARE REFERENCES TO THE "TELEPATHIC," "HOLY," "TANTRIC," "PSYCHEDELIC" QUALITIES OF BIRTHS. AS IN:
THINGS WERE GETTING REALLY PSYCHEDELIC AND HEAVY.
ROSEANN'S RUSHES WERE COMING ON PRETTY STRONG AND HOLY.
BABY ERNEST LOOKED AT ALL OF US.
SQUEEZE
SQUEEZE
IT WAS TELEPATHIC.
RANDALL SQUEEZED MY BREASTS TO GET THE RUSHES GOING. IT GOT VERY TANTRIC.

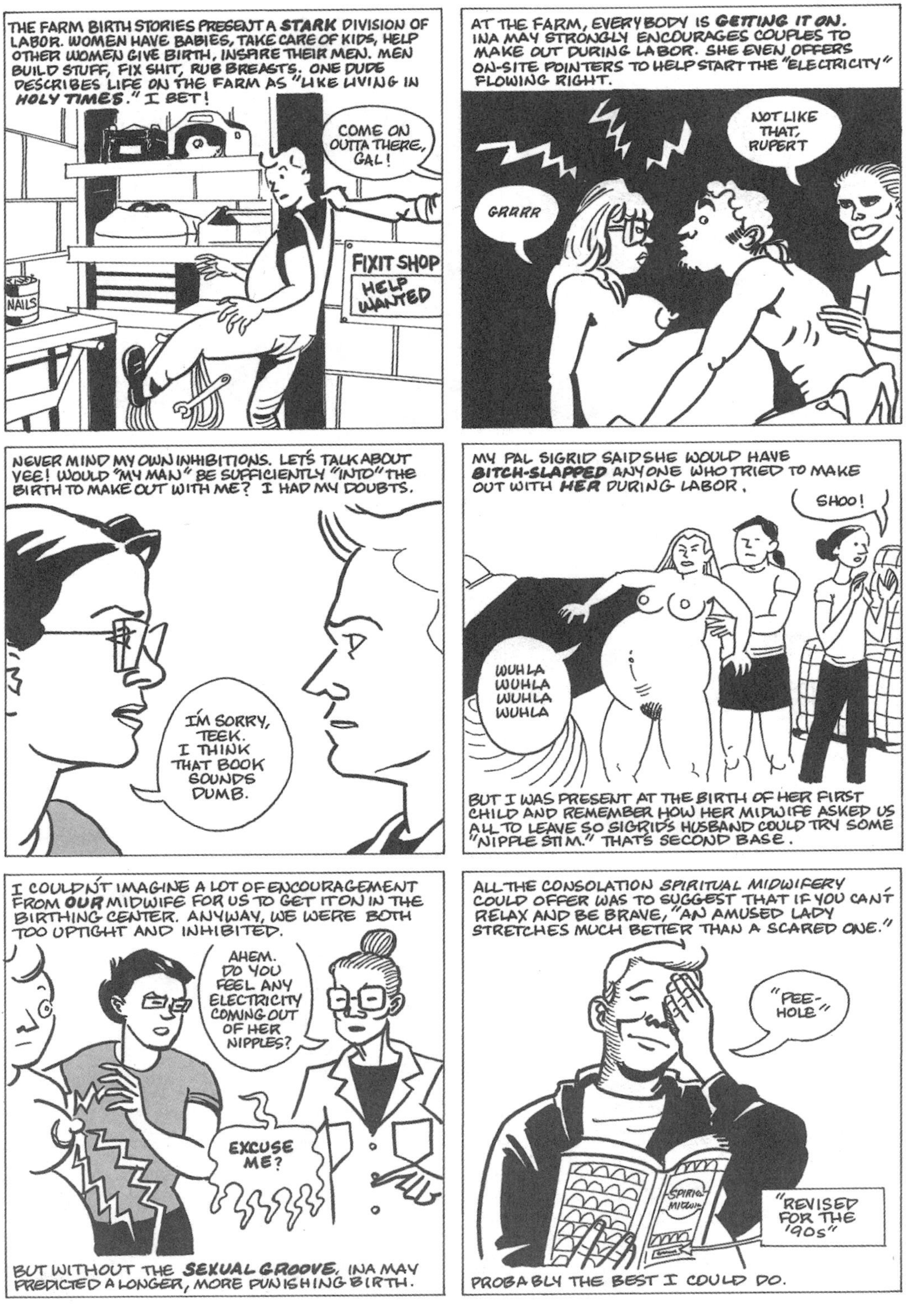
THE FARM BIRTH STORIES PRESENT A STARK DIVISION OF LABOR. WOMEN HAVE BABIES, TAKE CARE OF KIDS, HELP OTHER WOMEN GIVE BIRTH, INSPIRE THEIR MEN. MEN BUILD STUFF, FIX SHIT, RUB BREASTS. ONE DUDE DESCRIBES LIFE ON THE FARM AS "LIKE LIVING IN HOLY TIMES." I BET!
COME ON OUTTA THERE, GAL!
NAILS
FIXIT SHOP
HELP WANTED
AT THE FARM, EVERYBODY IS GETTING IT ON. INA MAY STRONGLY ENCOURAGES COUPLES TO MAKE OUT DURING LABOR. SHE EVEN OFFERS ON-SITE POINTERS TO HELP START THE "ELECTRICITY" FLOWING RIGHT.
GRRRR
NOT LIKE THAT, RUPERT
NEVER MIND MY OWN INHIBITIONS. LET'S TALK ABOUT YEE! WOULD "MY MAN" BE SUFFICIENTLY "INTO" THE BIRTH TO MAKE OUT WITH ME? I HAD MY DOUBTS.
I'M SORRY, TEEK. I THINK THAT BOOK SOUNDS DUMB.
MY PAL SIGRID SAID SHE WOULD HAVE BITCH-SLAPPED ANYONE WHO TRIED TO MAKE OUT WITH HER DURING LABOR.
SHOO!
WUHLA WUHLA WUHLA WUHLA
BUT I WAS PRESENT AT THE BIRTH OF HER FIRST CHILD AND REMEMBER HOW HER MIDWIFE ASKED US ALL TO LEAVE SO SIGRID'S HUSBAND COULD TRY SOME "NIPPLE STIM." THAT'S SECOND BASE.
I COULDN'T IMAGINE A LOT OF ENCOURAGEMENT FROM OUR MIDWIFE FOR US TO GET IT ON IN THE BIRTHING CENTER. ANYWAY, WE WERE BOTH TOO UPTIGHT AND INHIBITED.
AHEM. DO YOU FEEL ANY ELECTRICITY COMING OUT OF HER NIPPLES?
EXCUSE ME?
BUT WITHOUT THE SEXUAL GROOVE, INA MAY PREDICTED A LONGER, MORE PUNISHING BIRTH.
ALL THE CONSOLATION SPIRITUAL MIDWIFERY COULD OFFER WAS TO SUGGEST THAT IF YOU CAN'T RELAX AND BE BRAVE, "AN AMUSED LADY STRETCHES MUCH BETTER THAN A SCARED ONE."
"PEE-HOLE"
"REVISED FOR THE '90s"
PROBABLY THE BEST I COULD DO.

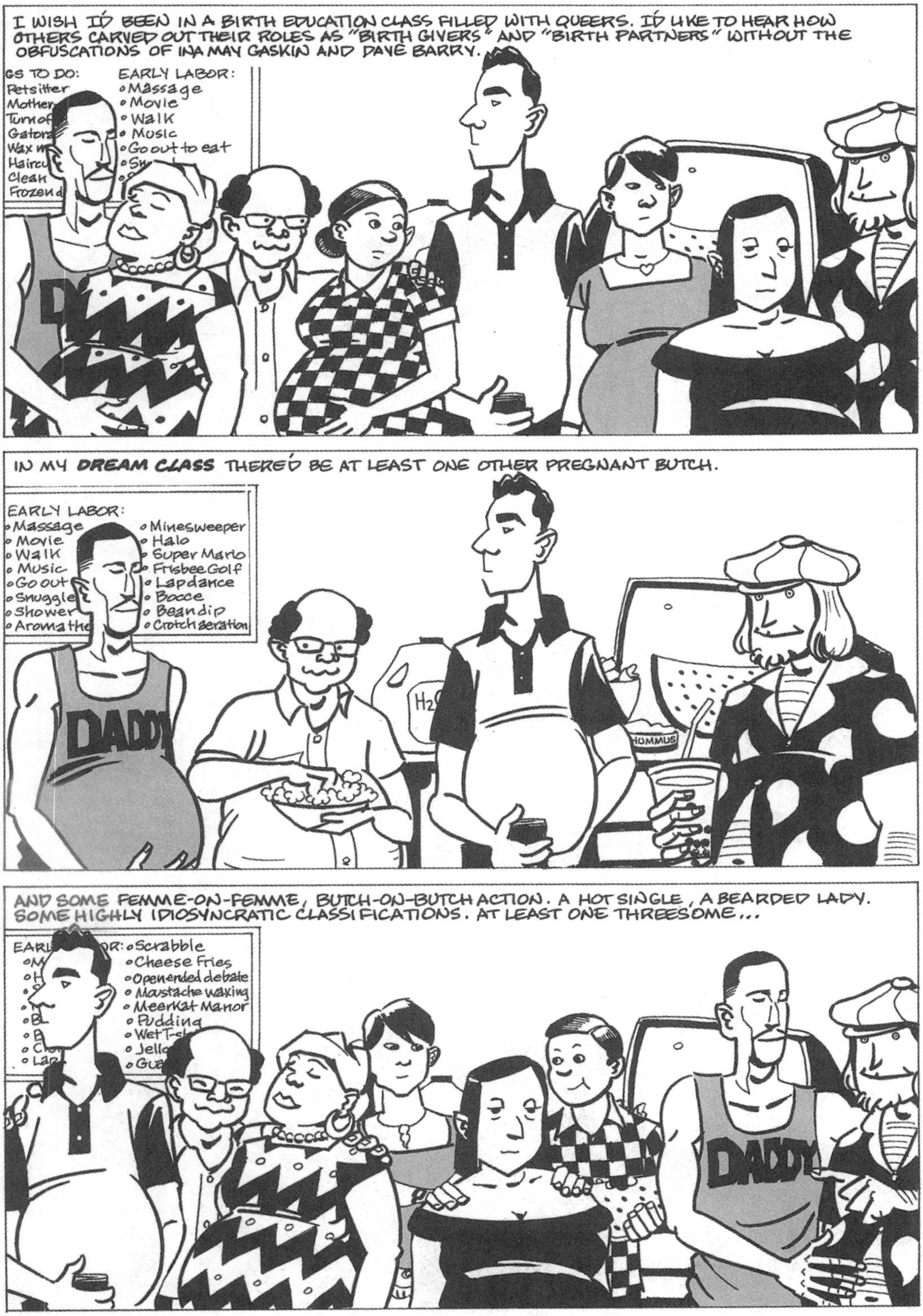
I WISH I'D BEEN IN A BIRTH EDUCATION CLASS FILLED WITH QUEERS. I'D LIKE TO HEAR HOW OTHERS CARVED OUT THEIR ROLES AS "BIRTH GIVERS" AND "BIRTH PARTNERS" WITHOUT THE OBFUSCATIONS OF INA MAY GASKIN AND DAVE BARRY.
EARLY LABOR:
Massage
Movie
Walk
Music
Go out to eat
IN MY DREAM CLASS THERE'D BE AT LEAST ONE OTHER PREGNANT BUTCH.
EARLY LABOR:
Massage
Movie
Walk
Music
Minesweeper
Halo
Super Mario
Frisbee Golf
Lapdance
Bocce
Beandip
Crotch aeration
DADDY
HUMMUS
AND SOME FEMME-ON-FEMME, BUTCH-ON-BUTCH ACTION. A HOT SINGLE, A BEARDED LADY. SOME HIGHLY IDIOSYNCRATIC CLASSIFICATIONS. AT LEAST ONE THREESOME...
Scrabble
Cheese Fries
Openended debate
Moustache waxing
MeerKat Manor
Pudding
DADDY

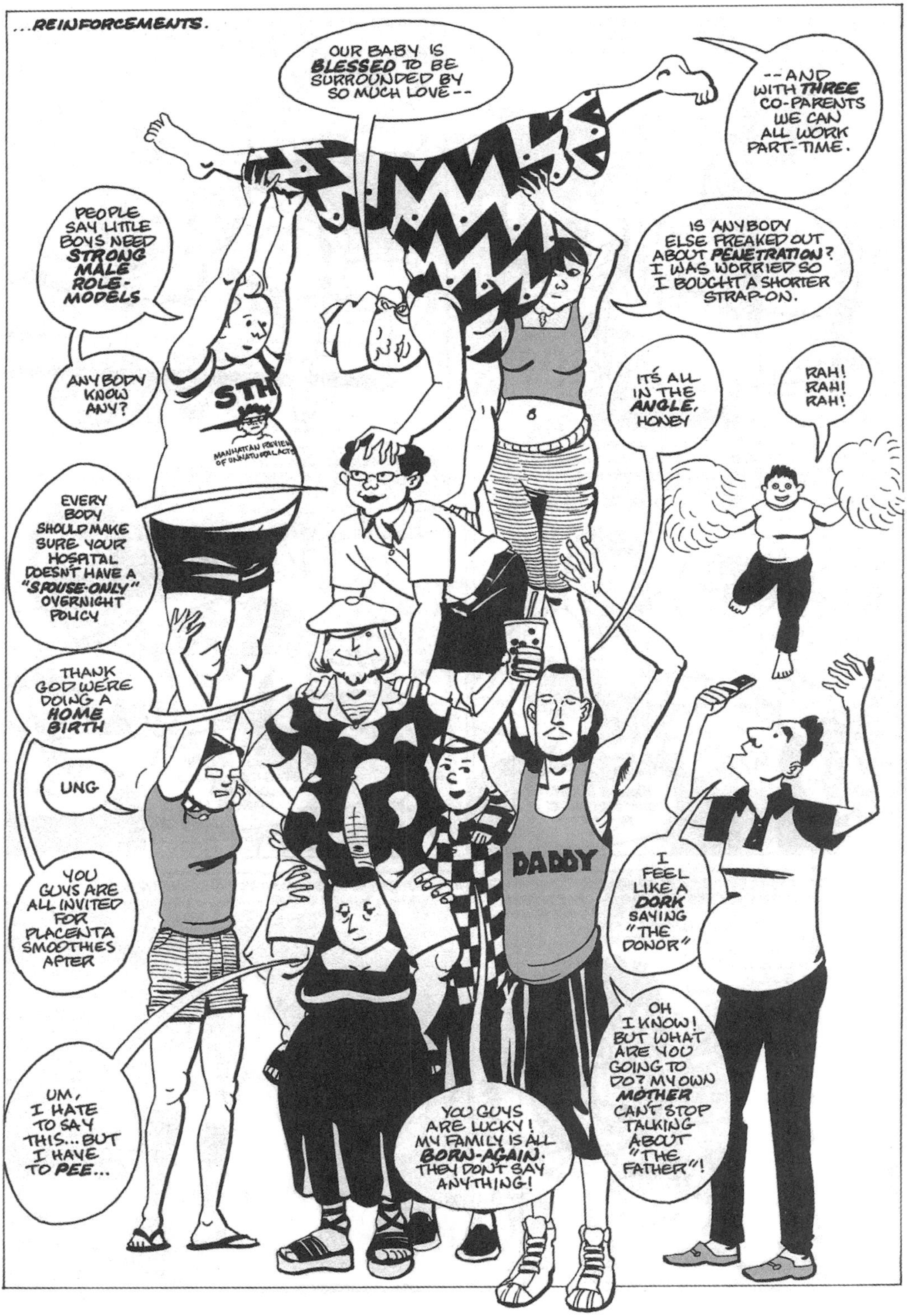
...REINFORCEMENTS.
OUR BABY IS BLESSED TO BE SURROUNDED BY SO MUCH LOVE--
--AND WITH THREE CO-PARENTS WE CAN ALL WORK PART-TIME.
PEOPLE SAY LITTLE BOYS NEED STRONG MALE ROLE-MODELS
ANYBODY KNOW ANY?
IS ANYBODY ELSE FREAKED OUT ABOUT PENETRATION? I WAS WORRIED SO I BOUGHT A SHORTER STRAP-ON.
STH
MANHATTAN REVIEW OF UNNATURAL ACTS
IT'S ALL IN THE ANGLE, HONEY
RAH! RAH! RAH!
EVERY BODY SHOULD MAKE SURE YOUR HOSPITAL DOESN'T HAVE A "SPOUSE-ONLY" OVERNIGHT POLICY
THANK GOD WE'RE DOING A HOME BIRTH
UNG
DADDY
YOU GUYS ARE ALL INVITED FOR PLACENTA SMOOTHIES AFTER
I FEEL LIKE A DORK SAYING "THE DONOR"
OH I KNOW! BUT WHAT ARE YOU GOING TO DO? MY OWN MOTHER CAN'T STOP TALKING ABOUT "THE FATHER"!
UM, I HATE TO SAY THIS... BUT I HAVE TO PEE...
YOU GUYS ARE LUCKY! MY FAMILY IS ALL BORN-AGAIN. THEY DON'T SAY ANYTHING!

EXCERPT FROM

Pushing Back: A Home Birth Story

(2017)

Bethany Doane

EARLY LABOR WAS RELATIVELY UNEVENTFUL. I'D HAD SOME "FALSE" LABOR FOR A FEW WEEKS, SO WHEN I HAD SOME STRONG CONTRACTIONS THE NIGHT BEFORE MY "OFFICIAL" DUE DATE, MY MIDWIFE SAID NOT TO WORRY.

I HAD A GLASS OF WINE, WALKED THROUGHOUT THE DAY, AND THE CONTRACTIONS CAME AND WENT SLOWLY. THE NEXT EVENING AND INTO THE MORNING, THEY CAME ON STRONG AGAIN.

IT FELT VERY REAL TO ME, BUT KAREN SAID TO WAIT, THAT SHE DIDN'T THINK IT WOULD CONTINUE.

IT DID.

WE WENT TO THE MALL, OF ALL PLACES, BUT LABOR CONTINUED TO PICK UP SO WE HAD TO HEAD BACK.

BACK AT HOME, JEFF CALLED THE MIDWIFE, AROUND 4 PM.

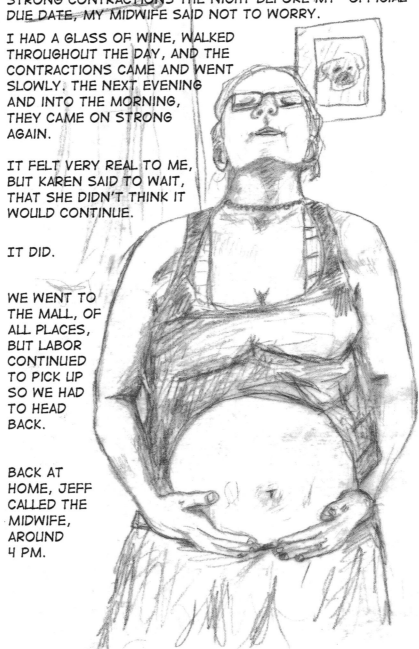

THE BEST POSITION TO LABOR IN
WAS LEANING OVER THE BACK OF
AN OLD CHAIR THAT HAD BEEN MY
GRANDFATHER'S.

I ROCKED MY HIPS BACK AND
FORTH DURING THE CONTRACT-
IONS, WHICH FELT PRETTY
GOOD.

I ALSO LABORED
OVER ONE OF
THOSE EXERCISE
BALLS FOR A
WHILE.

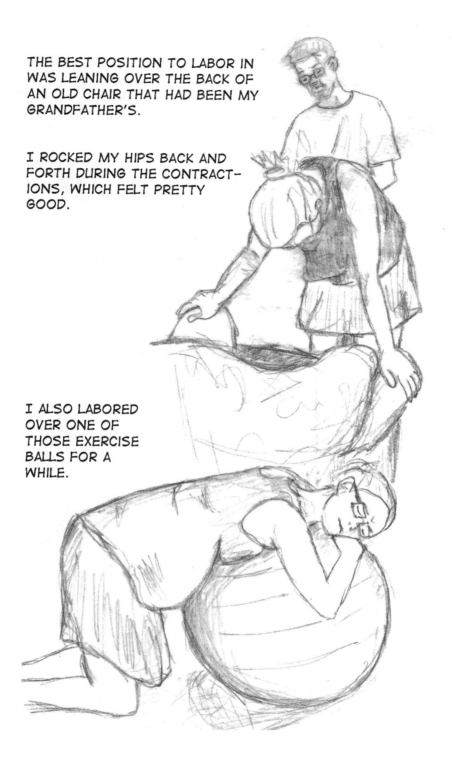

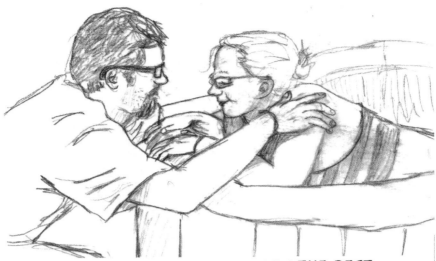

BUT GETTING INTO THE BIRTH POOL FELT *THE BEST*.

IT IS SERIOUSLY A CRIME THAT EVERY LABORING WOMAN DOESN'T GET TO CLIMB INTO A BIRTHING TUB. IT FELT THAT GOOD. (AND WHEN I SAY "GOOD," I MEAN A LOT LESS BAD, BECAUSE THOSE FOLKS WHO SAY BIRTH CAN BE PAINLESS ARE EITHER DAMNED LIARS OR THE LUCKIEST BUGGERS ON EARTH. THEY SAY IT'S JUST "INTENSE," BUT YOU KNOW WHAT'S INTENSE? A BUTTLOAD OF PAIN.)

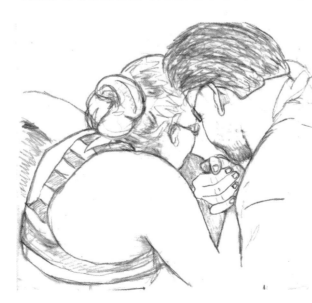

THINGS STARTED TO GET REALLY INTENSE. JEFF CALLED KAREN AGAIN, AND SHE SAID SHE WAS ON HER WAY.

SHE ARRIVED AROUND 9PM, BUT I BARELY NOTICED.

BY THE TIME KAREN CHECKED ME FOR THE FIRST TIME (EVER), SHE SAID, "WOW, THE HEAD'S RIGHT THERE! REACH DOWN AND FEEL THAT!"

SURE ENOUGH, I COULD FEEL A FUZZY LITTLE HEAD. AND EVEN THOUGH I WAS PUKING OUT MY NOSE AND WANTING TO CRY AND BITING JEFF'S PANTS LEG, I GOT REALLY EXCITED AND HAPPY, BECAUSE I KNEW BABY WAS COMING SO SOON!

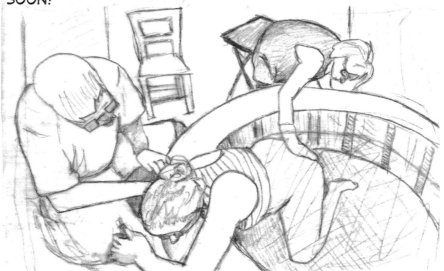

MY MOM WAS THERE TAKING PICTURES, AND WE HAD THE BEATLES "BEST OF" 1967-70 PLAYING ON A LOOP (I WOULDN'T LET ANYONE CHANGE IT).

KAREN AND MY MOM SANG ALONG TO THE SONGS.

JEFF AND I ALWAYS MAKE FUN OF THE SONG "OCTOPUS'S GARDEN" (EVEN THOUGH I LOVE IT). AT ONE POINT, WHEN I KNEW BABY WAS REALLY COMING BECAUSE THE HEAD WAS ON ITS WAY OUT, THAT SONG CAME ON, AND HE SAID "OH! THE BABY HAS TO BE BORN TO THIS SONG!"

BUT ALAS, THE SONG ENDED, AND I WAS STILL PUSHING LIKE A MADWOMAN. TWO SONGS LATER, THOUGH, I FELT THE HEAD POP OUT. THEN ONE MORE PUSH, AND KAREN SAID, "HERE, REACH DOWN AND TAKE THIS..."

AND THEN, THERE WAS JUST THIS LITTLE BABY IN MY ARMS, BLUISH, BUT PINKING UP QUICKLY. ONE OF THE FIRST THINGS I SAID WAS, "IT CAME OUT!"

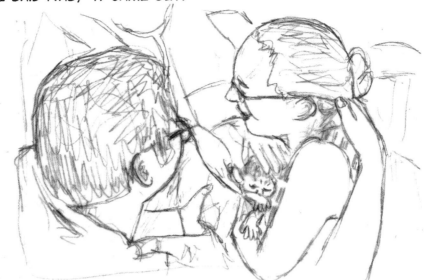

KAREN AND HER ASSISTANT CHECKED THE HEARTBEAT EVERY FEW MINUTES AND LOOKED ON TO MAKE SURE EVERYTHING WAS OKAY.

EVENTUALLY, I REMEMBERED THAT SEX/GENDER THING AND WE LOOKED UNDER THE BLANKET.

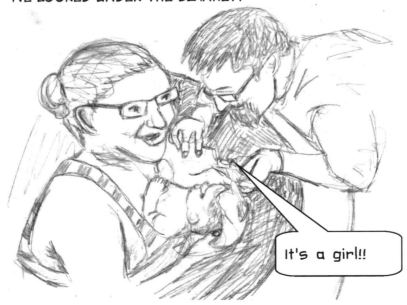

It's a girl!!

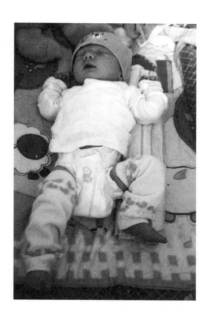

JOSEPHINE RIVER DOANE

BORN AT HOME

10:05 PM, SUNDAY AUGUST 12, 2012

6 LBS, 15 OZ

SHE WAS A FEISTY LITTLE MONSTER ALREADY.

4

AFTER BIRTH

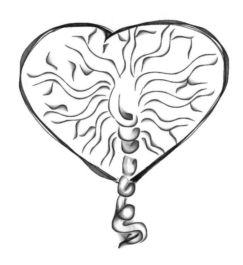

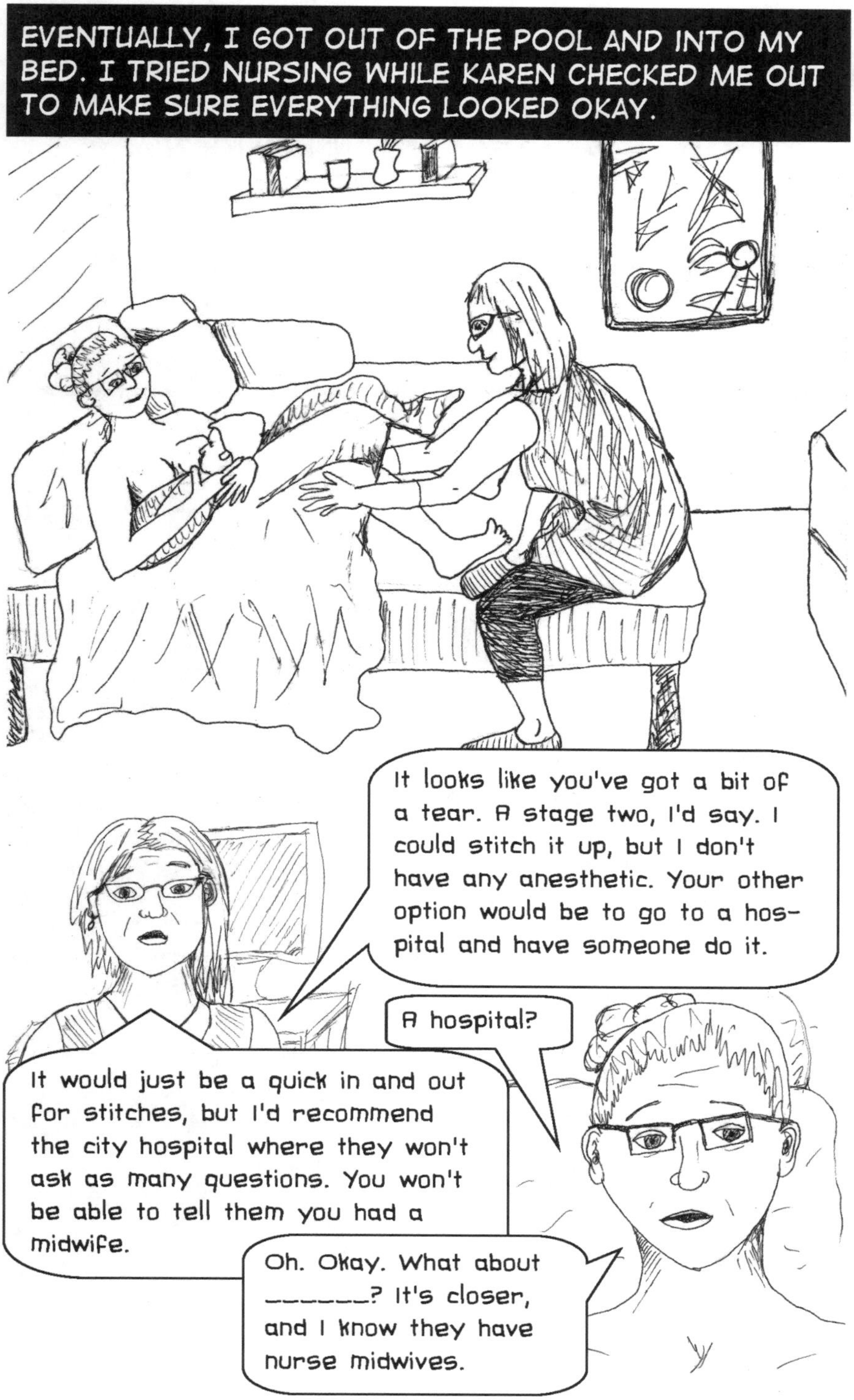
EVENTUALLY, I GOT OUT OF THE POOL AND INTO MY BED. I TRIED NURSING WHILE KAREN CHECKED ME OUT TO MAKE SURE EVERYTHING LOOKED OKAY.
It looks like you've got a bit of a tear. A stage two, I'd say. I could stitch it up, but I don't have any anesthetic. Your other option would be to go to a hospital and have someone do it.
A hospital?
It would just be a quick in and out for stitches, but I'd recommend the city hospital where they won't ask as many questions. You won't be able to tell them you had a midwife.
Oh. Okay. What about ______? It's closer, and I know they have nurse midwives.

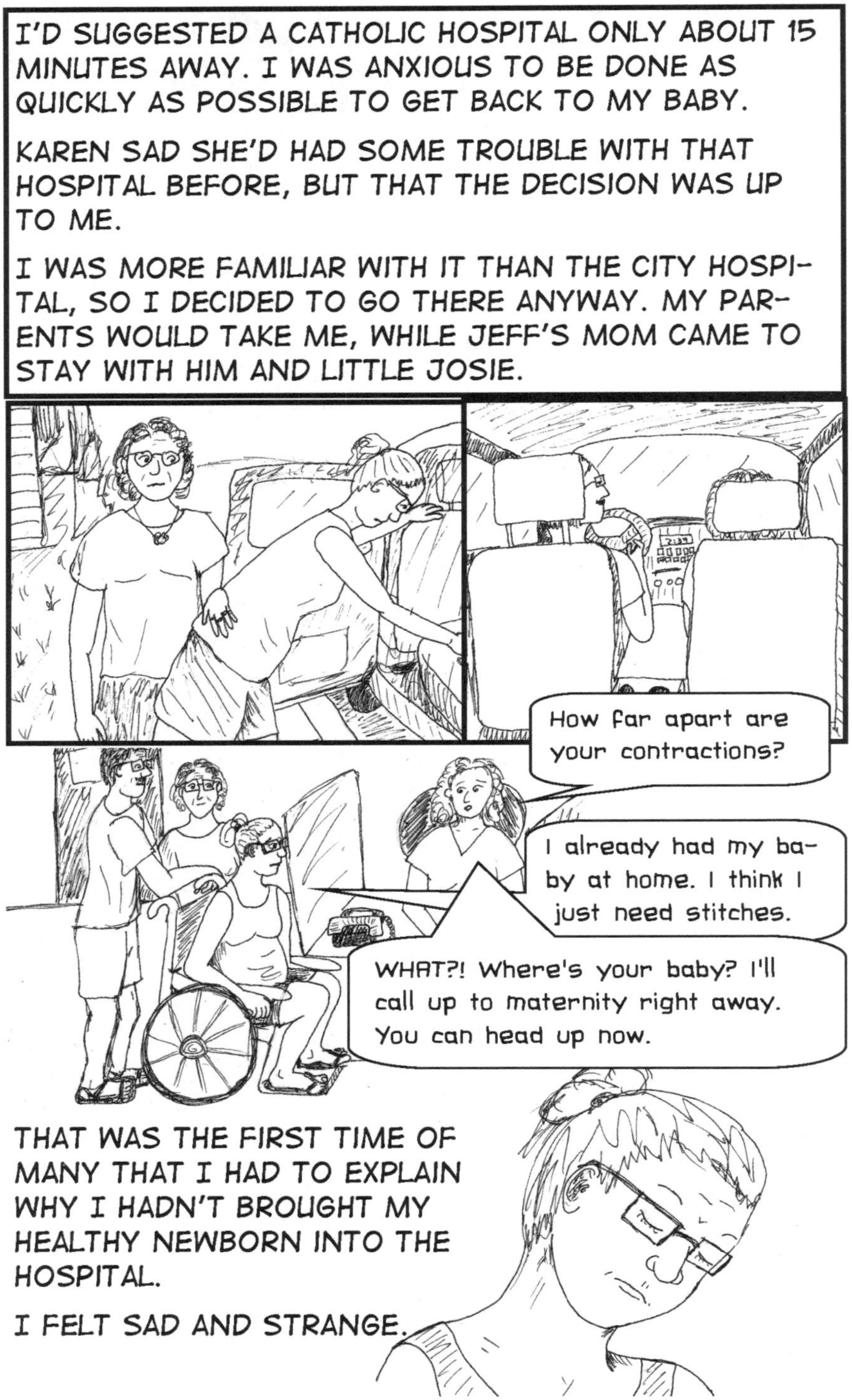
I'D SUGGESTED A CATHOLIC HOSPITAL ONLY ABOUT 15 MINUTES AWAY. I WAS ANXIOUS TO BE DONE AS QUICKLY AS POSSIBLE TO GET BACK TO MY BABY.
KAREN SAD SHE'D HAD SOME TROUBLE WITH THAT HOSPITAL BEFORE, BUT THAT THE DECISION WAS UP TO ME.
I WAS MORE FAMILIAR WITH IT THAN THE CITY HOSPITAL, SO I DECIDED TO GO THERE ANYWAY. MY PARENTS WOULD TAKE ME, WHILE JEFF'S MOM CAME TO STAY WITH HIM AND LITTLE JOSIE.
How far apart are your contractions?
I already had my baby at home. I think I just need stitches.
WHAT?! Where's your baby? I'll call up to maternity right away. You can head up now.
THAT WAS THE FIRST TIME OF MANY THAT I HAD TO EXPLAIN WHY I HADN'T BROUGHT MY HEALTHY NEWBORN INTO THE HOSPITAL.
I FELT SAD AND STRANGE.

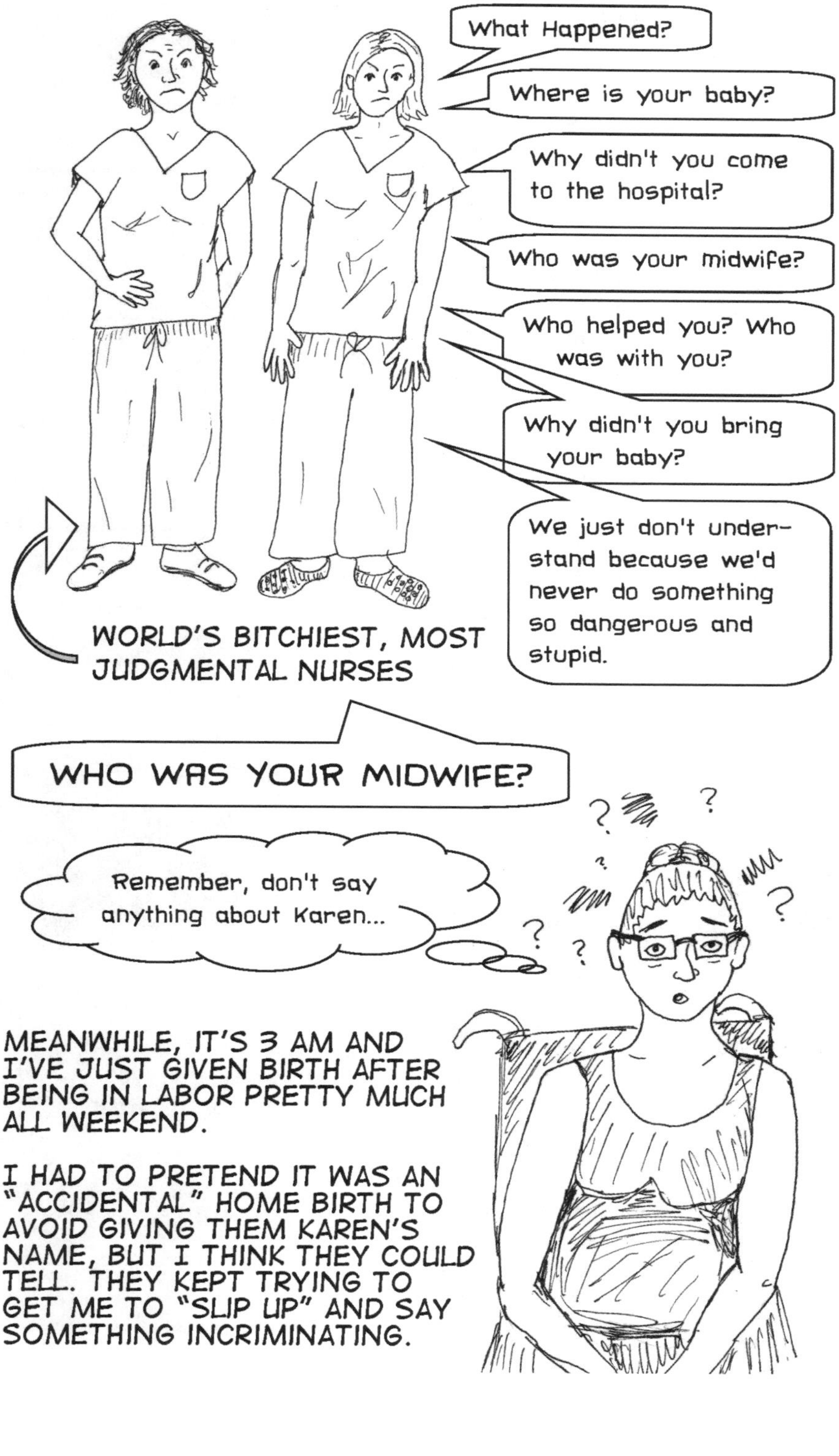
What Happened?
Where is your baby?
Why didn't you come to the hospital?
Who was your midwife?
Who helped you? Who was with you?
Why didn't you bring your baby?
We just don't under-stand because we'd never do something so dangerous and stupid.
WORLD'S BITCHIEST, MOST JUDGMENTAL NURSES
WHO WAS YOUR MIDWIFE?
Remember, don't say anything about Karen...
MEANWHILE, IT'S 3 AM AND I'VE JUST GIVEN BIRTH AFTER BEING IN LABOR PRETTY MUCH ALL WEEKEND.
I HAD TO PRETEND IT WAS AN "ACCIDENTAL" HOME BIRTH TO AVOID GIVING THEM KAREN'S NAME, BUT I THINK THEY COULD TELL. THEY KEPT TRYING TO GET ME TO "SLIP UP" AND SAY SOMETHING INCRIMINATING.

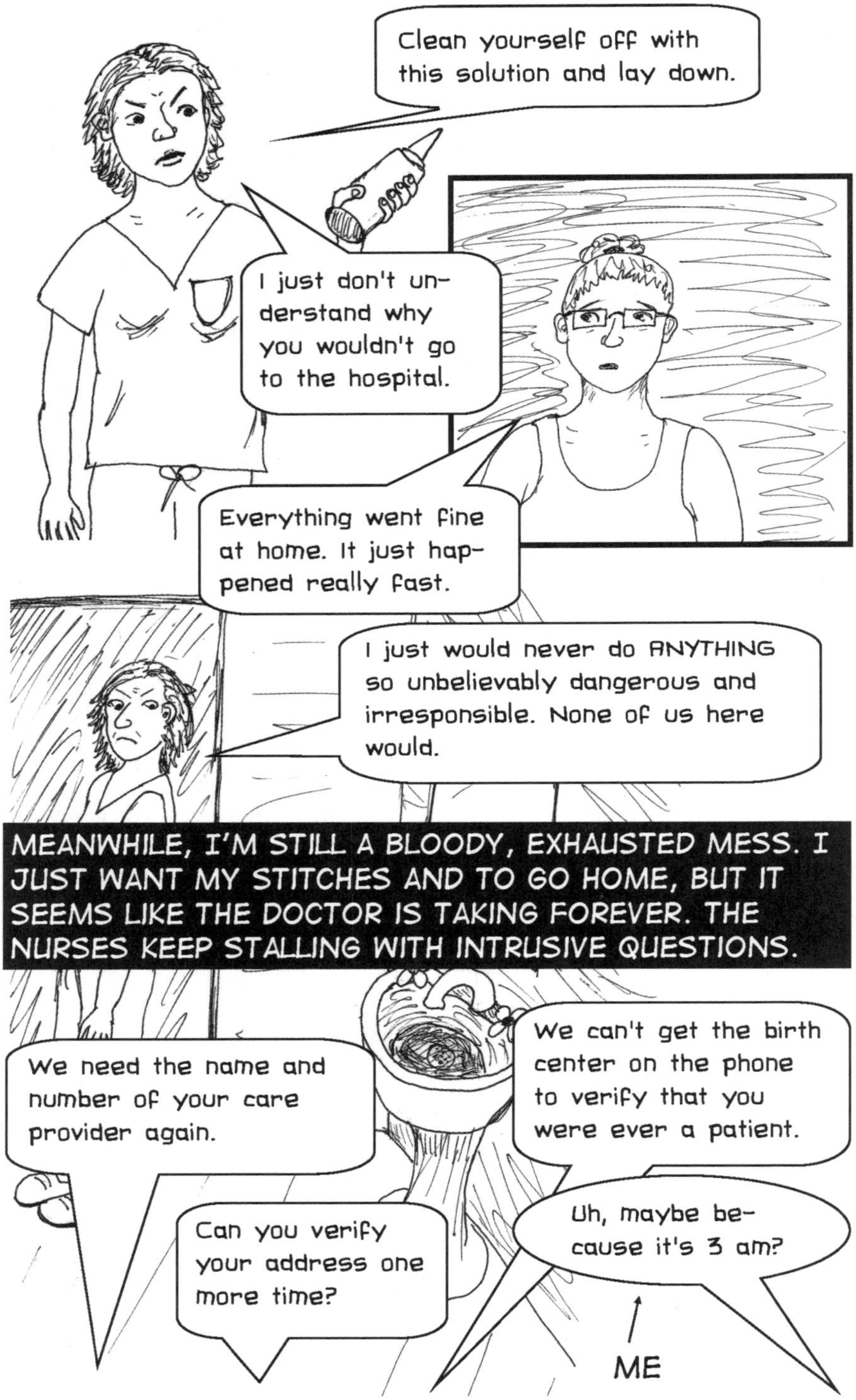
Clean yourself off with this solution and lay down.
I just don't understand why you wouldn't go to the hospital.
Everything went fine at home. It just happened really fast.
I just would never do ANYTHING so unbelievably dangerous and irresponsible. None of us here would.
MEANWHILE, I'M STILL A BLOODY, EXHAUSTED MESS. I JUST WANT MY STITCHES AND TO GO HOME, BUT IT SEEMS LIKE THE DOCTOR IS TAKING FOREVER. THE NURSES KEEP STALLING WITH INTRUSIVE QUESTIONS.
We need the name and number of your care provider again.
We can't get the birth center on the phone to verify that you were ever a patient.
Can you verify your address one more time?
Uh, maybe because it's 3 am?
ME

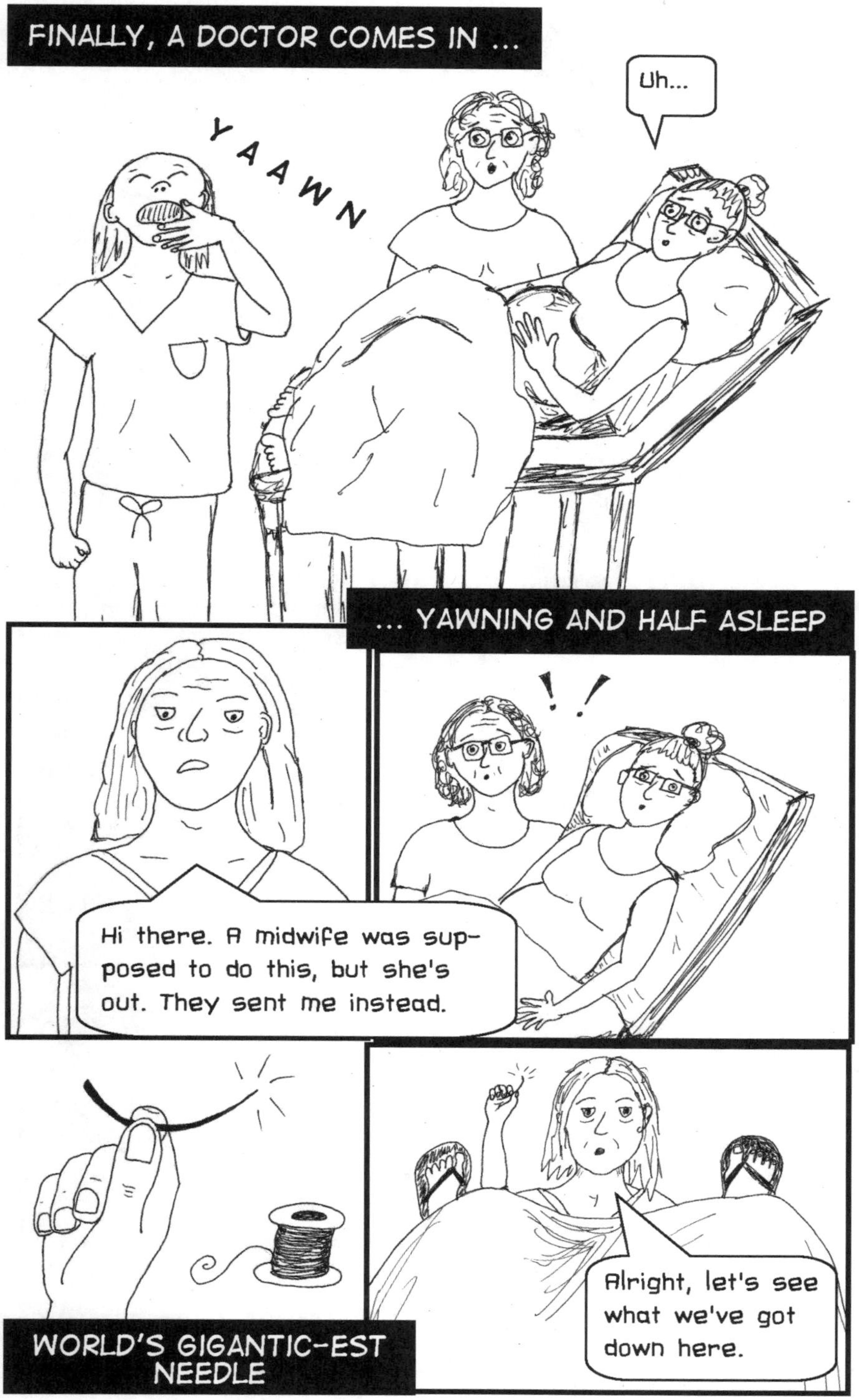
FINALLY, A DOCTOR COMES IN ...
YAAWN
Uh...
... YAWNING AND HALF ASLEEP
!!
Hi there. A midwife was supposed to do this, but she's out. They sent me instead.
WORLD'S GIGANTIC-EST NEEDLE
Alright, let's see what we've got down here.

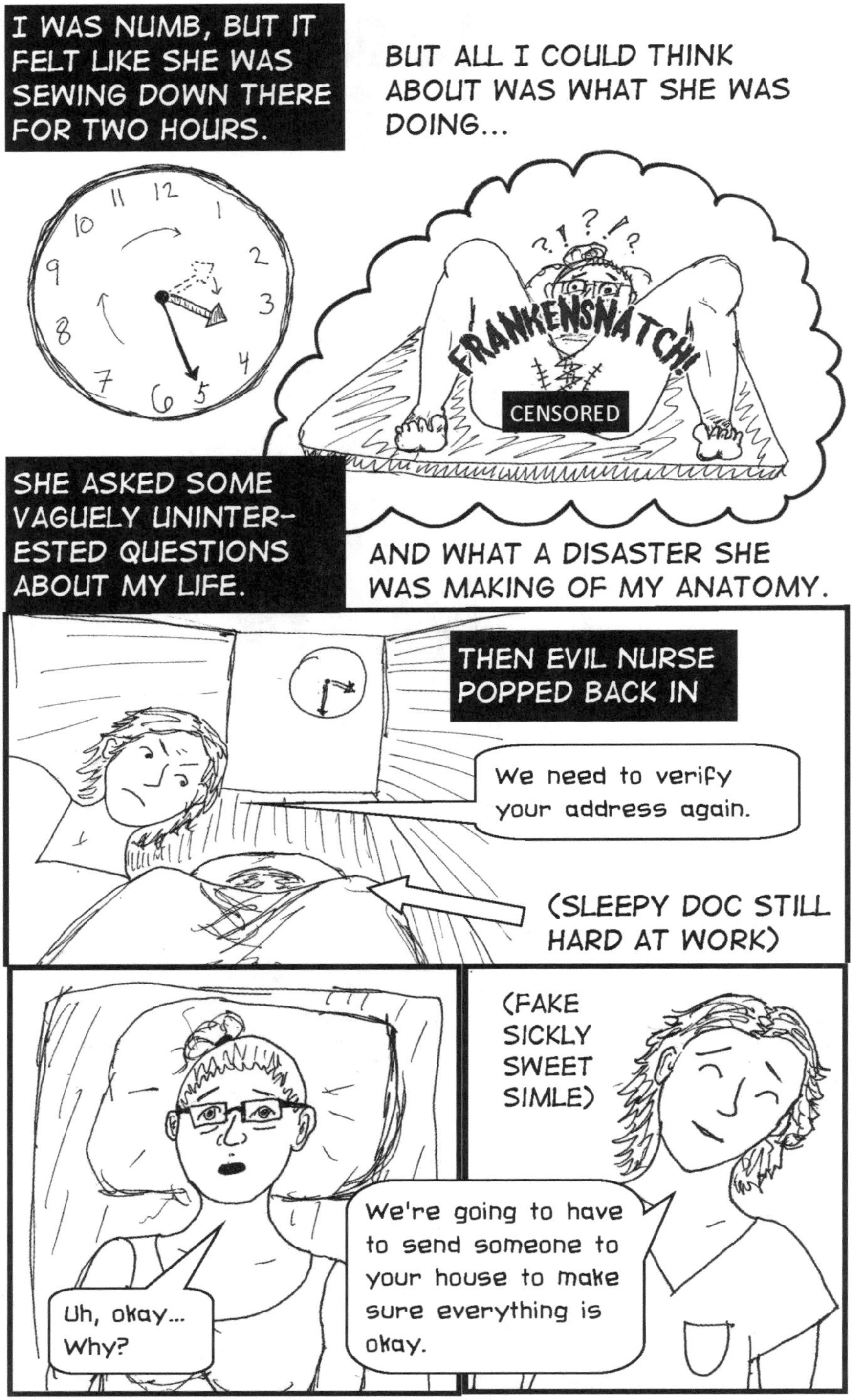
I WAS NUMB, BUT IT FELT LIKE SHE WAS SEWING DOWN THERE FOR TWO HOURS.
BUT ALL I COULD THINK ABOUT WAS WHAT SHE WAS DOING...
?!?!?
FRANKENSNATCH!
CENSORED
SHE ASKED SOME VAGUELY UNINTER-ESTED QUESTIONS ABOUT MY LIFE.
AND WHAT A DISASTER SHE WAS MAKING OF MY ANATOMY.
THEN EVIL NURSE POPPED BACK IN
We need to verify your address again.
(SLEEPY DOC STILL HARD AT WORK)
(FAKE SICKLY SWEET SIMLE)
We're going to have to send someone to your house to make sure everything is okay.
Uh, okay... Why?

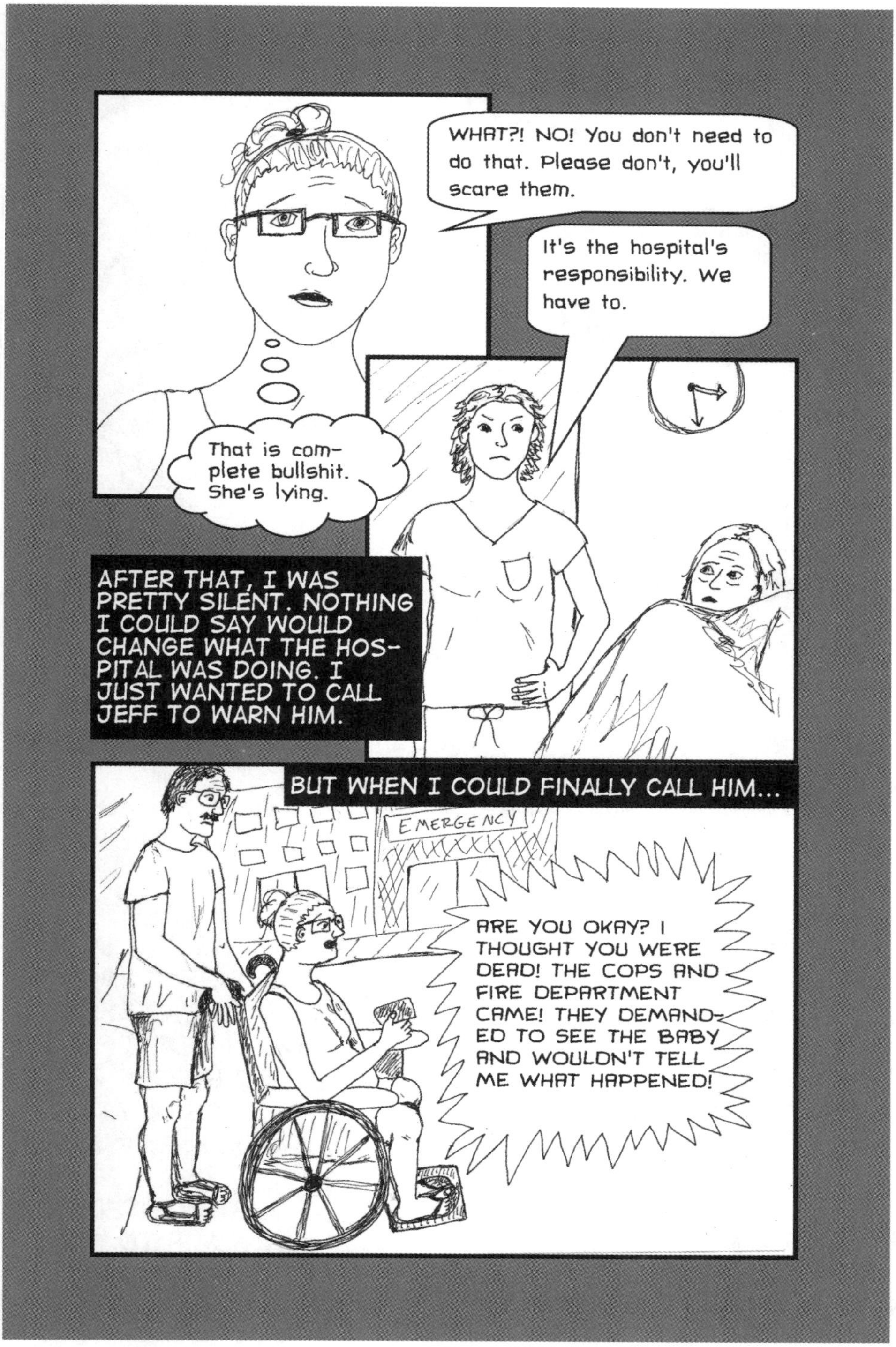
WHAT?! NO! You don't need to do that. Please don't, you'll scare them.
That is complete bullshit. She's lying.
It's the hospital's responsibility. We have to.
AFTER THAT, I WAS PRETTY SILENT. NOTHING I COULD SAY WOULD CHANGE WHAT THE HOSPITAL WAS DOING. I JUST WANTED TO CALL JEFF TO WARN HIM.
BUT WHEN I COULD FINALLY CALL HIM...
EMERGENCY
ARE YOU OKAY? I THOUGHT YOU WERE DEAD! THE COPS AND FIRE DEPARTMENT CAME! THEY DEMANDED TO SEE THE BABY AND WOULDN'T TELL ME WHAT HAPPENED!

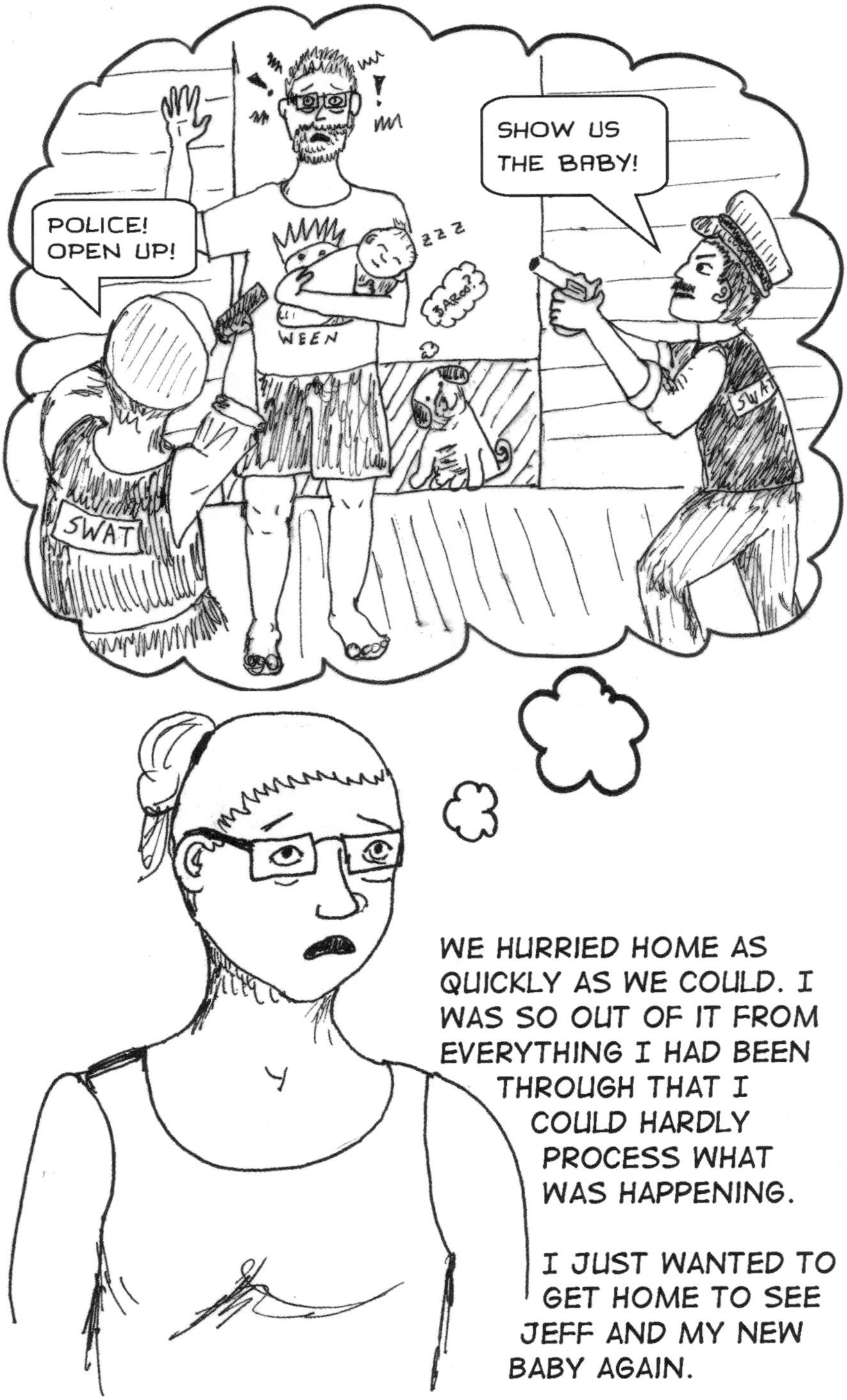
POLICE! OPEN UP!
SHOW US THE BABY!
WEEN
SWAT
SWAT
WE HURRIED HOME AS QUICKLY AS WE COULD. I WAS SO OUT OF IT FROM EVERYTHING I HAD BEEN THROUGH THAT I COULD HARDLY PROCESS WHAT WAS HAPPENING.
I JUST WANTED TO GET HOME TO SEE JEFF AND MY NEW BABY AGAIN.

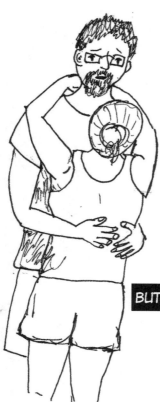

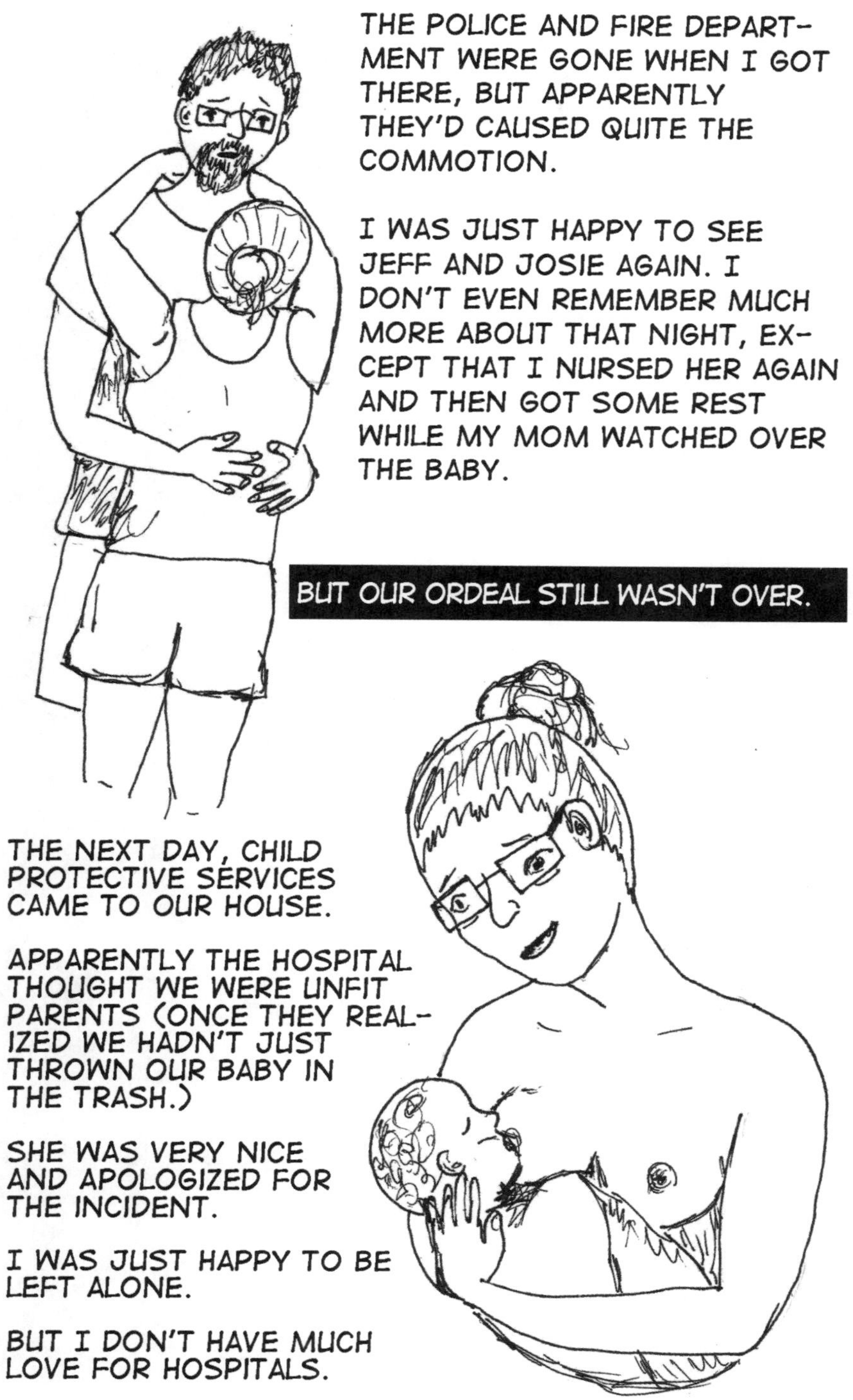

THE POLICE AND FIRE DEPART-
MENT WERE GONE WHEN I GOT
THERE, BUT APPARENTLY
THEY'D CAUSED QUITE THE
COMMOTION.

I WAS JUST HAPPY TO SEE
JEFF AND JOSIE AGAIN. I
DON'T EVEN REMEMBER MUCH
MORE ABOUT THAT NIGHT, EX-
CEPT THAT I NURSED HER AGAIN
AND THEN GOT SOME REST
WHILE MY MOM WATCHED OVER
THE BABY.

BUT OUR ORDEAL STILL WASN'T OVER.

THE NEXT DAY, CHILD
PROTECTIVE SERVICES
CAME TO OUR HOUSE.

APPARENTLY THE HOSPITAL
THOUGHT WE WERE UNFIT
PARENTS (ONCE THEY REAL-
IZED WE HADN'T JUST
THROWN OUR BABY IN
THE TRASH.)

SHE WAS VERY NICE
AND APOLOGIZED FOR
THE INCIDENT.

I WAS JUST HAPPY TO BE
LEFT ALONE.

BUT I DON'T HAVE MUCH
LOVE FOR HOSPITALS.

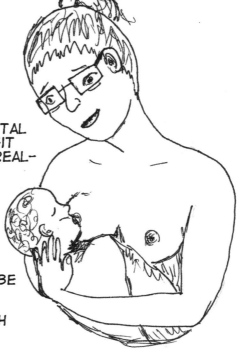

Overwhelmed, Anxious, and Angry: Navigating Postpartum Depression

(2015)

Ryan Alexander-Tanner

and Jessica Zucker

OVERWHELMED, ANXIOUS, AND ANGRY: NAVIGATING POSTPARTUM DEPRESSION

WRITTEN BY JESSICA ZUCKER, PH.D. CLINICAL PSYCHOLOGIST   ILLUSTRATED BY RYAN ALEXANDER-TANNER

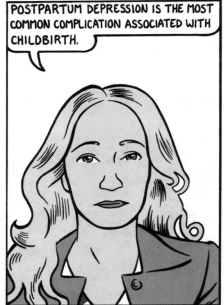

POSTPARTUM DEPRESSION IS THE MOST COMMON COMPLICATION ASSOCIATED WITH CHILDBIRTH.

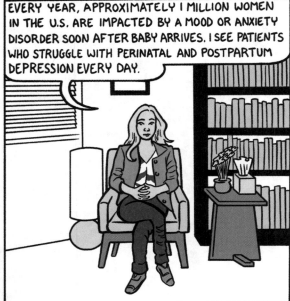

EVERY YEAR, APPROXIMATELY I MILLION WOMEN IN THE U.S. ARE IMPACTED BY A MOOD OR ANXIETY DISORDER SOON AFTER BABY ARRIVES. I SEE PATIENTS WHO STRUGGLE WITH PERINATAL AND POSTPARTUM DEPRESSION EVERY DAY.

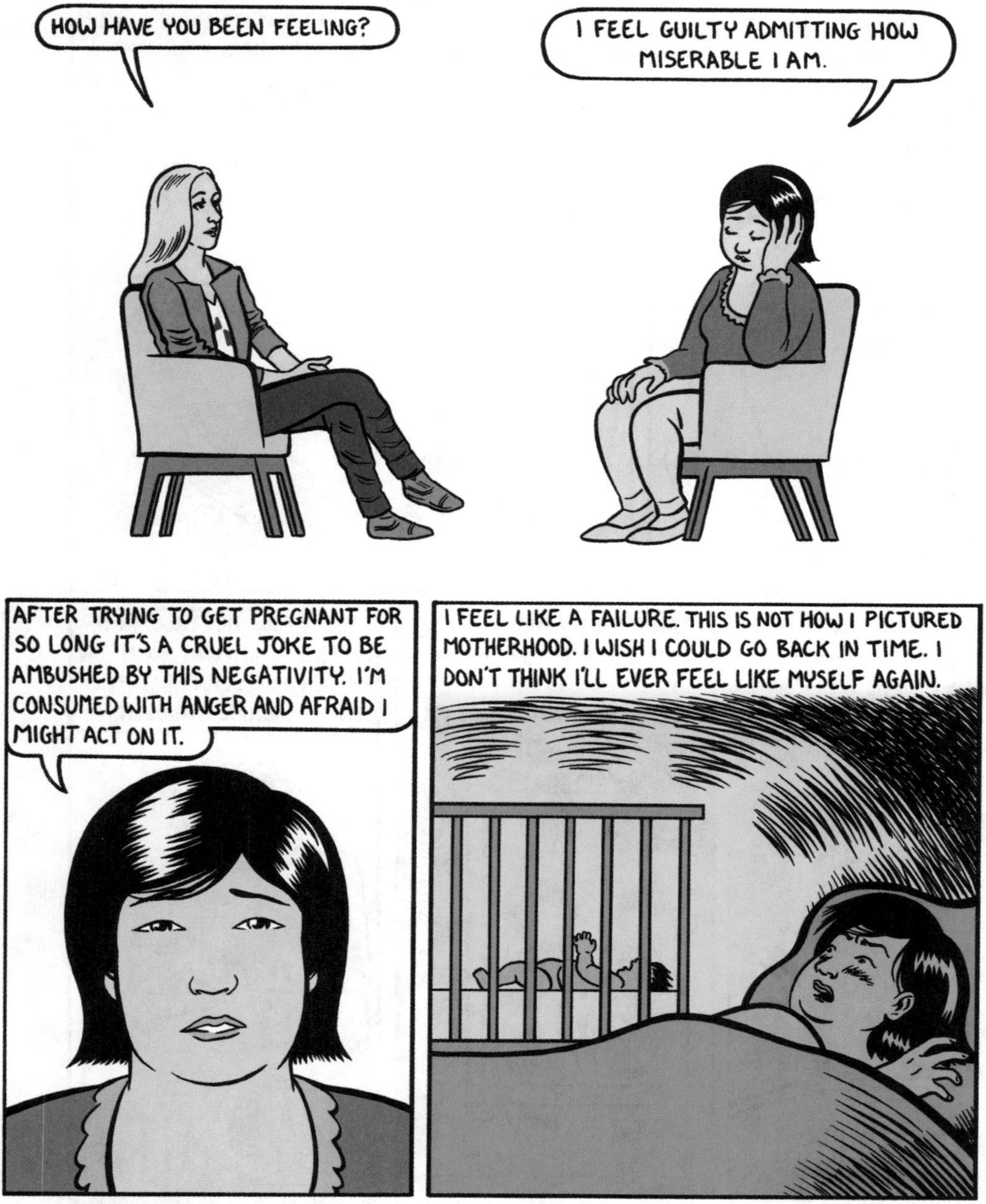
HOW HAVE YOU BEEN FEELING?
I FEEL GUILTY ADMITTING HOW MISERABLE I AM.
AFTER TRYING TO GET PREGNANT FOR SO LONG IT'S A CRUEL JOKE TO BE AMBUSHED BY THIS NEGATIVITY. I'M CONSUMED WITH ANGER AND AFRAID I MIGHT ACT ON IT.
I FEEL LIKE A FAILURE. THIS IS NOT HOW I PICTURED MOTHERHOOD. I WISH I COULD GO BACK IN TIME. I DON'T THINK I'LL EVER FEEL LIKE MYSELF AGAIN.

THE POSTPARTUM CONUNDRUM RAVAGES ONE IN SEVEN WOMEN. THE EMOTIONAL PAIN THAT ACCOMPANIES NEW MOTHERHOOD IN THE MIDST OF POSTPARTUM DEPRESSION IS TERRIFYING AND ISOLATING.

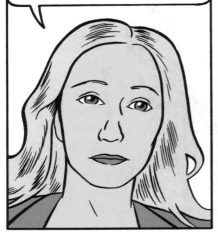

WOMEN ARE ASHAMED AND SHOCKED TO FEEL THE OPPOSITE OF WHAT THEY THOUGHT BECOMING A MOTHER MIGHT FEEL LIKE.

I THINK I'M GOING CRAZY. YESTERDAY I THOUGHT I WAS FEELING BETTER BUT BETTER DOESN'T LAST.

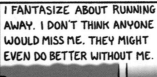

I'M ANXIOUS AND I CAN'T SLEEP. I'M NUMB AND DISCONNECTED. MY FAMILY MUST BE DISAPPOINTED IN ME.

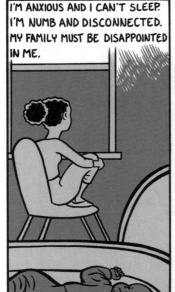

I FANTASIZE ABOUT RUNNING AWAY. I DON'T THINK ANYONE WOULD MISS ME. THEY MIGHT EVEN DO BETTER WITHOUT ME.

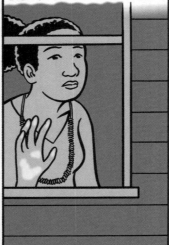

I DIDN'T FEEL THIS BADLY AFTER MY FIRST CHILD WAS BORN...OR MAYBE I DID? I CAN'T REMEMBER, I'M NOT THINKING STRAIGHT.

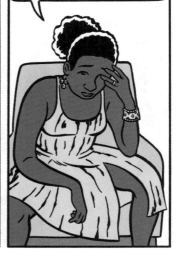

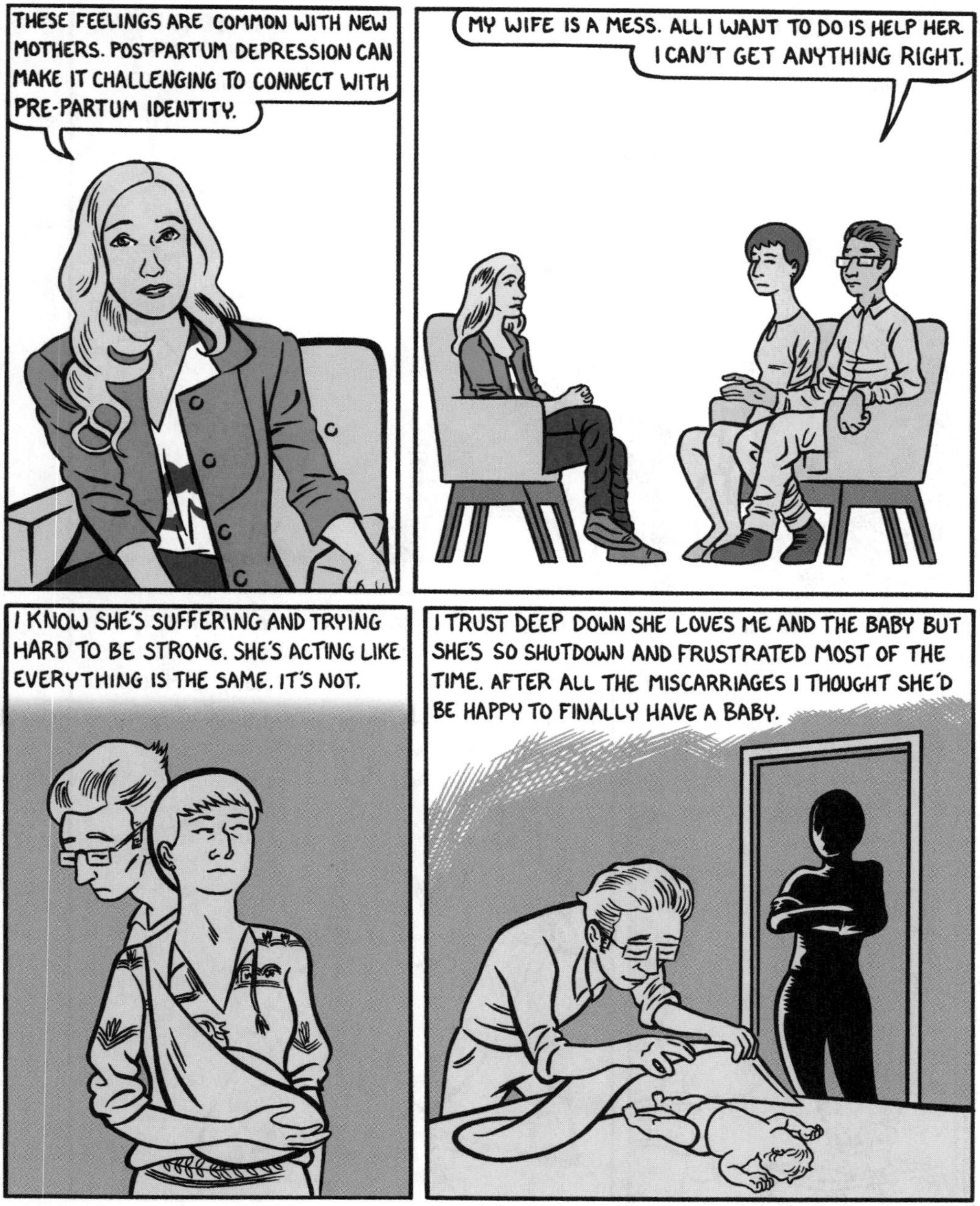
THESE FEELINGS ARE COMMON WITH NEW MOTHERS. POSTPARTUM DEPRESSION CAN MAKE IT CHALLENGING TO CONNECT WITH PRE-PARTUM IDENTITY.
MY WIFE IS A MESS. ALL I WANT TO DO IS HELP HER. I CAN'T GET ANYTHING RIGHT.
I KNOW SHE'S SUFFERING AND TRYING HARD TO BE STRONG. SHE'S ACTING LIKE EVERYTHING IS THE SAME. IT'S NOT.
I TRUST DEEP DOWN SHE LOVES ME AND THE BABY BUT SHE'S SO SHUTDOWN AND FRUSTRATED MOST OF THE TIME. AFTER ALL THE MISCARRIAGES I THOUGHT SHE'D BE HAPPY TO FINALLY HAVE A BABY.

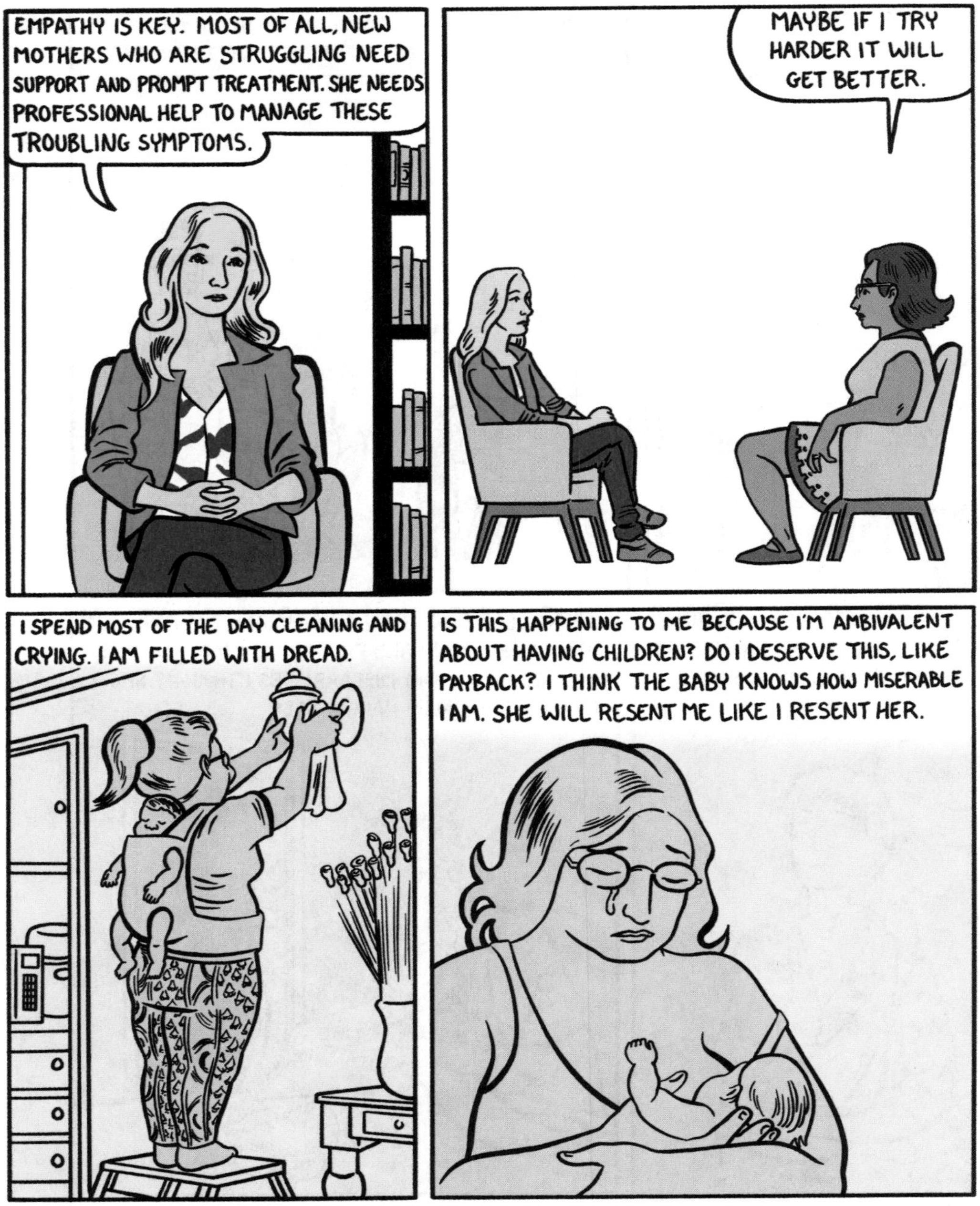
EMPATHY IS KEY. MOST OF ALL, NEW MOTHERS WHO ARE STRUGGLING NEED SUPPORT AND PROMPT TREATMENT. SHE NEEDS PROFESSIONAL HELP TO MANAGE THESE TROUBLING SYMPTOMS.
MAYBE IF I TRY HARDER IT WILL GET BETTER.
I SPEND MOST OF THE DAY CLEANING AND CRYING. I AM FILLED WITH DREAD.
IS THIS HAPPENING TO ME BECAUSE I'M AMBIVALENT ABOUT HAVING CHILDREN? DO I DESERVE THIS, LIKE PAYBACK? I THINK THE BABY KNOWS HOW MISERABLE I AM. SHE WILL RESENT ME LIKE I RESENT HER.

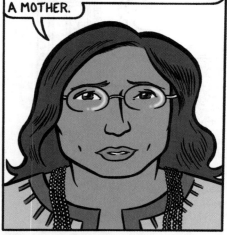

I'M HAUNTED BY THE TRAUMATIC BIRTH. BY THE TIME MY DAUGHTER CAME INTO THE WORLD I WAS SO DEBILITATED BY THE LABOR. I DON'T WANT TO BE NEAR HER. I LOVE HER BUT, SO FAR, I DON'T LIKE BEING A MOTHER.

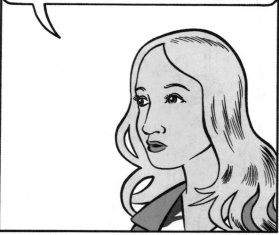

THE MOTHER'S MENTAL HEALTH TYPICALLY SETS THE STAGE FOR THE FAMILY, HAVING AN IMPACT ON ATTACHMENT AND BONDING AS WELL AS HOW HER CHILD WILL COME TO FEEL ABOUT INTERPERSONAL RELATIONSHIPS AND THE WORLD MORE GENERALLY.

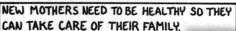
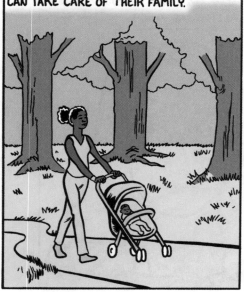

NEW MOTHERS NEED TO BE HEALTHY SO THEY CAN TAKE CARE OF THEIR FAMILY.

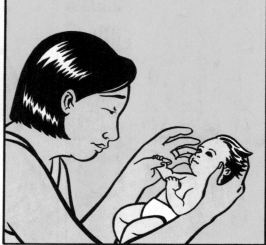

EVEN IF YOU DON'T HAVE THE MOTHER-CHILD RELATIONSHIP YOU HOPED FOR, WITH TREATMENT YOU AND YOUR BABY CAN BE MORE CONNECTED.

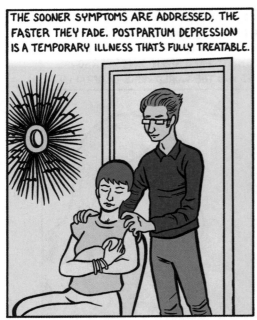

THE SOONER SYMPTOMS ARE ADDRESSED, THE FASTER THEY FADE. POSTPARTUM DEPRESSION IS A TEMPORARY ILLNESS THAT'S FULLY TREATABLE.

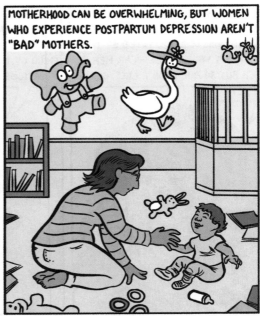

MOTHERHOOD CAN BE OVERWHELMING, BUT WOMEN WHO EXPERIENCE POSTPARTUM DEPRESSION AREN'T "BAD" MOTHERS.

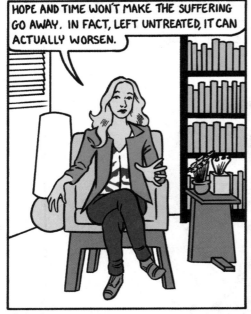

HOPE AND TIME WON'T MAKE THE SUFFERING GO AWAY. IN FACT, LEFT UNTREATED, IT CAN ACTUALLY WORSEN.

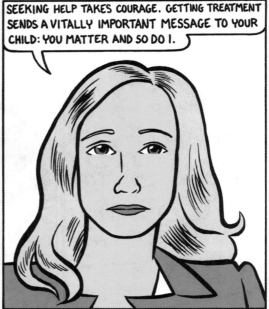

SEEKING HELP TAKES COURAGE. GETTING TREATMENT SENDS A VITALLY IMPORTANT MESSAGE TO YOUR CHILD: YOU MATTER AND SO DO I.

THIS IS A FICTIONALIZED ACCOUNT OF WOMEN'S EXPERIENCES DURING THE POSTPARTUM PERIOD.

"Anatomy of a New Mom"

(1988)

Carol Tyler

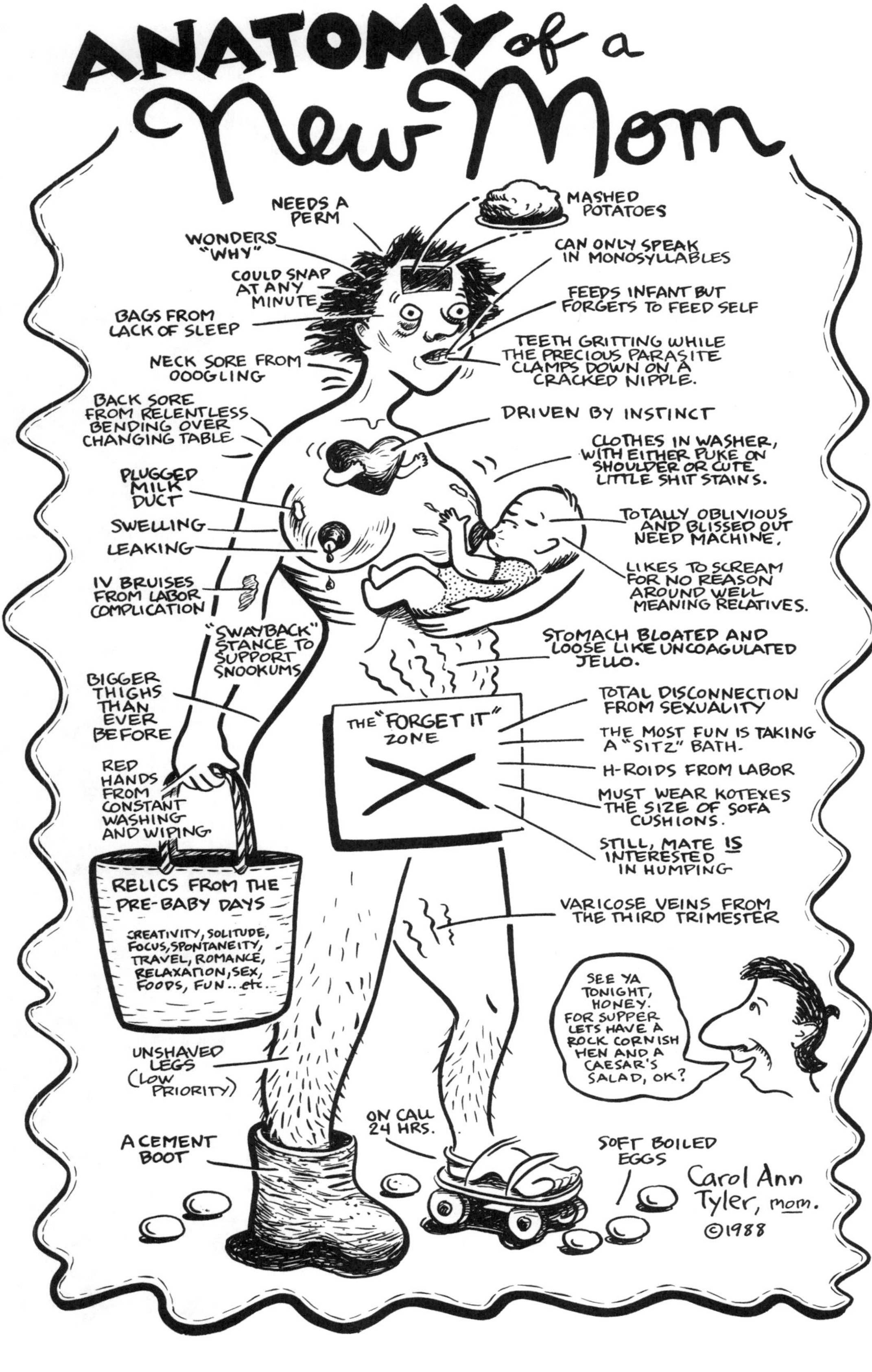

ANATOMY of a New Mom
NEEDS A PERM
MASHED POTATOES
WONDERS "WHY"
CAN ONLY SPEAK IN MONOSYLLABLES
COULD SNAP AT ANY MINUTE
FEEDS INFANT BUT FORGETS TO FEED SELF
BAGS FROM LACK OF SLEEP
TEETH GRITTING WHILE THE PRECIOUS PARASITE CLAMPS DOWN ON A CRACKED NIPPLE.
NECK SORE FROM OOOGLING
BACK SORE FROM RELENTLESS BENDING OVER CHANGING TABLE
DRIVEN BY INSTINCT
CLOTHES IN WASHER, WITH EITHER PUKE ON SHOULDER OR CUTE LITTLE SHIT STAINS.
PLUGGED MILK DUCT
SWELLING
LEAKING
TOTALLY OBLIVIOUS AND BLISSED OUT NEED MACHINE.
LIKES TO SCREAM FOR NO REASON AROUND WELL MEANING RELATIVES.
IV BRUISES FROM LABOR COMPLICATION
"SWAYBACK" STANCE TO SUPPORT SNOOKUMS
STOMACH BLOATED AND LOOSE LIKE UNCOAGULATED JELLO.
BIGGER THIGHS THAN EVER BEFORE
THE "FORGET IT" ZONE
TOTAL DISCONNECTION FROM SEXUALITY
THE MOST FUN IS TAKING A "SITZ" BATH.
H-ROIDS FROM LABOR
MUST WEAR KOTEXES THE SIZE OF SOFA CUSHIONS.
STILL, MATE IS INTERESTED IN HUMPING
RED HANDS FROM CONSTANT WASHING AND WIPING
RELICS FROM THE PRE-BABY DAYS
CREATIVITY, SOLITUDE, FOCUS, SPONTANEITY, TRAVEL, ROMANCE, RELAXATION, SEX, FOODS, FUN...etc.
VARICOSE VEINS FROM THE THIRD TRIMESTER
SEE YA TONIGHT, HONEY. FOR SUPPER LETS HAVE A ROCK CORNISH HEN AND A CAESAR'S SALAD, OK?
UNSHAVED LEGS (LOW PRIORITY)
ON CALL 24 HRS.
A CEMENT BOOT
SOFT BOILED EGGS
Carol Ann Tyler, mom.
©1988

Spawn of Dykes to Watch Out For

(1993)

Alison Bechdel

IN THE KITCHEN...
IT'S SO WILD, ONE OF US HAVING A KID!
YEAH. I LOVE TONI, BUT I DON'T GET IT. I HAVE THE MATERNAL INSTINCT OF A DOORKNOB.
USED TO BE, BEING A DYKE GOT YOU OFF THE HOOK. NO ONE EXPECTED YOU TO MAKE BABIES.
TELL ME ABOUT IT. EVER SINCE MY MAMA SAW LESBIAN MOTHERS ON 'OPRAH', I'VE BEEN UP TO MY EYEBALLS IN CLIPPINGS ABOUT SPERM BANKS.
YEAH, WELL... WHAT I WANT TO KNOW IS, HOW MUCH IS THIS LESBIAN BABY BOOM JUST A TICKET TO BEING SOCIALLY ACCEPTABLE-- A WAY FOR DYKES TO PROVE THEY'RE "REAL WOMEN" IN A CULTURE THAT EQUATES WOMANHOOD WITH MOTHERHOOD.
OH, MO! HAVEN'T YOU EVER THOUGHT ABOUT GIVING BIRTH? MARVELLED AT THE MIRACULOUS POWER OUR BODIES HAVE TO REPRODUCE? YEARNED TO EXPERIENCE THAT PROFOUND, PRIMAL CONNECTION WITH THE UNIVERSE?

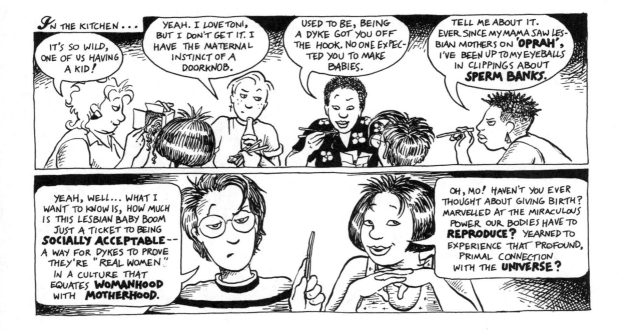

NO.
HEY, DOES YOUR NEW GIRL-FRIEND KNOW YOU WANT KIDS, SPARROW?
GIRLFRIEND?! DO TELL!
NAME'S JUNE. VERY CUTE. A REAL SCREAMER.
AANNH!
CAN YOU TELL US HOW IT FEELS, TONI?

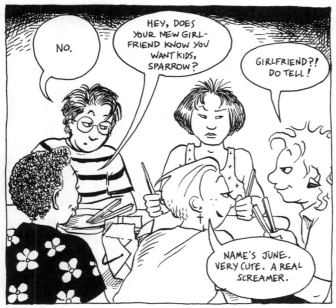

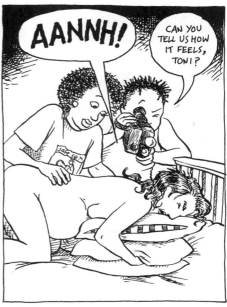

MALIKA, GET THAT THING OUT OF MY FACE!
GIVE IT A REST! WE'RE TRYING TO CONCENTRATE!
MO? CAN YOU DESCRIBE WHAT IT'S LIKE, BEING HERE WITH TONI IN LABOR?
IT'S WILD! I DON'T UNDERSTAND HOW THIS... THIS LARGE THING IS GOING TO SQUEEZE OUT OF HER BODY!
ARE YOU GONNA ENTER THIS IN THE SAN FRANCISCO QUEER FILM FESTIVAL? WANT ME TO UNDRESS?

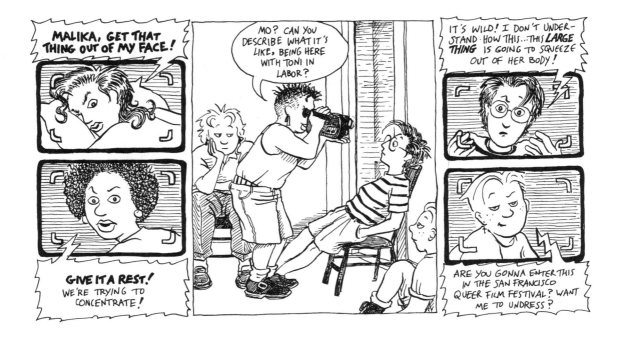

WAIT... TELL ME AGAIN WHAT A FULL HOUSE IS...
OH MY GOD!
PATHUMPATHUMPATHUMPA

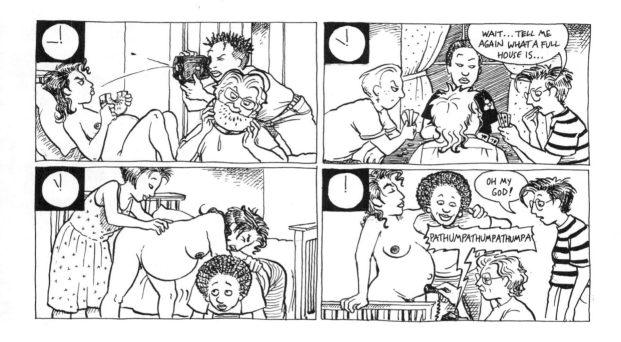

HOW MUCH LONGER? I DON'T KNOW IF I CAN DO THIS.
BUT YOU ARE DOING IT! QUITE BEAUTIFULLY!
safe sex
WANT A DRINK, BABE?
CLARICE, YOU SMELL LIKE SQUID! GO BRUSH YOUR TEETH!
SPARROW, QUIT TOUCHING ME!
MIRIAM, I THINK I HAVE TO GO TO THE BATHROOM.
YOU MIGHT BE SEN-SING THE BABY MOVING DOWN. YOU'RE FULLY DILATED... WHY DON'T YOU START PUSHING AND SEE HOW THAT FEELS?

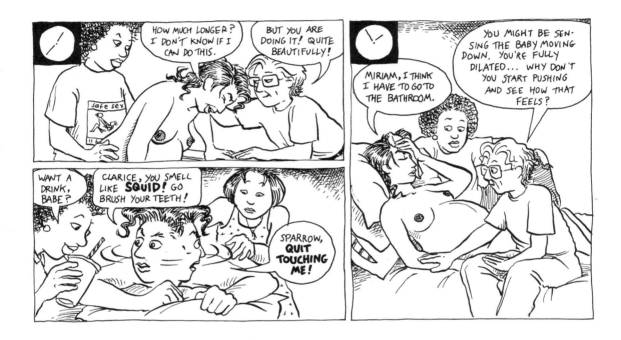

AYYY!
OH, BABY... I WISH I COULD HELP YOU! I WISH I COULD FEEL THE PAIN FOR YOU!
safe sex
DID YOU KNOW THAT IN THE HUICHOL INDIAN TRADITION, THE FATHER SQUATTED ON A PLATFORM ABOVE THE WOMAN IN LABOR, WITH ROPES TIED TO HIS BALLS? WHEN THE MOTHER HAD A CONTRACTION, SHE YANKED THE ROPES, SO THE GUY COULD SHARE THE EXPERIENCE.
THAT'S IT... BREATHE IT OPEN. YOU'RE DOING GREAT!
UNGGH!

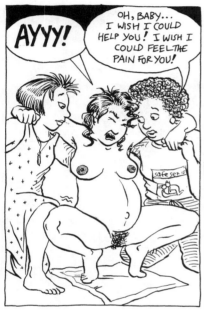

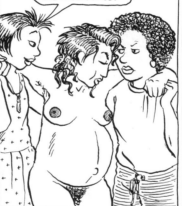

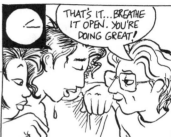

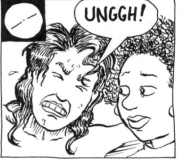

IT'S BURNING!
BABY'S CROWNING! THE BURNING MEANS GO SLOW SO YOU DON'T TEAR. I'M MASSAGING YOU WITH OLIVE OIL TO HELP YOU STRETCH.
XTRA VIR-GIN
CLARICE, IF YOU WANT TO CATCH THE BABY, GET DOWN HERE. SPARROW, WHY DON'T YOU PULL UP A CHAIR AND SUPPORT TONI FROM BEHIND.
IF YOU PUT YOUR HAND DOWN, YOU CAN FEEL THE HEAD.
IT'S RIGHT HERE!

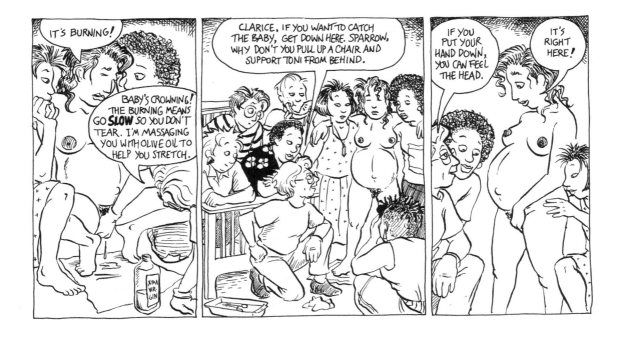

I CAN SEE IT!
I LOVE YOU.
ANH!..ANH!..ANH!
NGHH!
BEAUTIFUL! THE HEAD IS OUT! LET ME CHECK FOR THE CORD... CLARICE, PASS ME THAT GAUZE SO I CAN CLEAR THE MUCUS FROM THE FACE.
OKAY, TONI... NEXT CONTRACTION JUST GIVE A LITTLE PUSH.

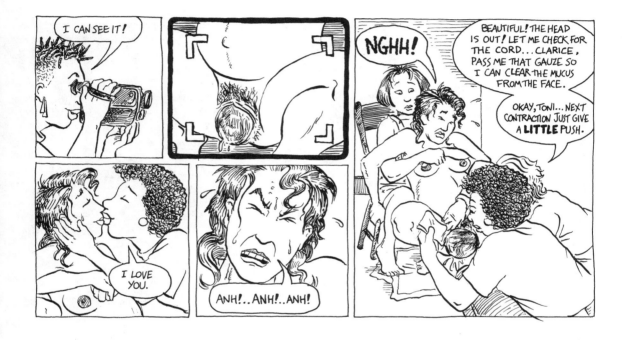

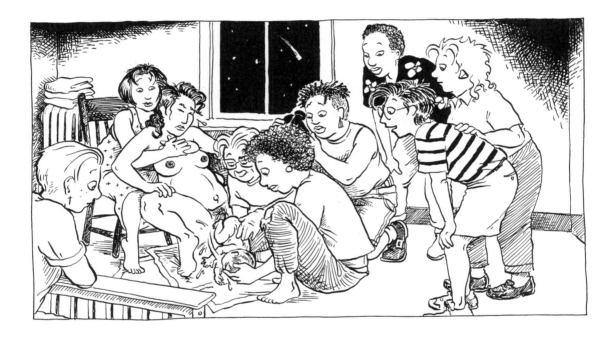

OH MY GOD! IT'S A BABY!
I CAN'T BELIEVE IT!
SLEP SLEP
JEEZIZ!
TONI, LOOK!

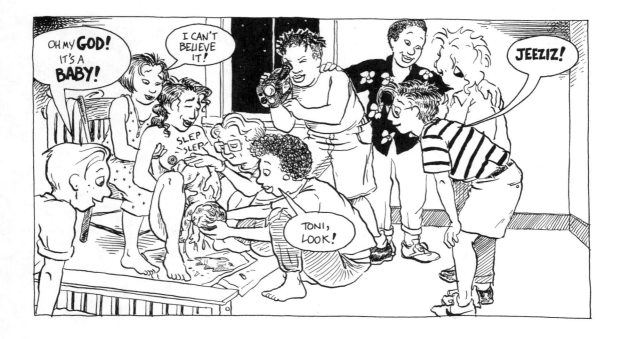

IT'S A BOY!
EHHH...
HELLO, BABY! COME ON!
A BOY!
WAAAAH!
THERE WE GO!
A MINUTE LATER...
OKAY, CLARICE. CUT THE CORD HERE BETWEEN THESE CLAMPS, CLOSE TO WHERE I'M HOLDING IT.
SNIP!

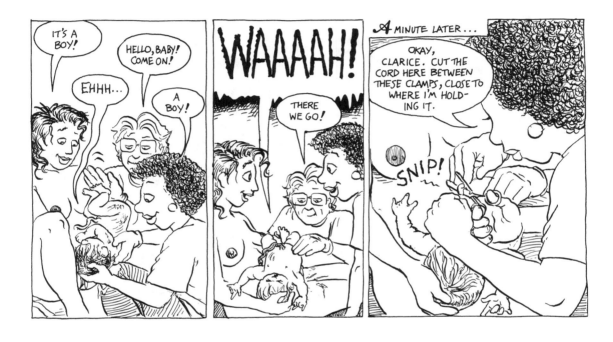

LOOKIT HIS JUG EARS! AND HE'S GOT FUR ALL OVER HIM!
WOW, HE'S GLOWING!
CLARICE, WHY DON'T YOU HOLD HIM WHILE WE DELIVER THE PLACENTA? TAKE OFF YOUR SHIRT SO HE CAN HAVE SKIN CONTACT.
CAREFUL, CLARICE. HE LOOKS HUNGRY.
SORRY, JUNIOR. WRONG MAMA
OKAY, GIVE A PUSH.

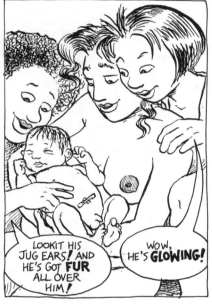

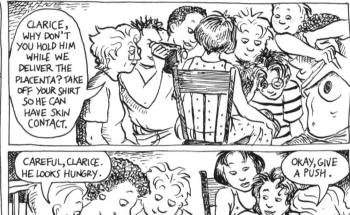

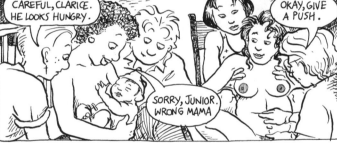

OW, WOW! LOOK AT THE SIZE OF THAT THING!
COOL.
YOU SHOULD SAVE THE PLACENTA, TONI, AND BURY IT IN YOUR BACK YARD!
OR BETTER YET, FREEZE IT AND EAT IT. IT'S A GREAT CURE FOR POST-PARTUM DEPRESSION!
OKAY, TONI. YOU HAVEN'T LOST MUCH BLOOD. LET'S GET YOU INTO BED.

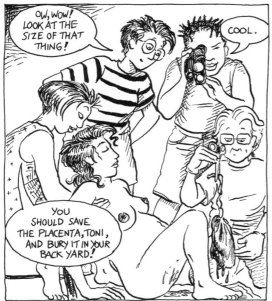

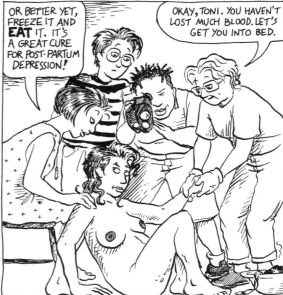

JUST THINK! THESE ARE THE MOST INTENSELY FORMATIVE MOMENTS OF THIS PERSON'S LIFE! WHAT A WONDERFUL ATMOSPHERE TO BE BORN INTO! HE MIGHT NOT EVEN NEED THERAPY WHEN HE GROWS UP!
WHAT ARE YOU GONNA CALL HIM?
RAFAEL, AFTER MY GRANDMOTHER RAFAELA.
I'LL BE BACK IN A BIT TO DO A MORE THOROUGH EXAM.

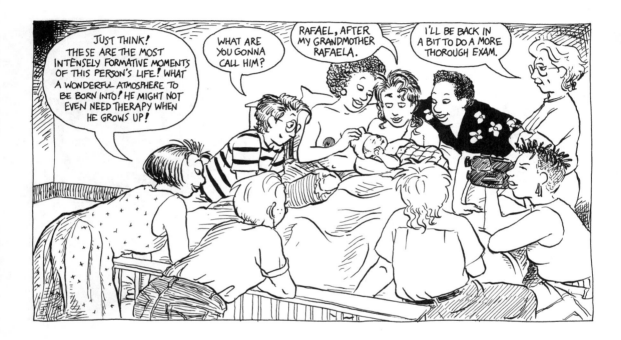

WOW, IT'S GOING ON FIVE. I GUESS WE SHOULD START MOVING OUT.
CON-GRATU-LATIONS, GIRLS.
THANKS, MO. THANK YOU EVERYONE. I LOVE YOU GUYS!
G'NIGHT, BEAUTIFUL.
I GOT SOME GREAT FOOTAGE, YOU TWO. I'LL BRING YOU A COPY LATER.
SEE YA LATER, BABY. WELCOME TO THE WORLD.

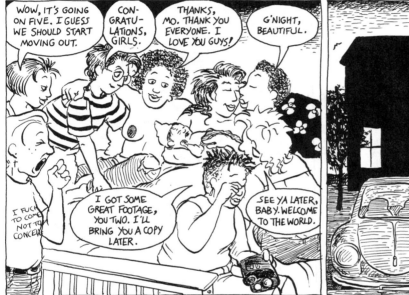

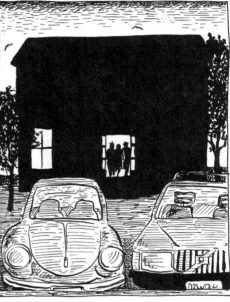

Afterword

Susan Merrill Squier

In the introduction to *Graphic Reproduction*, Jenell Johnson points out that most of the comics in this collection challenge the medicalization of reproduction, although of course "pregnancy is not de facto an illness, and childbirth is not de facto a medical emergency." We are pleased to welcome this comics anthology to our Graphic Medicine series not only because it voices the reproductive experiences of patients, friends, and family members, but also because it contests the narrow understanding of reproduction, presenting instead a wide range of experiences and subjects usually excised from the cheerily commodified "what to expect when you're expecting" narrative. The works included in *Graphic Reproduction* are able to frame reproduction with greater insight and complexity because they incorporate strategies integral to the medium of comics and to the genre of graphic medicine: intermedia references; the use of visual imagery to convey complex information wordlessly; an appreciation of performance as a mode of knowledge production; and an embrace of complexity befitting what has been called "an art of tension."[1]

Some of the pieces in this collection reveal the position of comics as one medium among other media—television, film, music recordings, photographs, the internet—which enables the cartoonist to lend resonance to the narrative. So Jenell Johnson's witty and moving *Present / Perfect* offers in quick succession allusions to the film *Charlotte's Web*, to the TV shows *Battlestar Galactica* and *Friday Night Lights*, and to the music of Bruce Springsteen, Skid Row, and the Shins. While positioning readers temporally, these intermedia allusions also provide a sociocultural context for the protagonists and an implicit sound track for their story. The medium of the internet opens the way to support groups for Johnson in this comic and for Endrené Shepherd in *A Significant Loss*, as they struggle with infertility and miscarriage. Finally, there's Malika's incessant filming of the birth in *Spawn of Dykes to Watch Out For*, which performs what Elisabeth El Refaie would call an act of "authentication."[2]

Comics rely on visual images as well as text, providing information through nonverbal cues as diverse as hair and clothing styles, car models, and medical equipment. *Abortion Eve* situates its story in the 1970s by showing granny gowns and hiking boots, turtleneck sweaters, bell bottoms, and Mark Spitz moustaches.

The images of a Volvo and a Volkswagen signal the comfortably left-leaning community into which Toni and Clarice's baby is born in *Spawn of Dykes to Watch Out For*. The contrast between the suction machine in *Abortion Eve* and the home pregnancy tests, biopsy needle, petri dishes, and ultrasound wand in *Present / Perfect* testify to the role of technological developments in the history of medicalized reproduction. And the wonderful variety of bodies, clothing styles, hairstyles, and reproductive plans in *Pregnant Butch* speaks to our contemporary openness to nonbinary gender roles and diverse parenting strategies. All of these visual images communicate implicitly rather than explicitly or didactically, setting the scene wordlessly even as the text propels the narrative.

"Talking, Thinking, Drawing," the section of classroom exercises with which this volume concludes, draws on a core principle of graphic medicine: that drawing is, in itself, a powerful mode of knowledge production. Or to put it more simply: drawing is a mode of thinking. KC Councilor and Jenell Johnson argue that in order to appreciate how the comics of *Graphic Reproduction* express their wide array of reproductive practices and meanings we must move from writing to drawing. Their performative approach to the teaching of comics studies repurposes a classic method of medical education: SODOTO, see one, do one, teach one. Having *seen* comics, now we should *do* comics, so we can *teach* comics.

On the opening page of the exercises, Johnson appears again as a comic avatar, along with KC Councilor, whose rainbow and unicorn T-shirt (and shades) is part of his social and cultural context. Tiny, naively drawn figures dance and cartwheel around the circled title above them. This whole page, like what follows, reflects the style and insights of two major figures in cartooning and graphic medicine: Lynda Barry, who in a celebrated series of comics and workbooks has taught people to access "what it is," to summon and express the sea of images within; and MK Czerwiec, aka Comic Nurse, who in the *Graphic Medicine Manifesto* argues that those of us who gave up drawing in fourth grade can rediscover our own visual style and our creativity by experimenting with "the power of the crayon."[3] As we pick up crayons again and draw ourselves reading the comics, share them with friends, copy them to notice their nuances, redraw them in our own style to express how we feel about them, and insert our own panels to elaborate on the ideas these comics spark in us, we can learn to become active, agential comics readers, cartoonists, and even inspired comics teachers.

Councilor and Johnson's questions in this teaching guide pull not for unanimity but for complexity. In "Exploring the Gutters," they ask, "Did you find yourself relating to . . . or resisting! . . . any of the comics?" They suggest, "Draw a satirical tabloid magazine cover that takes a more critical view" of the narrative that glorifies motherhood. Just as comics themselves can contain multiple meanings in one panel, this approach to comics education forges teachers who are not afraid of conflict or controversy. Crucially, both the critical view and the challenging questions are part of an ongoing conversation rather than being detached observations. That continuing engagement marks the volume as a whole: it accepts complexity, even conflict, as part of the process of engaged understanding. "This book does *not* seek to resolve the tension that arises among the stories," Johnson points out in the introduction, and this shouldn't surprise us, for the comics genre, as already mentioned, is an art of tensions.

Indeed, there is one zone of tension in the treatment of reproduction in comics that does not appear in *Graphic Reproduction* but should certainly be explored in the future. I have mentioned how the embodied aspects of *Abortion Eve* (hairstyles, clothing, facial hair) index the early 1970s, when the *Roe v. Wade* decision had newly affirmed women's access to legal abortions. "Every human body is a marker in time," artist Riva Lehrer observes in an essay that appeared in the *New York Times* the week I drafted this afterword.[4] Yet the embodied time markers that Lehrer considers in "Where All Bodies Are Exquisite" calibrate not the increasing access to legal abortion but the increasingly sophisticated surgeries she has undergone since her birth as a person with spina bifida. I have said that the comics in *Graphic Reproduction* encourage us to expand continually the ways we understand reproduction, rather than sticking with the conventional story, or myth, that is peddled by normative Western culture. In the same spirit as that message, we now need to ask: Whose voices have not been included? Whose bodies are still unseen? When we do so, we will recognize the tension between the range of reproductive narratives this volume explores, including abortion, infertility, miscarriage, stillbirth, postpartum exhaustion, postpartum depression, and varieties of home birth, and the various experiences of disability that Lehrer's essay brilliantly illuminates.[5]

Lehrer's essay, which begins with a visit to the Mütter Museum's collection of fetal specimens with spina bifida, "historical artifacts marking a moment when medicine had nothing to offer," goes on to detail the different surgeries she experienced between her birth in 1958, "just as surgeons found a way to close the spina bifida lesion," and her fifth year, by which she had experienced several dozen operations. These surgeries gave her the ability to walk and yet left her with "organ damage, an asymmetrical body, mobility problems, and a limp," all marks on her body testifying to the medicalization of disability and to the effects of new surgical techniques.[6] But it was not these surgical interventions that shaped her decisively, Lehrer writes: "Nothing changes a disabled person's sense of self like another disabled person. I am a painter, and . . . I was invited to join a group of artists, writers and performers who were building disability culture. Their work was daring, edgy, funny and dark; it rejected old tropes that defined us as pathetic, frightening and worthless. They insisted that disability was an opportunity for creativity and resistance."[7] Just as the cartoonists in this volume have challenged the limits of reproduction, so the group of artists and creators Lehrer met "stretched the boundaries of what it meant to be human." She began to interview them, and then to paint them with exquisite, precise specificity. The resulting group of portraits, *Circle Stories*, is featured on the Graphic Medicine website.[8] Circles within circles, the site also includes a documentary film of Lehrer creating a stunning portrait of cartoonist Alison Bechdel.

Two more quick points to conclude the conversation I have been staging between the works in *Graphic Reproduction* and Riva Lehrer's stunning visual and textual exploration of the experience of disability. First, although many of the comics in this collection resist the medicalization of reproduction, it is important to point out that people with disability have a complex engagement with medicine, viewing it as something to be affirmed when it offers benefit to people with painful or problematic embodiment, but seeing medicine as something to be contested when it leaves that person labeled as "pathetic, frightening, and worthless." Like disability studies, graphic medicine does important work at that intersection, since comics have a remarkable ability to embrace and reveal experiential ambivalence and complexity because of their multilayered, visual and verbal, linear and looping narrative capacity.

Second, just as works of graphic medicine affirm the agency of patients and family members as they tell their own stories of illness and medical treatment, so too we should abide by the disability studies motto "Nothing about us without us," and look for comics that speak from the perspectives of people with disability. I am thinking of such works as Kaisa Leka's *I Am Not These Feet* with its image of the in utero Kaisa as an embryonic Minnie Mouse, and of Al Davidson's graphic memoir about his own spina bifida, *The Spiral Cage*, with its powerful images of the dreaming infant flying as a merman above his hospital crib.[9] In these works neither reproduction nor disability is a simple, linear, or univocal experience. Instead, as both comics show, an exquisite creative potential resides at the intersection of reproduction and disability.

NOTES

1. Charles Hatfield, "Comics as an Art of Tension," in *A Comics Studies Reader*, ed. Jeet Heer and Kent Worcester (Jackson: University Press of Mississippi, 2009), 132–48.

2. Elisabeth El Refaie, "Visual Authentication Strategies in Autobiographical Comics," November 30, 2012, https:// comicsforum.org/ 2012/11/30/visual-authentication -strategies-in-autobiographical-comics -by-elisabeth-el-refaie.

3. Lynda Barry, *What It Is: The Formless Thing Which Gives Things Form* (Montreal: Drawn and Quarterly, 2008); MK Czerwiec, Ian Williams, Susan Merrill Squier, Michael J. Green, Kimberly R. Myers, and Scott T. Smith, *Graphic Medicine Manifesto* (University Park: Penn State University Press, 2015).

4. Riva Lehrer, "Where All Bodies Are Exquisite," *New York Times*, August 9, 2017.

5. This tension is central to another comic in our Graphic Medicine series, Henny Beaumont's *Hole in the Heart: Bringing Up Beth* (University Park: Penn State University Press, 2016).

6. Lehrer, "Where All Bodies Are Exquisite."

7. Lehrer, "Where All Bodies Are Exquisite."

8. See "A Conversation with Riva Lehrer," *Graphic Medicine*, May 30, 2012, https:// www.graphicmedicine.org/a -conversation-with-riva-lehrer.

9. Kaisa Leka, *I Am Not These Feet* (Helsinki: Absolute Truth Press, 2003); Al Davidson, *The Spiral Cage* (Los Angeles: Active Images and Astral Gypsy Press, 2003).

TALKING
THINKING
DRAWING
CLASSROOM EXERCISES
by
KC COUNCILOR
&
JENELL JOHNSON

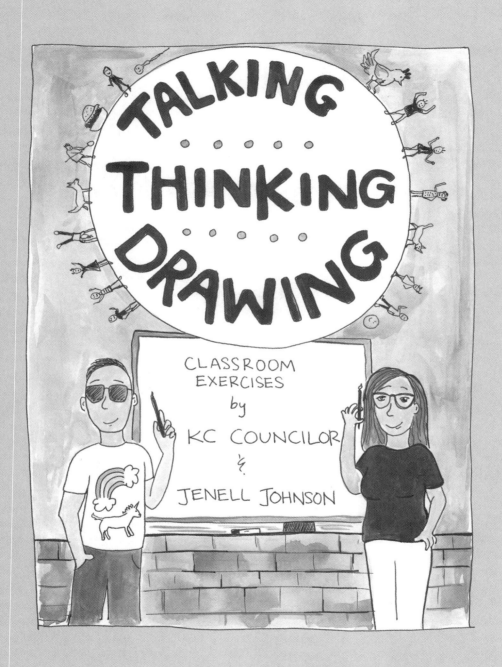

Discussion Questions

1. As Johnson explains in the introduction, comics often challenge dominant narratives of human experience. How do conception, pregnancy, and birth typically get presented in film, television, literature, and art? Come up with some examples and compare them. What narrative features do they share? What emotions do they allow (and disallow)? Whose bodies do they portray? Whose bodies are left out? What endings do they offer? How do the comics in this book challenge these narratives? How do they reproduce them?

2. Do some research on the women's health movement of the 1960s and 1970s. How does it fit within the women's movement more generally? How do you understand Farmer and Chevli's *Abortion Eve* as a part of that movement? How does it depart from that movement? Why do you think Planned Parenthood resisted distributing this comic?

3. As the name of the genre suggests, comics sometimes take a humorous approach to serious subjects. Where are the moments of humor in this collection? What narrative role do they serve?

4. Look through the comics to find what they *don't* show. What experiences fall into the gutters? What happens between panels? What is the effect of these absences in the comic narrative?

5. How do the artists' depictions of their selves/characters change according to the emotions in the panels? What happens to the light and shadow? Facial expressions? Line width? How else do the artists represent emotions in their comics?

6. How do gender and sexuality function in these comics? How do the artists represent issues of gender and sexuality? What is left out?

7. What assumptions do you find in the comics about the medicalization of conception, pregnancy, and childbirth? How do the artists challenge those assumptions, and where do they reproduce them?

8. How do the different comics represent the embryo/fetus and its connection to the pregnant person? How do these different representations shift your experience of each narrative?

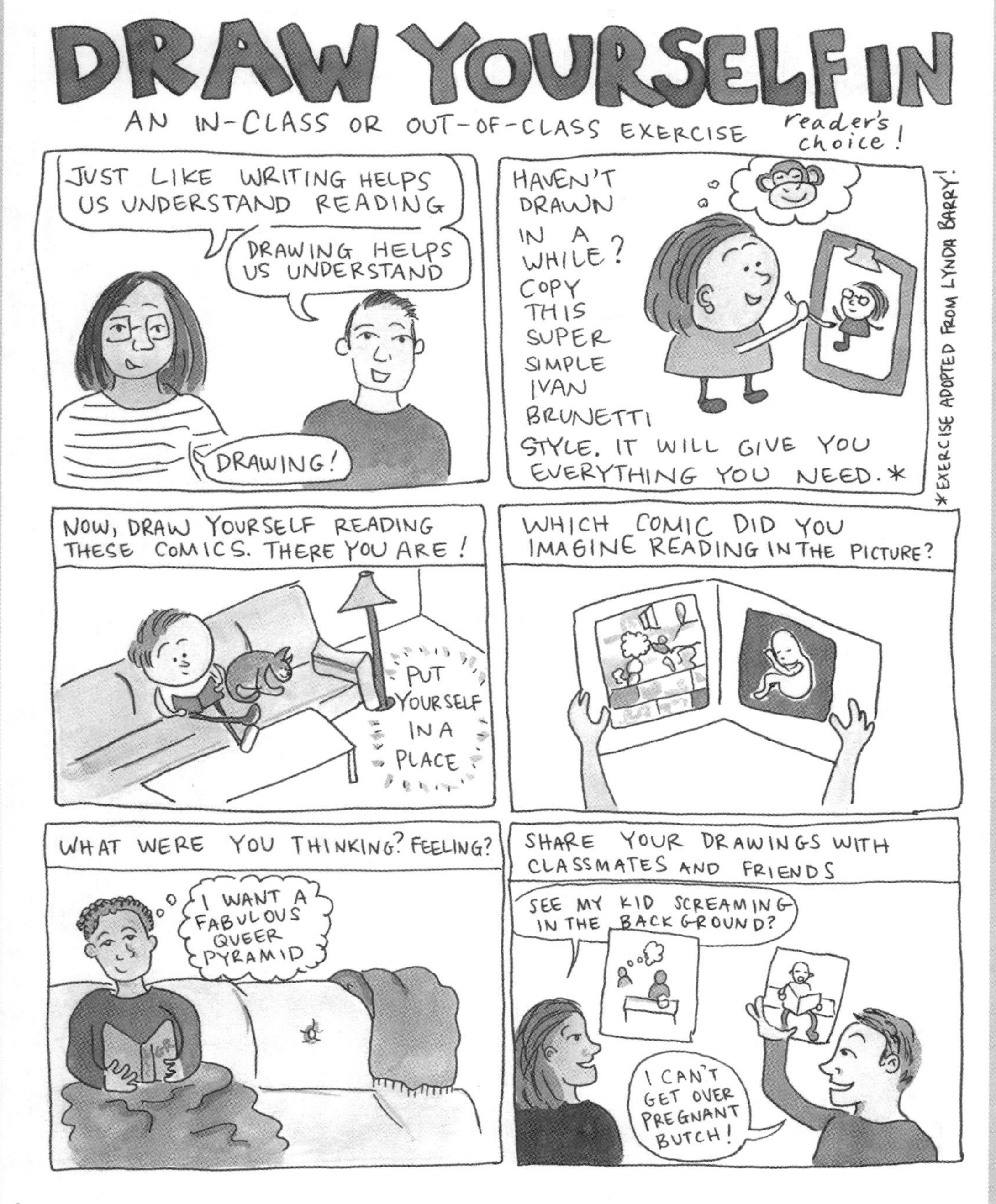
DRAW YOURSELF IN
AN IN-CLASS OR OUT-OF-CLASS EXERCISE
reader's choice!
JUST LIKE WRITING HELPS US UNDERSTAND READING
DRAWING HELPS US UNDERSTAND
DRAWING!
HAVEN'T DRAWN IN A WHILE? COPY THIS SUPER SIMPLE IVAN BRUNETTI STYLE. IT WILL GIVE YOU EVERYTHING YOU NEED.*
*EXERCISE ADOPTED FROM LYNDA BARRY!
NOW, DRAW YOURSELF READING THESE COMICS. THERE YOU ARE!
PUT YOURSELF IN A PLACE
WHICH COMIC DID YOU IMAGINE READING IN THE PICTURE?
WHAT WERE YOU THINKING? FEELING?
I WANT A FABULOUS QUEER PYRAMID
SHARE YOUR DRAWINGS WITH CLASSMATES AND FRIENDS
SEE MY KID SCREAMING IN THE BACKGROUND?
I CAN'T GET OVER PREGNANT BUTCH!

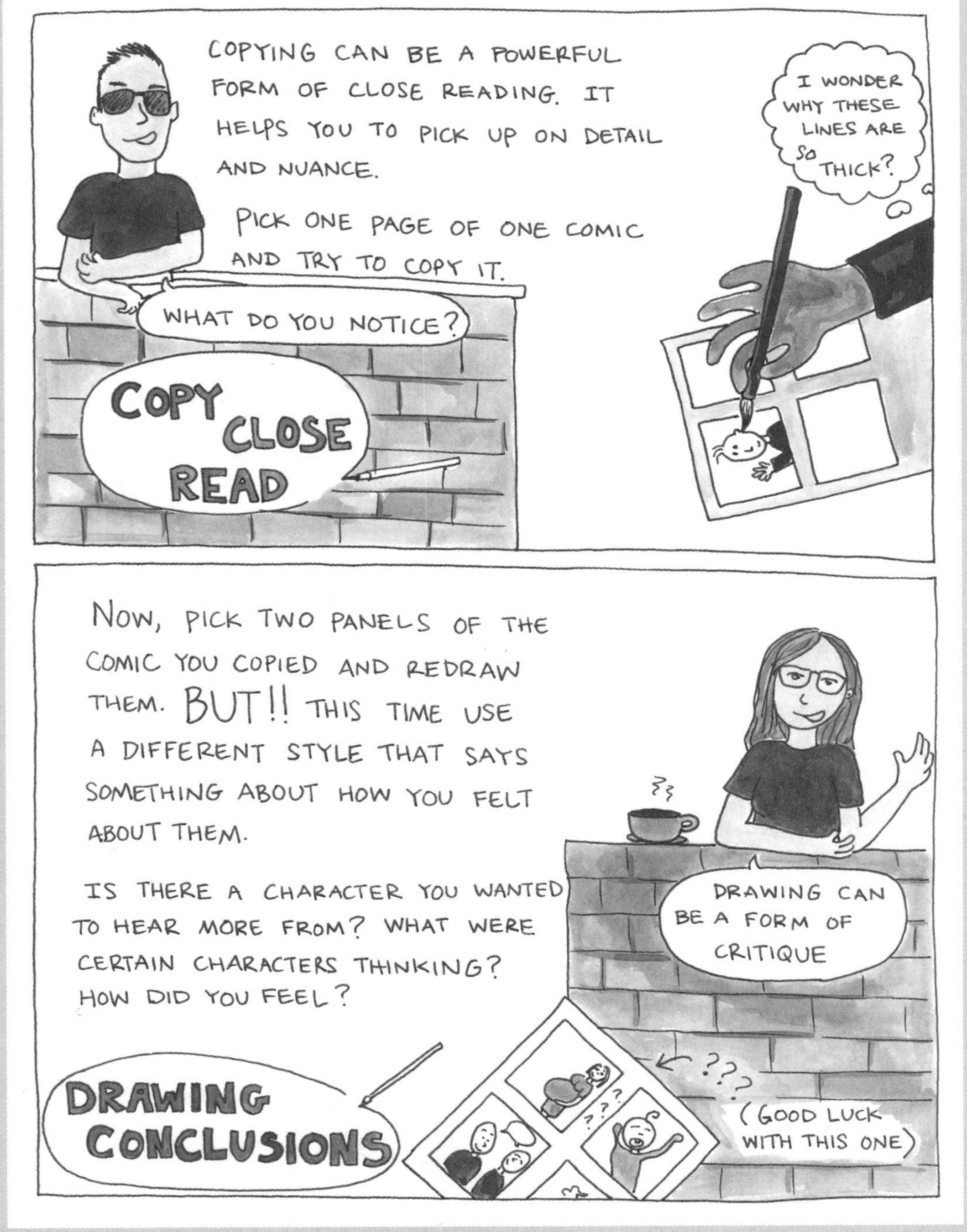
COPYING CAN BE A POWERFUL FORM OF CLOSE READING. IT HELPS YOU TO PICK UP ON DETAIL AND NUANCE.
PICK ONE PAGE OF ONE COMIC AND TRY TO COPY IT.
WHAT DO YOU NOTICE?
I WONDER WHY THESE LINES ARE SO THICK?
COPY CLOSE READ
NOW, PICK TWO PANELS OF THE COMIC YOU COPIED AND REDRAW THEM. BUT!! THIS TIME USE A DIFFERENT STYLE THAT SAYS SOMETHING ABOUT HOW YOU FELT ABOUT THEM.
IS THERE A CHARACTER YOU WANTED TO HEAR MORE FROM? WHAT WERE CERTAIN CHARACTERS THINKING? HOW DID YOU FEEL?
DRAWING CAN BE A FORM OF CRITIQUE
???
(GOOD LUCK WITH THIS ONE)
DRAWING CONCLUSIONS

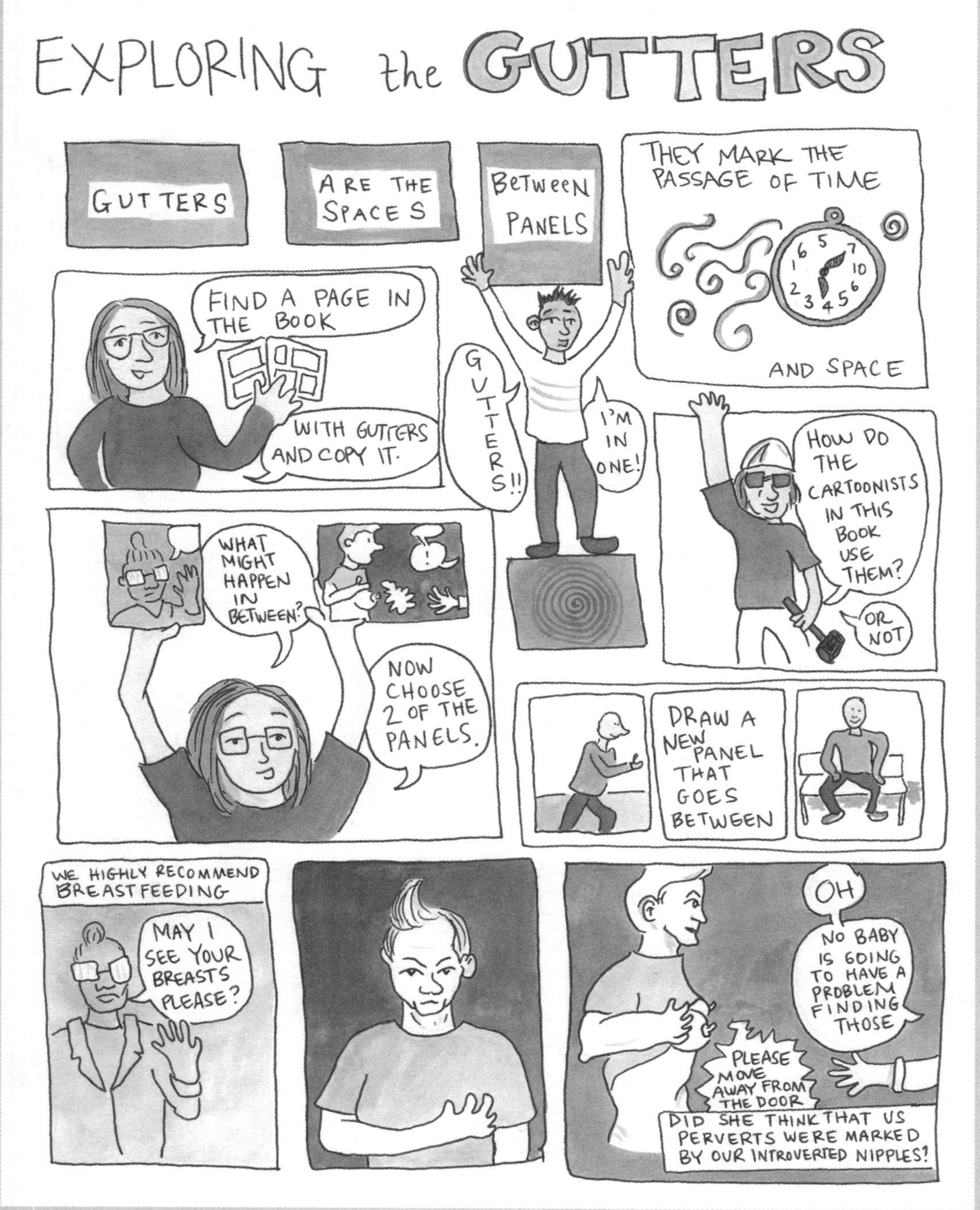
EXPLORING the GUTTERS
GUTTERS
ARE THE SPACES
BETWEEN PANELS
THEY MARK THE PASSAGE OF TIME
AND SPACE
FIND A PAGE IN THE BOOK
WITH GUTTERS AND COPY IT.
GUTTERS!!
I'M IN ONE!
HOW DO THE CARTOONISTS IN THIS BOOK USE THEM?
OR NOT
WHAT MIGHT HAPPEN IN BETWEEN?
NOW CHOOSE 2 OF THE PANELS.
DRAW A NEW PANEL THAT GOES BETWEEN
WE HIGHLY RECOMMEND BREASTFEEDING
MAY I SEE YOUR BREASTS PLEASE?
OH
NO BABY IS GOING TO HAVE A PROBLEM FINDING THOSE
PLEASE MOVE AWAY FROM THE DOOR
DID SHE THINK THAT US PERVERTS WERE MARKED BY OUR INTROVERTED NIPPLES?

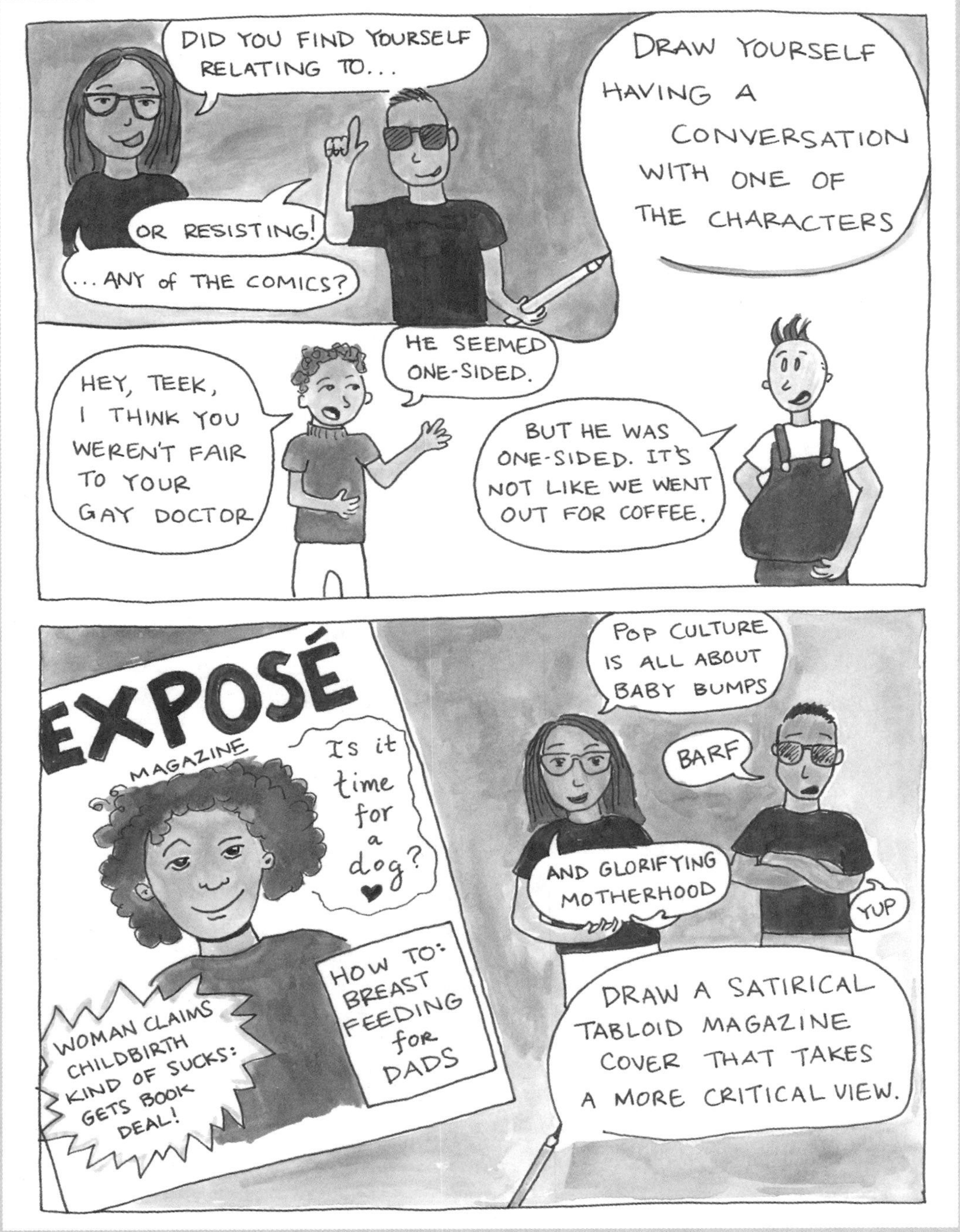
DID YOU FIND YOURSELF RELATING TO...
OR RESISTING!
...ANY of THE COMICS?
DRAW YOURSELF HAVING A CONVERSATION WITH ONE OF THE CHARACTERS
HEY, TEEK, I THINK YOU WEREN'T FAIR TO YOUR GAY DOCTOR
HE SEEMED ONE-SIDED.
BUT HE WAS ONE-SIDED. IT'S NOT LIKE WE WENT OUT FOR COFFEE.
EXPOSÉ
MAGAZINE
Is it time for a dog?
HOW TO: BREAST FEEDING for DADS
WOMAN CLAIMS CHILDBIRTH KIND OF SUCKS: GETS BOOK DEAL!
POP CULTURE IS ALL ABOUT BABY BUMPS
BARF
AND GLORIFYING MOTHERHOOD
YUP
DRAW A SATIRICAL TABLOID MAGAZINE COVER THAT TAKES A MORE CRITICAL VIEW.

Contributors

Ryan Alexander-Tanner is a cartoonist and educator living in Portland, Oregon. His work is heavily focused on using the medium of comics to invite audiences to engage with material they may not have otherwise. His website is www.oh yesverynice.com.

Alison Bechdel is the author of the graphic memoirs *Fun Home: A Family Tragicomic* (2006) and *Are You My Mother? A Comic Drama* (2012). For twenty-five years, she wrote and drew the comic strip *Dykes to Watch Out For*. She was the recipient of a 2014 MacArthur fellowship.

Lyn Chevli was an American cartoonist, writer, editor, publisher and pioneering participant in the underground comix movement; she died in 2016. She was best known for her work with Joyce Farmer on the *Tits and Clits Comix* series (1972–1987) and the pamphlet *Abortion Eve* (1973), which she published under the name Chin Lyvely.

KC Councilor is a cartoonist, teacher, and doctoral candidate in communication arts (rhetoric, politics, and culture) at the University of Wisconsin–Madison. He draws comics about the experience of being transgender and about being human. You can see more of his work at www.kccouncilor.com.

Bethany Doane is a Ph.D. candidate at Penn State University in English and women's, gender, and sexuality studies. Her research areas are critical theory, contemporary fiction, film, and feminist theory. Her current project works to develop new feminist and antiracist reading practices by looking at horror fiction and film in the "weird" tradition.

Joyce Farmer (aka Joyce Sutton) is an American cartoonist and a major participant in the underground comix movement. With Lyn Chevli, she created and published the first all-women's comic book, *Tits and Clits Comix*, in 1972. In 2011, her graphic novel *Special Exits* (2010) won the National Cartoonists Society's Reuben Award and was nominated for an Eisner at Comic-Con.

Leah Hayes is an illustrator, musician, cartoonist, songwriter, and music producer. She has published several books with Fantagraphics, including *Holy Moly* (2005), *Funeral of the Heart* (2008), and *Not Funny Ha-Ha* (2015). She also has several albums out with her band, Scary Mansion, and produces beats for pop and hip-hop artists.

Jenell Johnson is the Mellon-Morgridge Professor of the Humanities and an associate professor of communication arts at the University of Wisconsin–Madison. She is the author of *American Lobotomy: A Rhetorical History* (2014), co-editor of *The Neuroscientific Turn: Transdisciplinarity in the Age of the Brain* (2012), and co-editor of *Biocitizenship: The Politics of Bodies, Governance, and Power* (2018).

Paula Knight is an author, illustrator, and comics creator working in the United Kingdom. Her first graphic memoir, *The Facts of Life*, was published in 2017. She has presented her work at literary events, comics festivals, universities, and conferences such as Graphic Medicine, Laydeez Do Comics, and Fertility Fest 2016.

Endrené Shepherd is a Canadian artist hailing from Penticton, British Columbia. She learned how to handle watercolors from her grandfather and has made art the focal point of her life for as long as she has existed. Shepherd lives with her partner, Dave, their son, and a rotund and opinionated cat.

Susan Merrill Squier is the Brill Professor Emerita of English and Women's, Gender, and Sexuality Studies at Penn State University and the Einstein Visiting Fellow at Freie Universität, Berlin, where she is part of the PathoGraphics Project. One of the authors of *Graphic Medicine Manifesto* and a co-editor of the Graphic Medicine book series at Penn State Press, she is also the author of *Babies in Bottles: Twentieth-Century Visions of Reproductive Technology* (1994); *Liminal Lives: Imagining the Human at the Frontiers of Biomedicine* (2003); and *Poultry Science, Chicken Culture: A Partial Alphabet* (2010). Her most recent book, which features a chapter on graphic embryos, is *Epigenetic Landscapes: Drawings as Metaphor* (2017).

A. K. Summers began working on *Pregnant Butch* in 2005, following the birth of her son, and in 2012 serialized it on the webcomics site www.activatecomix .com. A longtime artist, Summers is the creator of *Negativa: Chicago's Astute Lezbo Fantasy Mag* and was included in Dennis Cooper's *Discontents: New Queer Writers* (1992). Summers lives with her son in Providence, Rhode Island.

Carol Tyler is a master cartoonist and a pioneer of the auto-bio comics genre. Her work includes the books *The Job Thing* (1993), *Late Bloomer* (2005), *Soldier's Heart* (2015), and *Fab4 Mania* (2018) and the trilogy *You'll Never Know* (2009,

2010, 2012). She also teaches comics at the University of Cincinnati. These days, Tyler works out of her Ink Farm in northern Kentucky, which offers an annual summer camp experience for cartoonists.

Marcus B. Weaver-Hightower is a professor of educational foundations and research at the University of North Dakota. His research focuses on boys and masculinity; the use of comics and graphic novels in qualitative methods and in education; food politics; and the politics and sociology of education and policy. He is the author of *The Politics of Policy in Boys' Education: Getting Boys "Right"* (2008), numerous articles, and chapters in edited collections.

Jessica Zucker, Ph.D., is a Los Angeles–based psychologist specializing in women's reproductive and maternal mental health. Her writing has appeared in the *New York Times*, the *Washington Post*, the *Guardian*, and *Time*, among other publications. She is the creator of the #IHadAMiscarriage campaign. Website: www.drjessicazucker.com, IG: @ihadamiscarriage.